Chronic Total Occlusions
A Guide to Recanalization

Commissioning Editor: Oliver Walter
Development Editor: Kate Newell

Chronic Total Occlusions

A Guide to Recanalization

EDITED BY

Ron Waksman, MD, FACC

Washington Hospital Centre
Washington, DC
USA

Shigeru Saito, MD, FACC, FSCAI, FJCC

Shonan Kamakura General Hospital
Kamakura
Japan

WILEY-BLACKWELL

A John Wiley & Sons, Ltd., Publication

This edition first published 2009, © 2009 by Blackwell Publishing Ltd
Blackwell Publishing was acquired by John Wiley & Sons in February 2007. Blackwell's publishing program
has been merged with Wiley's global Scientific, Technical and Medical business to form Wiley-Blackwell.

Registered office:
John Wiley & Sons Ltd, The Atrium, Southern Gate, Chichester, West Sussex, PO19 8SQ, UK

Editorial offices:
9600 Garsington Road, Oxford, OX4 2DQ, UK
The Atrium, Southern Gate, Chichester, West Sussex, PO19 8SQ, UK
111 River Street, Hoboken, NJ 07030-5774, USA

For details of our global editorial offices, for customer services and for information about how to apply for
permission to reuse the copyright material in this book please see our website at www.wiley.com/wiley-
blackwell

Library of Congress Cataloging-in-Publication Data
Chronic total occlusions / edited by Ron Waksman, Shigeru Saito.
     p. ; cm.
  Includes bibliographical references and index.
  ISBN 978-1-4051-5703-2 (alk. paper)
  1. Coronary heart disease. 2. Arterial occlusions. I. Waksman, Ron. II. Saito, Shigeru, 1950, Feb. 15-
[DNLM: 1. Coronary Occlusion. 2. Chronic Disease. 3. Coronary Angiography--methods.
  WG 300 C557 2009]
RC685.C6C485 2009
616.1′23–dc22

                                                                                                2008042836
A catalogue record for this book is available from the British Library.

Set in 9.5/12pt Minion by Newgen Imaging Systems Pvt. Ltd., Chennai, India
Printed and bound in Malaysia by Vivar Printing Sdn Bhd

1   2009

Contents

Contributors

Lutz Buellesfeld, MD
Department of Cardiology & Angiology, HELIOS Heart
Center, Siegburg, Germany

Nicholas Burke, MD
Minneapolis Heart Institute and Foundation, Minneapolis,
MN, USA

Antonio Colombo, MD
Cardiovascular Research Foundation, New York, NY, USA
and
Columbia University Medical Center, New York, NY, USA
and
Cardiac Cath Lab and Interventional Cardiology, EMO
Centro Cuore Columbus, Milan, Italy

Brian Courtney, MD
Sunnybrook Health Sciences Center, Schulich Heart
Program, University of Toronto, Toronto, Canada

George Dangas, MD, PhD
Cardiovascular Research Foundation, New York, NY, USA
and
Columbia University Medical Center, New York,
NY, USA

Eberhard Grube, MD
Department of Cardiology & Angiology, HELIOS Heart
Center, Siegburg, Germany

Luis Gruberg, MD, FACC
Division of Cardiology Stony Brook University Medical
Center, Stony Brook, New York, NY, USA

Hidehiko Hara, MD
Minneapolis Heart Institute and Foundation, Minneapolis,
MN, USA

**Richard Heuser, MD, FACC, FACP,
FESC, FASCI**
St. Luke's Medical Center, University of Arizona College of
Medicine, Phoenix, AZ, USA

Ronen Jaffe, MD
Sunnybrook Health Sciences Center, Schulich Heart
Program, University of Toronto, Toronto, Canada

David E. Kandzari, MD
Duke University Medical Center, Durham, NC, USA

Hideaki Kaneda, MD, PhD
Cardiology and Catheterization Laboratories, Shonan
Kamakura General Hospital, Kanagawa, Japan

Osamu Katoh, MD
Toyohashi Heart Center, Toyohashi, Japan

Masashi Kimura, MD, PhD
Cardiovascular Research Foundation, New York,
NY, USA
and
Columbia University Medical Center, New York,
NY, USA
and
Department of Cardiology, Toyohashi Heart Center, Aichi,
Japan

Chad Kliger, MD
New York University School of Medicine, New York,
NY, USA
and
VA New York Harbor Healthcare System, New York
Campus, NY, USA

Axel de Labriolle, MD
Washington Hospital Center, Washington, DC, USA

Thierry Lefèvre, MD, FESC, FSCAI
Institut Cardiovasculaire Paris Sud, Massy, France

John R. Lesser, MD
Minneapolis Heart Institute and Foundation, Minneapolis,
MN, USA

Jeffrey D. Lorin, MD, FACC
New York University School of Medicine, New York,
NY, USA
and
VA New York Harbor Healthcare System, New York
Campus, NY, USA

Yves Louvard, MD, FSCAI
Institut Cardiovasculaire Paris Sud, Massy, France

Robin Mathews, MD
Stony Brook University Medical Center, Stony Brook,
New York, NY, USA

Lampros K. Michalis, MD,
MRCP, FESC
Medical School, University of Ioannina, Ioannina, Greece

Marie-Claude Morice, MD, FACC, FESC
Institut Cardiovasculaire Paris Sud, Massy, France

Eugenia Nikolsky, MD, PhD
Cardiovascular Research Foundation, New York, NY, USA
and
Columbia University Medical Center, New York, NY, USA

Steve Ramcharitar, BMBCh, DPhil
The Thoraxcenter, Erasmus Medical Center,
The Netherlands

Nicolaus Reifart, MD, PhD, FESC,
FACC, RANS
Johann Wolfgang Goethe University Frankfurt and Main
Taunus Kliniken, Bad Soden, Germany
and
Chefarzt Kardiologie Main Taunus Kiliniken, Kardioligische
Praxis Prof. Reifart & Partner, Bad Soden, Germany

Shigeru Saito, MD, FACC, FSCAI, FJCC
Shonan Kamakura General Hospital, Kamakura, Japan

Mickey Scheinowitz, PhD
Neufeld Cardiac Research Institute and Department of
Biomedical Engineering Tel-Aviv University, Israel

Mirko Schiemann, MD
University Hospital Frankfurt, Frankfurt, Germany

Robert S. Schwartz, MD
Minneapolis Heart Institute and Foundation, Minneapolis,
MN, USA

Steven P. Sedlis, MD, FACC, FSCAI
New York University School of Medicine, New York,
NY, USA

Patrick Serruys, MD, PhD
The Thoraxcenter, Erasmus Medical Center,
The Netherlands

Tina L. Pinto Slottow, MD
Division of Cardiology, Washington Hospital Center,
Washington, DC, USA

Bradley H. Strauss, MD, PhD
Sunnybrook Health Sciences Center, Schulich Heart
Program, University of Toronto, Toronto, Canada
and
The Heart Institute, Chaim Sheba Medical Center,
Tel Hashomer, Israel

Jean-François Surmely, MD
District General Hospital, Aarau, Switzerland

Takahiko Suzuki, MD
Toyohashi Heart Center, Toyohashi, Japan

Hideo Tamai, MD
Kusatsu Heart Center, Shiga, Japan

On Topaz, MD
McGuire Veterans Affairs Medical Center, Richmond,
VA, USA
and
Virginia Commonwealth University, VA, USA

Etsuo Tsuchikane, MD, PhD
Cardiovascular Research Foundation, New York, NY, USA
and
Columbia University Medical Center, New York, NY, USA
and
Department of Cardiology, Toyohashi Heart Center, Aichi,
Japan

Takafumi Tsuji, MD
Kusatsu Heart Center, Shiga, Japan

Ron Waksman, MD, FACC
Washington Hospital Center, Washington, DC, USA

Preface

With the recent advances in the growing field of interventional cardiology, one of the last frontiers left to be conquered is the treatment of chronic total occlusion (CTO). Over the past 20 years, CTO lesions have represented the most difficult anatomy for treatment – with lower success rates and higher complication rates. The procedure duration has exceeded records for conventional percutaneous coronary intervention (PCI) and the increased exposure to radiation and contrast has made CTO a major challenge for the interventional cardiology community. Meanwhile, the indication of when to intervene on CTOs is a debated topic especially for asymptomatic patients. During the past few years we have experienced tremendous advances in imaging by utilizing CT angiography and intravascular ultrasound (IVUS) to assist in the procedure. In addition, new wires, devices, and techniques have evolved to conquer the challenges of recanalizing CTOs.

CTOs provide interventionalists insight into the world of CTOs with introductory chapters that describe the pathology and indications of CTOs along with a review of clinical trials. Subsequent chapters introduce imaging modalities including CT angiography, magnetic navigation wire, and IVUS-guided recanalization of CTO.

You will then find information on new wires technology and devices for CTOs. The newest technical approaches employ novel support catheters such as the Tornus catheter, vibrating penetrating catheter guidewire systems, and combinations of new material guidewires. Our Japanese colleagues have shared with us their knowledge and expertise on the innovative technique tips and tricks they've developed, including chapters on the ASAHI family of wires, wire control handling, and the parallel wire technique.

The increased interest in treating CTOs has come from the development of the subspecialty wires previously discussed and the use of drug-eluting stents (DES). The impact of DES implantation for the treatment of CTOs has been shown to reduce the subsequent rate of restenosis compared with bare metal stents. Details on DES use, along with other device technology such as vibrational angioplasty and radio frequency, are then presented. Finally, avoiding and treatment of complications and interesting cases are discussed.

It is our hope that *CTOs* will prove useful to the medical community in its effort to serve as a comprehensive guide to understanding the multiple complexities of treating CTOs. As an instructional tool, *CTOs* presents information to help fine-tune techniques and provides various tips and tricks to physicians interested in embarking on this subset of interventional cardiology.

Many thanks to all of our contributors recognized and respected worldwide for their work with chronic total occlusions. We hope you find the book useful for day-to-day practice in the cath lab.

Ron Waksman, MD, FACC
Shigeru Saito, MD, FACC, FSCAI, FJCC

Foreword

What is the relevance of chronic total occlusions of the coronary arteries? From an examination of interventional practice behavior one might conclude that they are not important because the rate of attempting to open them is very low. The reasons for this are several including the fact that they are difficult to open and stenting stenoses seems a much more productive use of one's time. After all, if the artery is already closed, can it pose a threat? The answer is that it does pose a threat in the form of untreated ischemia which in many cases is much more marked, even with collaterals, than subtotal stenosis. Examination of the New York State Registry of Percutaneous Coronary Interventions shows that leaving chronic total occlusions unrevascularized poses a significant mortality threat over a three-year period compared to those patients who are completely revascularized. One solution is to perform coronary artery bypass graft surgery on those patients with chronic total occlusions, a frequent practice in the United States. Another approach pursued by our Japanese colleagues is to work diligently to open and stent chronic total occlusions. The aversion to surgery in Japan has enabled the chronic total occlusion envelope to be pushed and now techniques for improving success of chronic total occlusion therapy are spreading worldwide. This book, edited by Drs. Waksman and Saito, brings "east" and "west" together to examine the current state of chronic total occlusion technology. The editors have assembled the leading thinkers and "tinkerers" in technology to address chronic total occlusion. The authoritative authors produced chapters ranging from the pathologic expression and clinical results of chronic total occlusion trials to technology and devices to enable successful opening, and finally to methods for identifying and treating complications of the interventions. This effort will not only help highly experienced experts solve difficult problems, but will also make the approach clearer to many chronic total occlusions so that the average operator will consider the relevance of chronic total occlusions and open the ones that do indeed pose a threat to the patient, otherwise left with unrevascularized ischemic myocardium.

Spencer B. King, III, MD, MACC
President, Saint Joseph's Heart and
Vascular Institute
Professor of Medicine Emeritus
Emory University School of Medicine
Atlanta, GA

PART I

Pathology and Indications: Clinical Trials

CHAPTER 1

The Pathobiology of CTO

Ronen Jaffe, MD, *Brian Courtney,* MD, &
Bradley H. Strauss, MD, PhD

University of Toronto, Toronto, Canada

Introduction

Chronic total occlusions (CTOs), defined as occlusions more than 1 month old, are common in patients undergoing diagnostic coronary artery catheterization, with up to 20% of angiograms reported to have one or more CTO [1]. Despite its common occurrence, there is surprisingly little information about the pathophysiology of CTOs, and why some CTOs can be crossed, while in others, crossing is unsuccessful.

Current paradigm of CTO evolution

Composition of the CTO evolves over time and has remarkable spatial variability. Arterial occlusions may develop insidiously with minimal symptoms, or may present as an acute coronary syndrome. The initial acute event leading to the development of a CTO is a ruptured atherosclerotic plaque with bidirectional thrombus formation [2]. In patients with minimal or no symptoms, the timing of the occlusive event can not be clearly identified. In patients with ST-segment elevation myocardial infarction (MI) not treated with reperfusion therapy, an occluded infarct-related artery has been found in 87% of the patients within 4 hours, in 65% within 12–24 hours, and in 45% at 1 month [3,4]. As many as 30% of the patients treated with thrombolytic therapy alone have a chronically occluded artery 3–6 months after

Chronic Total Occlusions, 1st edition. Edited by R. Waksman and S. Saito. © 2009 Blackwell Publishing, ISBN: 978-1-4051-5703-2.

MI [5]. In patients treated with percutaneous coronary intervention (PCI) during evolving acute myocardial infarction (AMI), approximately 6–11% will have chronic occlusion of an infarct-related artery at 6 months due to either initial treatment failure or late re-occlusion [6].

The current understanding of CTO development is derived from autopsy studies, imaging in human subjects, and animal CTO models. Characterization of CTO development in human studies is problematic, since CTOs are often diagnosed after a prolonged maturation period, and data regarding initial stages in their evolution is lacking. Several animal models have been developed to systematically define the developmental stages of a CTO; however, these models have certain characteristics that could potentially limit their relevance to humans, such as the lack of underlying atherosclerosis or significant calcification. In this chapter we shall review the current understanding of CTO pathobiology.

Early stages of CTO development: Thrombus and inflammation

Our knowledge of thrombus organization is almost exclusively limited to veins. This process resembles the pattern of wound healing [7]. Initially, the freshly formed thrombus contains platelets and erythrocytes within a fibrin mesh, which is followed by invasion of acute inflammatory cells [8]. Neutrophils predominate at first but are later replaced with mononuclear cells [9,10]. Endothelial cells also invade the fibrin lattice and form tube-like structures and microvessels within the organizing thrombi [7,11]. Inflammatory cell infiltrates in CTOs consist of macrophages, foam cells, and lymphocytes. Inflammation may exist in the intima, media, and adventitia of CTOs, although it is most predominant in the intima, regardless of lesion age.

Extracellular matrix

Collagen is the major structural component of the extracellular matrix (ECM) [12] with predominance of types I and III (and minor amounts of IV, V, and VI) in the fibrous stroma of atherosclerotic plaques [13]. In an autopsy study, cholesterol and foam cell-laden plaque were more frequent in younger lesions, whereas fibrocalcific plaque increased with CTO age [14]. Proteoglycans are important components of the CTO within the first year. It is generally stated that the concentration of collagen-rich fibrous tissue is particularly dense at the proximal and distal ends of the lesion, contributing to a columnlike lesion of calcified, resistant fibrous tissue surrounding a softer core of organized thrombus and lipids. However, there is sparse human CTO histological data to support this concept (see Figure 1.1).

Neovascularization and angiogenesis

Presence of microvessels within the CTO may facilitate angioplasty success [15]. There are three

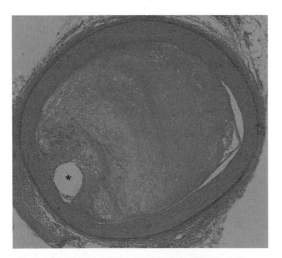

Figure 1.1 H&E stained cross-section of a fibrotic CTO (H&E) containing predominantly collagen-rich extracellular matrix (* indicates intraluminal microvessel).

types of microvessel formation in arteries with advanced atherosclerotic lesions. The first pattern occurs in the vasa vasorum, which is the fine network of microvessels in the adventitia and outer media. These vessels proliferate in atherosclerosis and in response to vascular injury such as angioplasty and stenting [16–18]. Hypoxia in the outer levels of the vessel wall appears to act as an important stimulus [18]. Occasionally in CTOs, these adventitial blood vessels are well developed and can be recognized as "bridging collaterals." Such microchannels, which can recanalize the distal lumen, may result from thrombus-derived angiogenic stimuli [19] and are suggested on an angiogram of an old CTO without a well-defined stump. Second, neovascularization can develop within occlusive atherosclerotic intimal plaques, predominantly in response to chronic inflammation [20]. The localization of plaque vessels in so-called "hot spots" in the shoulders of atheromas may predispose these plaques to rupture and acute coronary events [21,22]. The third type is the pattern of intraluminal microvessel formation (known as "recanalization") that occurs as part of the organization phase in CTO in which thrombus is replaced by fibrous tissue. These microvessels generally range in size from 100 to 200 μm, but can be as large as 500 μm (Figure 1.2) [14]. In contrast to the vasa vasorum which runs in radial directions, these intimal microvessels run within and parallel to the thrombosed parent vessel [8]. This is suggested by a tapered CTO on an angiogram. Such channels may serve as a route for a guidewire to reach the distal vessel and hence may have therapeutic value.

There is little published data on the process of intraluminal microvessel formation in thrombin within arterial occlusions. Inflammation may play a role since high concentrations of macrophages have been detected in regions of recanalization in spontaneous human thrombi and in experimental animal arterial thrombi [10,23]. Frequent co-localization of inflammation and neovascularization within the intimal plaque and adventitia suggests that these findings are closely related, although it is unclear whether inflammation is a cause or an effect of neovascularization in CTOs [14]. Lymphocytes and monocytes/macrophages may play an active role in both angiogenesis and atherosclerotic lesion progression

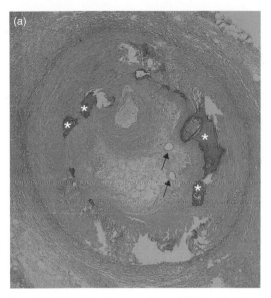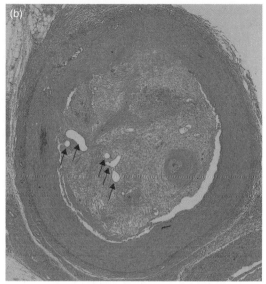

Figure 1.2 H&E stained cross-sections of CTOs containing prominent fibro-calcific tissue (a) and intraluminal microvessels (b) (* indicates calcium deposits and arrows identify microvessels).

by producing a variety of mitogenic and angiogenic actors [24]. The local ECM (extracellular matrix) environment is probably an additional important modifier, with specific matrix components exerting either pro-angiogenic (hyaluronan, fibronectin, perlecan, versican), or anti-angiogenic (type I collagen, decorin) effects.

Advanced CTO

Vessels with fibrotic CTO lesions typically undergo negative remodeling [25]. Intravascular ultrasound has demonstrated a positive correlation between degree of plaque calcification and duration of the occlusion [26]. These changes negatively impact the likelihood of successful angioplasty.

Current research in CTO pathobiology

Identification of specific components of the CTO at the various stages of development is critical to understanding CTO pathobiology and improving guidewire crossing success rates. Complementary information is required from the following areas of research.

Human CTO samples

Samples of CTOs collected during autopsies, amputations, endarterectomies, and transplants provide an important but very infrequent opportunity to study these highly heterogeneous lesions. Information regarding the three-dimensional (3D) architecture of occluded segments, the mechanical properties of their components, and changes in the integrity of the vessel wall layers over the natural history of CTO development are important areas of further study. Histological analysis provides an opportunity to assess a large range of features related to composition and structure.

Animal models of CTO

The optimal animal CTO model should be reproducible, contain fibro-calcific tissue, allow serial device evaluation and be able to be utilized with intravascular ultrasound or other technologies. A challenge in developing models of CTO is the lack of spontaneous atherosclerosis in animals. Different approaches have included external arterial constriction, thermal injury, gas-drying of the artery, injection of autologous blood above a stenosis, copper stents, stents with occluded outflow, alcohol injection, and insertion of polymer plugs. We have developed a rabbit CTO model in which thrombin is injected into an isolated femoral artery segment [27]. This model is being used to investigate the temporal and spatial evolution of CTO, and correlate histological findings with non-invasive imaging modalities.

Imaging techniques

Non-invasive imaging provides an opportunity to observe features of CTOs at several stages in their development in patients and experimental models. Magnetic resonance imaging (MRI) has spatial resolution down to 100–200 μm in plane and about 1 mm through the plane and can determine composition of atherosclerotic plaque components such as lipid, thrombus, fibrous tissue, and calcium based on signal intensities in T1-, T2-, and proton-density-weighted images. Administration of contrast agents (Gd-DTPA (gadolinium diethylenetriaminepentaacetic acid), Clariscan) permits calculations of relative extracellular volume and blood volume within regions of the CTO. Sequential MRI scans can follow the evolution of CTO at different time points. In human studies, CT angiography can provide insight into the presence of calcifications, vessel tortuosity, lesion length, and bridging collaterals [28]. Micro computerized tomography (micro-CT) performed on *ex vivo* specimens (and therefore limited to autopsy material or animal models) has a spatial resolution of 17 μm and can be used to visualize specific microchannels within the CTO. Direct magnetic resonance direct thrombus imaging (MRDTI) can help estimate the presence and age of thrombus in occluded segments [29].

Pilot studies with human tissue and animal models have shown the potential of invasive optical coherence tomography (OCT) and ultrasound (in forward-looking configurations) to identify the layers of the vessel wall. OCT has sufficient resolution to identify microchannels *in vivo* [30]. These techniques are being adapted for *in vivo* use to enable nondestructive serial assessment of composition at the proximal entry point of CTOs. The ability to understand and non-invasively characterize the specific histologic and spatial features of CTOs, particularly online during revascularization, may dramatically impact on procedural success rates, particularly in complex CTOs.

See Plate 1 in the color plate section.

References

1 Baim DS, Ignatius EJ. Use of percutaneous transluminal coronary angioplasty: results of a current survey. *Am J Cardiol* 1988; **61**: 3G–8G.

2 Stone GW, Kandzari DE, Mehran R *et al*. Percutaneous recanalization of chronically occluded coronary arteries: a consensus document: Part I. *Circulation* 2005; **112**: 2364–2372.

3 DeWood MA, Spores J, Notske R *et al*. Prevalence of total coronary occlusion during the early hours of transmural myocardial infarction. *N Engl J Med* 1980; **303**: 897–902.

4 Betriu A, Castaner A, Sanz GA *et al*. Angiographic findings 1 month after myocardial infarction: a prospective study of 259 survivors. *Circulation* 1982; **65**: 1099–1105.

5 Veen G, Meyer A, Verheugt FW *et al*. Culprit lesion morphology and stenosis severity in the prediction of reocclusion after coronary thrombolysis: angiographic results of the APRICOT study. Antithrombotics in the prevention of reocclusion in coronary thrombolysis. *J Am Coll Cardiol* 1993; **22**: 1755–1762.

6 Stone GW, Grines CL, Cox DA *et al*. Comparison of angioplasty with stenting, with or without abciximab, in acute myocardial infarction. *N Engl J Med* 2002; **346**: 957–966.

7 Wakefield TW, Linn MJ, Henke PK *et al*. Neovascularization during venous thrombosis organization: a preliminary study. *J Vasc Surg* 1999; **30**: 885–892.

8 Dible JH. Organisation and canalisation in arterial thrombosis. *J Pathol Bacteriol* 1958; **75**: 1–7.

9 Burnand KG, Gaffney PJ, McGuinness CL, Humphries J, Quarmby JW, Smith A. The role of the monocyte in the generation and dissolution of arterial and venous thrombi. *Cardiovasc Surg* 1998; **6**: 119–125.

10 McGuinness CL, Humphries J, Waltham M, Burnand KG, Collins M, Smith A. Recruitment of labelled monocytes by experimental venous thrombi. *Thromb Haemost* 2001; **85**: 1018–1024.

11 Sevitt S. Organic canalisation and vascularisation of deep vein thrombi studied with dyed-micropaque injected at necropsy. *J Pathol* 1970; **100**: Pi.

12 Hosoda Y, Kawano K, Yamasawa F, Ishii T, Shibata T, Inayama S. Age-dependent changes of collagen and elastin content in human aorta and pulmonary artery. *Angiology* 1984; **35**: 615–621.

13 Katsuda S, Okada Y, Minamoto T, Oda Y, Matsui Y, Nakanishi I. Collagens in human atherosclerosis. Immunohistochemical analysis using collagen type-specific antibodies. *Arterioscler Thromb* 1992; **12**: 494–502.

14 Srivatsa SS, Edwards WD, Boos CM *et al.* Histologic correlates of angiographic chronic total coronary artery occlusions: influence of occlusion duration on neovascular channel patterns and intimal plaque composition. *J Am Coll Cardiol* 1997; **29**: 955–963.

15 Katsuragawa M, Fujiwara H, Miyamae M, Sasayama S. Histologic studies in percutaneous transluminal coronary angioplasty for chronic total occlusion: comparison of tapering and abrupt types of occlusion and short and long occluded segments. *J Am Coll Cardiol* 1993; **21**: 604–611.

16 Kwon HM, Sangiorgi G, Ritman EL *et al.* Enhanced coronary vasa vasorum neovascularization in experimental hypercholesterolemia. *J Clin Invest* 1998; **101**: 1551–1556.

17 Kwon HM, Sangiorgi G, Ritman EL *et al.* Adventitial vasa vasorum in balloon-injured coronary arteries: visualization and quantitation by a microscopic three-dimensional computed tomography technique. *J Am Coll Cardiol* 1998; **32**: 2072–2079.

18 Cheema AN, Hong T, Nili N *et al.* Adventitial microvessel formation after coronary stenting and the effects of SU11218, a tyrosine kinase inhibitor. *J Am Coll Cardiol* 2006; **47**: 1067–1075.

19 Sakuda H, Nakashima Y, Kuriyama S, Sueishi K. Media conditioned by smooth muscle cells cultured in a variety of hypoxic environments stimulates *in vitro* angiogenesis. A relationship to transforming growth factor-beta 1. *Am J Pathol* 1992; **141**: 1507–1516.

20 De Martin R, Hoeth M, Hofer-Warbinek R, Schmid JA. The transcription factor NF kappa B and the regulation of vascular cell function. *Arterioscler Thromb Vasc Biol* 2000; **20**: E83–E88.

21 de Boer OJ, van der Wal AC, Teeling P, Becker AE. Leucocyte recruitment in rupture prone regions of lipid-rich plaques: a prominent role for neovascularization? *Cardiovasc Res* 1999; **41**: 443–449.

22 Jeziorska M, Woolley DE. Local neovascularization and cellular composition within vulnerable regions of atherosclerotic plaques of human carotid arteries. *J Pathol* 1999; **188**: 189–196.

23 Singh I, Burnand KG, Collins M *et al.* Failure of thrombus to resolve in urokinase-type plasminogen activator gene-knockout mice: rescue by normal bone marrow-derived cells. *Circulation* 2003; **107**: 869–875.

24 Sueishi K, Yonemitsu Y, Nakagawa K, Kaneda Y, Kumamoto M, Nakashima Y. Atherosclerosis and angiogenesis. Its pathophysiological significance in humans as well as in an animal model induced by the gene transfer of vascular endothelial growth factor. *Ann N Y Acad Sci* 1997; **811**: 311–324.

25 Burke AP, Kolodgie FD, Farb A, Weber D, Virmani R. Morphological predictors of arterial remodeling in coronary atherosclerosis. *Circulation* 2002; **105**: 297–303.

26 Suzuki T, Hosokawa H, Yokoya K *et al.* Time-dependent morphologic characteristics in angiographic chronic total coronary occlusions. *Am J Cardiol* 2001; **88**: 167–169, A5–A6.

27 Strauss BH, Goldman L, Qiang B *et al.* Collagenase plaque digestion for facilitating guide wire crossing in chronic total occlusions. *Circulation* 2003; **108**: 1259–1262.

28 Yokoyama N, Yamamoto Y, Suzuki S *et al.* Impact of 16-slice computed tomography in percutaneous coronary intervention of chronic total occlusions. *Catheter Cardiovasc Interv* 2006; **68**: 1–7.

29 Moody AR, Murphy RE, Morgan PS *et al.* Characterization of complicated carotid plaque with magnetic resonance direct thrombus imaging in patients with cerebral ischemia. *Circulation* 2003; **107**: 3047–3052.

30 Munce NR, Yang VX, Standish BA *et al.* Ex vivo imaging of chronic total occlusions using forward-looking optical coherence tomography. *Lasers Surg Med* 2007; **39**: 28–35.

CHAPTER 2

Indication and Outcome of PCI for CTO

Ron Waksman, MD, FACC

Washington Hospital Center, Washington, DC, USA

Chronic total occlusions (CTOs) are found in approximately one-third of the patients with significant coronary disease who undergo angiography. Despite the introduction of novel technologies, newer guidewires, and a tremendous advancement of technical skills, percutaneous coronary intervention (PCI) for CTO remains a challenge. Indeed, the most common reason for referral to bypass surgery or exclusion from clinical studies comparing outcomes of angioplasty to bypass surgery has been the presence of a CTO [1,2].

Anatomically, CTOs typically consist of a hard fibro-calcific proximal cap, a distal cap with generally less fibrotic material, and a central area of organized thrombus. Indications for opening CTOs include relief of angina, evidence of ischemia in asymptomatic patients, improved left ventricular (LV) function, and improved long-term survival. Recently the focus has been shifted to patients with documented ischemia, and reconsideration of the need for recanalyzing CTOs that do not contribute to ischemia. The fibro-calcific nature of these CTOs is responsible for the somewhat lower success rates in opening these lesions, predominantly by increasing the difficulty in passing the occlusion with a guidewire. Newer technology, primarily new wires, has improved the ability to cross these previously uncrossable lesions, thereby improving the acute success rates of opening them. Stenting has

improved long-term patency rates for these lesions, and now drug-eluting stents (DESs) have made the late restenosis rates similar to those seen for non-occluded arteries. Therefore, the clinical imperative for opening these arteries has increased. CTOs are defined as occlusions in the coronary arteries with thrombolysis in myocardial infarction (TIMI) 0 flow or functional occlusions with TIMI 1 flow (penetration of contrast without filling of the distal vessel) of at least 1-month duration. Some extend the definition to 3 months of occlusion. Age criteria for total occlusion vary among studies – from 2 weeks to 3 months – but are difficult to assess unless serial angiograms are available. Thus, age is often difficult to define and is dependent on clinical history [3–6]. A prior history of myocardial infarction (MI) was present in 42–68% of the patients who had angiographically documented CTOs [1,7–10]. Not surprisingly, the incidence of CTOs seems to increase with patient age, especially in the left anterior descending (LAD) coronary artery distribution [11]. The presence of one or more CTOs was an angiographic exclusion for randomization in 43% of patients ineligible for the German Angioplasty Bypass Investigation (GABI) [12] and for 35% of the patients who had angiographic exclusions for the Balloon Angioplasty Revascularization Investigation (BARI) trials [2]. Accordingly, although CTOs represented 30–40% of the patients listed in the National Cardiovascular Registry of the American College of Cardiology, CTO angioplasty accounted for only 12% of the procedures between January 1998 and September 2000 in 139 United States hospitals [13].

Chronic Total Occlusions, 1st edition. Edited by R. Waksman and S. Saito. © 2009 Blackwell Publishing, ISBN: 978-1-4051-5703-2.

Clinical indications for treating CTOs

The rationale for treating CTOs follows several lines of evidence; the strongest include improved survival with successful procedures. The Mid-America Heart Institute published the results of a 10-year retrospective analysis of 2007 patients who had CTOs in whom PCI was attempted and matched those patients with 2007 patients undergoing PCI for non-occlusive disease between 1980 and 1999. There was a 74.4% success rate in the CTO group. Better in-hospital outcomes were associated with a successful procedure (major adverse coronary event [MACE] rate of 3.2% versus 5.4%; $p = 0.02$) [14] (Figure 2.1). Several other registries

	CTO success (n = 1491)	CTO failure (n = 514)	p value
Death	15 (1.0%)	12 (2.3%)	0.024
Q-wave MI	6 (0.4%)	4 (0.8%)	0.3
Non-Q-wave MI	22 (1.5%)	16 (3.1%)	0.02
Urgent repeat PCI	29 (1.9%)	1 (0.2%)	0.005
Any dissection	255 (17.1%)	102 (19.8%)	0.16
Cerebrovascular accident	0	1 (0.2%)	0.2
Vascular complications	29 (1.9%)	5 (1.0%)	0.1
MACE	48 (3.2%)	28 (5.4%)	0.023

Source: Suero *et al.* [14]

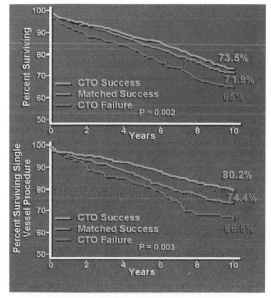

Figure 2.1 Re-opening CTOs: 20 years experience at the Mid-American Heart Institute.

have shown similar results. There was a 56% ($p < 0.001$) reduction in relative risk for mortality over 7 years' follow-up in the British Columbia Cardiac Registry in which 1458 patients with CTO were treated [15]. The Total Occlusion Angioplasty Study-Societa Italiana di Cardiologia Invasiva (TOAST-GISE) showed a similar result in a smaller cohort of patients (369 patients) over a shorter follow-up (1 year), with a reduced incidence of cardiac death or MI with successful procedures (1.1% versus 6.2%; $p = 0.005$) [7]. In the only study incorporating stent use to a significant degree, the Thorax Center reported 5-year follow-up of 885 consecutive patients who had CTO treated from 1992 through 2002. There was a 65.1% success rate in these patients. Successful procedures were again associated with improved 5-year survival (93.5% versus 88.0%; $p = 0.02$) [16].

Besides a survival benefit seen from of treating CTOs, improvements in clinical symptoms, improvements in LV function, and a reduced need for late coronary bypass surgery (CABG) have been associated with successful opening of CTOs. There was a greater freedom from angina in TOAST-GISE for successful procedures (88.7% versus 75.0%; $p = 0.008$) [7]. LV function improved in a series of 95 patients studied at baseline and at 6.7 ± 1.4 months. Left ventricular ejection fraction (LVEF) increased from $625 \pm 13\%$ to $675 \pm 11\%$ ($p < 0.001$) with the opening of these occluded arteries [17,18]. Chung and colleagues [19] showed a similar effect in a population of 75 patients who did not have known MI, demonstrating an improvement in ejection fraction from 59.5% to 67.3% ($p < 0.001$), but not in a similar group with a previously documented MI (48.9–50.5%; $p =$ not significant).

Patient selection

Certain angiographic and clinical features have been associated with higher success rates for opening totally occluded coronary arteries. Angiographic features include the presence of a tapered stump at the occlusion site and the presence of microchannels (subtotally occluded arteries). The features associated with a lower likelihood of success include the presence of a blunt or flush occlusion, the presence of the occlusion at a side branch, small vessel size, marked tortuosity, and heavy calcification. The presence of bridging collaterals also negatively impacts outcome with CTOs. Lesion length also predictably affects outcomes, with longer occlusions having worse results and short occlusions with a better chance of success. Nonvisualization of the distal bed remains a strong contraindication when attempting to recanalize CTOs using percutaneous techniques. CT angiography performed prior to the CTO recanalization was found to be helpful in determining the length of the total occlusion, the information on the runoff of the vessels, and the direction guide for the intervention.

From a clinical point of view, age, symptom severity, associated comorbidities (e.g., diabetes mellitus and chronic renal insufficiency), and overall functional status are major determinants of treatment strategy. Angiographically, the extent and complexity of coronary artery disease, likelihood for complete revascularization, and the presence and degree of valvular heart disease and LV dysfunction are all very important factors. The technical probability of achieving successful recanalization of the PCI without complications, as well as the anticipated restenosis rate, must also be heavily weighed in the decision-making process [20]. Another technical consideration for a successful procedure is the presence or absence of collaterals that can be utilized for a retrograde approach.

Long-term outcomes and impact on survival

Long-term success rates traditionally have been less than ideal, with high restenosis- and re-occlusion rates compared with PCI of non-occluded vessels. Various randomized trials comparing percutaneous transluminal coronary angioplasty with stenting have provided bare metal insight into these long-term outcomes. Restenosis rates for balloon angioplasty of CTOs have ranged from 33% to 74%. Additionally, the re-occlusion rates have been high, ranging from 7% to 34% in various studies. The use of stents has improved these outcomes markedly. Importantly, the Mid-America Heart Study reported that long-term survival was similar in patients with successful CTO recanalization compared with a matched cohort of patients undergoing successful angioplasty of non-occluded lesions, and significantly longer than in patients where attempted CTO revascularization failed (10-year survival 73.5% with CTO success versus 65.1% with CTO failure; $p < 0.001$) [14].

In the prospective, observational TOAST-GISE study of 390 CTOs (369 patients), a successful PCI was associated with a reduced 12-month incidence of cardiac death or MI (1.1% versus 7.2%), a reduced need for CABG (2.5% versus 15.7%), and greater freedom from angina (88.7% versus 75.0%). In the overall study population, the only factor associated with enhanced 1-year event-free survival was successful CTO recanalization (odds ratio = 0.24; $p < 0.018$) [7].

What mechanisms explain these benefits? Late reopening of an occluded infarct-related artery (IRA) may improve LV function provided viable myocardium is present within the zone supplied by the artery. Available data suggest that viable myocardium can survive only a few weeks after an acute event. However, collateral flow may prolong this time window due to the so-called "hibernating" myocardium. Recently, a team of investigators in Italy showed that late restoration of IRA patency (6 months after an acute event) improved LV function, prevented LV dilatation, and reduced cardiac death [21]. In the randomized Désobstruction Coronaire en Post-Infarctus (DECOPI) trial, Steg and others showed that routinely late (2–15 days after acute MI) recanalization of an IRA provided only little clinical benefit [22]. Yet patients with effective recanalization, persisting at 6 months' angiography had improved LVEF and reduced mortality.

The authors of the Italian study noted above concluded that there is probably little to gain in re-establishing flow in a chronically occluded IRA supplying a thin, scarred area of myocardium. However, if the IRA had occluded slowly, developed collaterals, and myocardial viability had been maintained by these collaterals, then re-establishing blood flow to that segment provides the opportunity for considerable benefit from a pathophysiological perspective. Although their data could not with certainty claim that reopening a chronically occluded IRA reduced death related to heart failure or major arrhythmias, the Italian team noted that 75% of cardiac deaths in their population were related to sudden death and acute heart failure.

Clinical and diagnostic efforts should be made to identify patients who may gain the most from a strategy of reopening a chronically occluded IRA. Most recent publications with the use of DESs also favor recanalizing of CTO. Among them are the results of the second Prospective Randomized Trial of Sirolimus-Eluting and Bare Metal Stents in Patients with Chronic Total Occlusions (The PRISON II trial) [23]. The first PRISON trial demonstrated a reduction in target lesion revascularization among CTOs treated with bare metal stents (BMSs) compared with balloon angioplasty. While registry data have reported on the use of DESs in CTOs, PRISON II appears to be the first randomized trial to compare the efficacy of sirolimus-eluting stents (SESs) with BMSs in this population, which has traditionally been excluded from the larger randomized studies of DESs.

Two hundred patients were evenly randomized to either SES or BMS after crossing the totally occluded lesion. Angiographic restenosis, the primary endpoint, occurred less often in the SES group. There was a similar significant advantage in terms of reduced frequency of MACE at 6 months, driven almost exclusively by a reduction in target lesion revascularization, with a similar reduction in target vessel revascularization. There was no difference in the two groups in regard to MI (2–3%) and no deaths in the trial. There were two cases of stent thrombosis in the SES group and none in the BMS group. This incidence of stent thrombosis (2%) in the SES group is higher than often seen in trials with lower-risk populations.

The impact of the OAT on ACC/AHA (American College of Cardiology/American Heart Association) PCI guidelines

The open artery hypothesis suggests that late patency of an infarct artery is associated with improved LV function, increased electrical stability, and provision of collateral vessels to other coronary beds for protection against future events. The Occluded Artery Trial (OAT) [24] tested the hypothesis that routine PCI for total occlusion 3–28 days after MI would reduce the composite of death, reinfarction, or Class IV heart failure. Stable patients with an occluded infarct artery after MI (about 20% of whom received fibrinolytic therapy for the index event) were randomized to optimal medical therapy and PCI with stenting or optimal medical therapy alone. The qualifying period of 3–28 days was based on calendar days; thus, the minimal time from symptom onset to angiography was just over 24 hours. Inclusion criteria included total occlusion of the infarct-related artery with TIMI grade 0 or 1 antegrade flow and LVEF <50% or proximal occlusion of a major epicardial artery with a large-risk region. Exclusion criteria included NYHA (New York Heart Association) Class III or IV heart failure, serum creatinine >2.5 mg/dL, left main or three-vessel disease, clinical instability, and severe inducible ischemia on stress testing if the infarct zone was not akinetic or dyskinetic. The 4-year cumulative end point was 17.2% in the PCI group and 15.6% in the medical therapy group (HR 1.16 [95% CI 0.92 to 1.45]; $p = 0.2$). Reinfarction rates tended to be higher in the PCI group, which may have attenuated any benefit in LV remodeling. There was no interaction between treatment effect and any subgroup variable. Preclinical studies have suggested that late opening of an occluded infarct artery may reduce adverse LV remodeling and preserve LV volumes. However, five previous clinical studies in 363 patients have demonstrated inconsistent improvement in LVEF or LV end-systolic and end-diastolic volumes after PCI. The largest of these, the DECOPI trial [22], found a higher LVEF at 6 months with PCI. TOSCA-2 [21] enrolled 381 stable patients in a mechanistic ancillary study of OAT and had the same eligibility criteria. The PCI procedure success rate was 92% and the complication rate was 3%, although 9% had periprocedural MI as measured by biomarkers. At 1 year, patency rates ($n = 332$) were higher with PCI (83% versus 25%; $p <0.0001$), but each group ($n = 286$) had equivalent improvement in LVEF (4.2% versus 3.5%; $p = 0.47$). There was modest benefit of PCI on preventing LV dilation over 1 year in a multivariate model, but only 42% had paired volume determinations, so it is unclear whether this finding extended to the whole cohort. The potential benefit of PCI in attenuating remodeling may have been decreased by periprocedural MI and the high rate of use of beta blockers and ACE inhibitors. There was no significant interaction between treatment effect and time, infarct artery, or infarct size. The most recent ACC/AHA guidelines recommend Class III for PCI to a totally occluded infarct artery >24 hours after STEMI (ST-segment elevation myocardial infarction) in an asymptomatic patient with one- or two-vessel disease if they are hemodynamically and electrically stable and do not have evidence of severe ischemia (Level of Evidence B). These revised recommendations will potentially reduce the level of enthusiasm of operators to perform PCI on patients with CTO who have a history of MI [25].

Over the last decade there have been major developments in understanding the pathology of CTO and in the tools available to recanalize CTO. Nevertheless, more clarity is needed to determine which patient population should be subjected to percutaneous intervention. There is a consensus that all patients with evidence of ischemia should be subject for intervention. The anatomy assessed by angiography or with CT can suggest whether this should be done percutaneously or by CABG. The open artery hypothesis is still controversial, with no hard data to support intervention in CTO post–acute MI in asymptomatic patients. The OAT trial was a landmark study which impacted the guidelines and challenged the open artery hypothesis. The impact of this theory on angiogenesis and protection of the myocardium with a subsequent MI remains unclear. Since CTO is a procedure involving high doses of radiation and contrast, selection of patients should be done carefully based on proven ischemia related to the occluded vessel and evidence of favorable anatomy, which can improve the success.

See Plate 2 in the color plate section.

References

1 King SB 3rd, Lembo NJ, Weintraub WS *et al.* A randomized trial comparing coronary angioplasty with coronary bypass surgery. Emory Angioplasty versus Surgery Trial (EAST). *N Engl J Med* 1994; **331**: 1044–1050.

2 Bourassa MG, Roubin GS, Detre KM *et al.* Bypass angioplasty revascularization investigation: patient screening, selection, and recruitment. *Am J Cardiol* 1995; **75**: 3C–8C.

3 Stone GW, Kandzari DE, Mehran R *et al.* Percutaneous recanalization of chronically occluded coronary arteries: a consensus document: Part I. *Circulation* 2005; **112**: 2364–2372.

4 Werner GS, Emig U, Mutschke O, Schwarz G, Bahrmann P, Figulla HR. Regression of collateral function after recanalization of chronic total coronary occlusions: a serial assessment by intracoronary pressure and Doppler recordings. *Circulation* 2003; **108**: 2877–2882.

5 Tamai H, Berger PB, Tsuchikane E, Suzuki T *et al.* Frequency and time course of reocclusion and restenosis in coronary artery occlusions after balloon angioplasty versus Wiktor stent implantation: results from the Mayo-Japan Investigation for Chronic Total Occlusion (MAJIC) trial. *Am Heart J* 2004; **147**: E9.

6 Zidar FJ, Kaplan BM, O'Neill WW *et al.* Prospective, randomized trial of prolonged intracoronary urokinase infusion for chronic total occlusions in native coronary arteries. *J Am Coll Cardiol* 1996; **27**: 1406–1412.

7 Olivari Z, Rubartelli P, Piscione F *et al.* Immediate results and one-year clinical outcome after percutaneous coronary interventions in chronic total occlusions: data from a multicenter, prospective, observational study (TOAST-GISE). *J Am Coll Cardiol* 2003; **41**: 1672–1678.

8 Höher M, Wöhrle J, Grebe OC *et al.* A randomized trial of elective stenting after balloon recanalization of chronic total occlusions. *J Am Coll Cardiol* 1999; **34**: 722–729.

9 Rubartelli P, Verna E, Niccoli L *et al.* Coronary stent implantation is superior to balloon angioplasty for chronic coronary occlusions: six-year clinical follow-up of the GISSOC trial. *J Am Coll Cardiol* 2003; **41**: 1488–1492.

10 Buller CE, Dzavik V, Carere RG *et al.* Primary stenting versus balloon angioplasty in occluded coronary arteries: the Total Occlusion Study of Canada (TOSCA). *Circulation* 1999; **100**: 236–242.

11 Cohen HA, Williams DO, Holmes DR Jr *et al.* Impact of age on procedural and 1-year outcome in percutaneous transluminal coronary angioplasty: a report from the NHLBI Dynamic Registry. *Am Heart J* 2003; **146**: 513–519.

12 Hamm CW, Reimers J, Ischinger T, Rupprecht HJ, Berger J, Bleifeld W. A randomized study of coronary angioplasty compared with bypass surgery in patients with symptomatic multivessel coronary disease. German Angioplasty Bypass Surgery Investigation (GABI). *N Engl J Med* 1994; **331**: 1037–1043.

13 Anderson HV, Shaw RE, Brindis RG *et al.* A contemporary overview of percutaneous coronary interventions. The American College of Cardiology-National Cardiovascular Data Registry (ACC-NCDR). *J Am Coll Cardiol* 2002; **39**: 1096–1103.

14 Suero JA, Marso SP, Jones PG *et al.* Procedural outcomes and long-term survival among patients undergoing percutaneous coronary intervention of a chronic total occlusion in native coronary arteries: a 20-year experience. *J Am Coll Cardiol* 2001; **38**: 409–414.

15 Ranmanathan K, Gao M, Nogareda G *et al.* Successful percutaneous recanalization of a non-acute colluded coronary artery predicts clinical outcome and survival. *Circulation* 2001; **104**: II-415a.

16 Hoye A, van Domburg RT, Sonnenschein K, Serruys PW. Percutaneous coronary intervention for chronic total occlusions: the Thoraxcenter experience 1992–2002. *Eur Heart J* 2005; **26**: 2630–2636.

17 Dzavik V, Carere RG, Mancini GB *et al.* Predictors of improvement in left ventricular function after percutaneous revascularization of occluded coronary arteries: a report from the Total Occlusion Study of Canada (TOSCA). *Am Heart J* 2001; 142: 301–308.

18 Sirnes PA, Myreng Y, Mølstad P, Bonarjee V, Golf S. Improvement in left ventricular ejection fraction and wall motion after successful recanalization of chronic coronary occlusions. *Eur Heart J* 1998; **19**: 273–281.

19 Chung CM, Nakamura S, Tanaka K *et al.* Effect of recanalization of chronic total occlusions on global and regional left ventricular function in patients with or without previous myocardial infarction. *Catheter Cardiovasc Interv* 2003; **60**: 368–374.

20 Stone GW, Reifart NJ, Moussa I *et al.* Percutaneous recanalization of chronically occluded coronary arteries: a consensus document: Part II. *Circulation* 2005; **112**: 2530–2537.

21 Dzavík V, Buller CE, Lamas GA *et al.* Randomized trial of percutaneous coronary intervention for subacute infarct-related coronary artery occlusion to achieve long-term patency and improve ventricular function: the Total Occlusion Study of Canada (TOSCA)-2 trial. *Circulation* 2006; **114**: 2449–2457.

22 Steg PG, Thuaire C, Himbert D *et al.* DECOPI (DEsobstruction COronaire en Post-Infarctus): a randomized multi-centre trial of occluded artery angioplasty after acute myocardial infarction. *Eur Heart J* 2004; **25**: 2187–2194.

23 Suttorp M. for the PRISON II Investigators. Prospective Randomized trial of sirolimus-eluting and bare metal stents in patients with chronic total occlusions (PRISON II). Results presented at TCT 2005, Washington, DC.

24 Hochman JS, Lamas GA, Buller CE *et al.* Coronary intervention for persistent occlusion after myocardial infarction. *N Engl J Med* 2006; **355**: 2395–2407.

25 King SB 3rd, Smith SC Jr, Hirshfeld JW Jr *et al.* 2007 focused update of the ACC/AHA/SCAI 2005 guideline update for percutaneous coronary intervention: a report of the American College of Cardiology/American Heart Association Task Force on Practice guidelines. *J Am Coll Cardiol* 2008; **51**: 172–209.

CHAPTER 3

CTO – Review of Trials

Tina L. Pinto Slottow, MD *& Ron Waksman,* MD, FACC

Division of Cardiology, Washington Hospital Center, Washington, DC, USA

Chronic total occlusions (CTO) are common, estimated to occur in approximately half of patients with obstructive coronary artery disease (CAD) [1]. These lesions are technically challenging to manage percutaneously, however, and comprised approximately 2% of all percutaneous coronary interventions (PCI) in the 1970s [2]. Success rates have improved from 40–50% to 70–75% [3–5] with improved techniques, equipment, and operator experience and led to increased attempts at recanalization. CTO-PCI now comprises about 10–20% of the total PCI volume [2,6,7]. There are a number of reasons why CTO-PCI may be beneficial to patients and worth attempting, including reduced need for coronary artery bypass grafting (CABG), reduced angina, improved ejection fraction, and improved long-term mortality. Stent deployment has improved vessel patency following PCI, and stents have been shown to be beneficial in CTO. Drug-eluting stents (DES) may provide even further benefit above and beyond the gains achieved with bare metal stenting in this setting. This chapter will discuss the available evidence in the field of CTO-PCI.

Factors associated with successful CTO-PCI

Procedural success

Many retrospective analyses have found a number of factors to be associated with procedural failure

in the setting of CTO-PCI including multivessel disease, presence of bridging collaterals, moderate to severe calcification, CTO length, and CTO duration.

A series of 480 patients with attempted CTO-PCI at Emory between 1980 and 1988 had a 66% success rate. Failure to recanalize was associated with multivessel disease, lack of distal vessel filling, and non-LAD (left anterior descending coronary artery) CTO [8]. The 312 CTO that underwent PCI attempts between 1981 and 1992 resulted in a 61.2% success rate with a 1.9% complication rate and found a number of factors to be independently associated with procedural failure: the presence of bridging collaterals, time of occlusion >3 months, and vessel diameter <3 mm ($p < 0.003$) [9].

A retrospective multivariate analysis of 226 consecutive patients who had attempted CTO-PCI between 1986 and 1996 resulted in 134 successes and 92 failures and found calcification, length of the occlusion, and multivessel disease to be associated with failure. In this series, duration of occlusion, specific vessel, and presence of collaterals were not associated with failure [3]. A retrospective analysis of 83 patients who had 26 CTO of <30 day duration and 59 CTO of >30 day duration found that successful recanalization was more frequent in the <30 day group (96% versus 81%, $p = 0.017$) [10].

Multiple logistic regression analysis of 253 patients with 283 CTO with a 85% rate of successful PCI found that a tapered morphology (OR 6.1, 95% CI 2.1–18.2, $p < 0.001$), ≤45° angulation of the target artery (OR 4.5, 95% CI 1.2–17.2, $p < 0.03$), length of occlusion <15 mm (OR 3.4, 95% CI 1.6–7.0, $p < 0.001$), and multiple lesions in the target artery (OR 2.2, 95% CI 1.1–4.4,

Chronic Total Occlusions, 1st edition. Edited by R. Waksman and S. Saito. © 2009 Blackwell Publishing, ISBN: 978-1-4051-5703-2.

$p < 0.003$) were independently associated with procedural success [11].

A multicenter analysis of 419 patients who were scheduled to undergo CTO-PCI, the TOAST-GISE study, was performed at 29 Italian centers between June 1999 and January 2000. A total of 390 CTOs were confirmed in 376 patients. Procedural success was 73%. Multivariate analysis revealed a number of factors associated with procedural failure: CTO length >15 mm, moderate to severe vessel calcification, CTO duration >6 months, and multivessel disease [12].

Sustained recanalization

The major factor found to affect subsequent restenosis and occlusion in the era of bare metal stents is stented length. Among 716 CTO following successful stent placement, 57% had 6-month angiographic follow-up and found a binary restenosis rate of 40% and a reocclusion rate of 11%. Multivariate analysis revealed the only factors associated with reocclusion to be stented length [13].

A retrospective review of 220 patients who underwent CTO stenting and stratified patients by stent length (<20 mm, $n = 113$ and >20 mm, $n = 107$) found a higher restenosis rate in patients who had a longer stented length (34% versus 19%). Multivariate analysis found the only independent factor associated with restenosis was minimal lumen diameter (MLD) following stent placement. If MLD was <3 mm, restenosis was significantly more common in the group with longer stented length (56% versus 29%, $p = 0.021$), while if MLD was >3 mm, there was no significant difference between groups (19% versus 12%, $p = ns$) [14].

Clinical benefits of CTO-PCI

Given the technical challenges of recanalizing chronically occluded vessels, the difficulty in maintaining patency, and the potential for causing catastrophic complications such as coronary perforations and dissections, the questions arises as to whether the benefits of CTO-PCI outweigh the risks. A number of case series have followed patients with successful and failed CTO-PCI procedures and looked at outcomes, specifically demonstrating

a reduction in need for CABG and an improvement in left ventricular function (Table 3.1).

Coronary artery bypass grafting

A series of 44 patients with attempted CTO angioplasty had a 59% success rate. Of the 26 patients who had their CTO opened, only 3 (12%) required CABG while 7 of the 18 patients (39%, $p = 0.04$) whose CTO could not be recanalized underwent CABG by 31-month follow-up [2]. Freedom from CABG was significantly higher among the 317 patients at Emory with successful CTO-PCI at 4-year follow-up when compared to the 163 patients with failed PCI (87% versus 64%, $p < 0.0001$) [8].

Among 100 CTO in patients with Canadian Cardiovascular Society (CCS) angina class III or IV despite medical therapy, 47 were successfully recanalized, and only 7 (15%) of these patients went on to undergo CABG. Among the 45 patients who had unsuccessful, uncomplicated procedures, 16 (36%) surgeries were required and among the 8 patients with complicated procedures, 3 (38%) required CABG [7]. Noguchi and colleagues' series of 226 patients found no difference at 4-year follow-up in the composite of death or MI based upon whether CTO-PCI was successful or not. There were fewer CABG in the success group, however (7% versus 28%, $p < 0.001$) [3].

In the TOAST-GISE study, 1-year follow-up was available on 99% of the patients. Patients who had successful CTO-PCI had a lower rate of the composite of cardiac death or MI (1% versus 7%, $p = 0.005$), a lower rate of CABG (2.5% versus 15.7%, $p < 0.0001$), and were more likely to be free of angina (89% versus 75%, $p = 0.008$). Multivariate analysis confirmed that the only characteristic associated with event-free survival was CTO-PCI success or failure [12].

Left ventricular ejection fraction

Ninety-five patients who underwent catheterization for angina and were found to have a CTO underwent successful recanalization, with 71% receiving stents. Angiographic follow-up including ventriculogram was completed in all of these patients at 6 months and ejection fraction (EF) was found to increase from 62% to 67% ($p < 0.001$). There was no change in EF among the 8 patients

Table 3.1 Clinical benefits of CTO-PCI

				CABG		
				Successful	Failed	
Trial	Follow-up (months)	n	Success rate	PCI, n (%)	PCI, n (%)	p
Warren et al. [2]	31	44	26 (59%)	3 (12)	7 (39)	0.04
Ivanhoe et al. [8]	48	480	317 (66%)	28 (8)	55 (34)	<0.0001
Stewart et al. [7]	12	100	47 (47%)	7 (15)	19 (36)	n/a
Noguchi et al. [3]	48	226	134 (59%)	n/a (7)	n/a (28)	<0.001
TOAST-GISE [12]	12	369	286 (73%)	7 (3)	13 (16)	<0.0001

			Ejection fraction			
Trial	Follow-up (months)	n	Pre-PCI	Post-PCI	p	Other findings
Sirnes et al. [15]	6	95	62%	67%	<0.001	No increase in EF if CTO reoccluded at follow-up.
TOSCA [16]	6	244	59%	61%	0.003	EF improved only if CTO ≤6 weeks old
Chung et al. [17]	6	44–CTO in area of MI	49	51	ns	
		31–CTO not in area of MI	60	67	<0.001	

n/a = not available; ns = non-significant.

who were found to have reocclusion of the CTO at angiographic follow-up [15].

A substudy of 244 patients in the Total Occlusion Study of Canada (TOSCA) study who had ventriculograms at baseline and 6-month follow-up found a significant improvement in EF over time (from 59% to 61%, $p = 0.003$) that did not vary based on whether the patient had PTCA or stenting. When divided by duration of CTO, patients with a CTO for >6 weeks had no improvement in EF while those whose CTO was ≤6 weeks old had a significant improvement in EF (+3%, $p = 0.0006$). Multivariate analysis revealed that baseline EF <60%, duration of occlusion ≤6 weeks, and CCS angina class I or II were independently associated with an improvement in EF following successful CTO-PCI [16].

A retrospective analysis of 75 patients who had successful CTO-PCI and ventriculograms at baseline and 6 months between 1998 and 2002 investigated change in EF based on whether the patient had a MI in the area of the CTO. Among the 44 patients whose CTO was supplying the area that had sustained a MI, there was no significant change

in EF (from 49% to 51%, $p = $ ns) or in regional wall motion. However, among the 31 patients whose CTO was not supplying an area of infarction, there was significant improvement in EF (from 60% to 67%, $p < 0.001$) and in regional wall motion [17].

Angioplasty versus stent placement

Eight randomized trials of PTCA (percutaneous transluminal coronary angioplasty) compared to bare metal stent (BMS) placement in CTO lesions have been published [18–27] (Table 3.2). These trials have varied in definition of CTO, antithrombotic regimen, and design, but the findings in all have trended the same way. Stent deployment consistently resulted in lower rates of restenosis, reocclusion, and revascularization compared to PTCA alone. Absolute rates of target lesion revascularization (TLR) were higher in these patients following stenting than among patients treated for non-occlusive native coronary lesions, however [28–30]. The high rates of restenosis and reocclusion, despite the significant improvements achieved

Table 3.2 RCT of PTCA compared to BMS for CTO-PCI

Trial	Follow-up (mos (%))	n, PTCA	n, BMS	Reocclusion			Restenosis			TVR		
				PTCA (%)	Stent (%)	p	PTCA (%)	Stent (%)	p	PTCA (%)	Stent (%)	p
SICCO (Stenting in Chronic Coronary Occlusion) [18,19]	6 (97) 33 (97)	57	57	26	12	0.058	74	32	<0.001	42 53	22 24	0.025 0.002
GISSOC (Gruppo Italiano di Studi sulla Stent nelle Occlusioni coronariche) [20,21]	9 (88) 72 (52)	54	56	34	8	0.004	68	32	0.0008	22 35	5 15	0.04 0.02
TCSCA (Total Occlusion Study of Canada) [22]	6 (96)	208	202	20	11	0.024	70	55	0.001	15	8	0.03
SARECCO (Stent or Angioplasty after Recanalization of chronic coronary Occlusions) [23]	4 (94)	55	55	14	2	0.05	62	26	0.01	55	24	0.05
SPACTO (Stent versus Percutaneous Angioplasty in Chronic Total Occlusion) [24]	6 (79)	43	42	24	3	0.01	64	32	0.01	40	25	ns
STOP (Stents in Total Occlusion for Restenosis Prevention) [25]	6 (72)	48	48	16	8	ns	71	42	0.032	42	25	ns
MAJIC (Mayo-Japan Investigation for Chronic Total Occlusion) [26]	6 (88)	111	110	9	2	<0.05	55	57	ns	50	31	<0.005
PRISON (Primary Stenting of Occluded Native Coronary Arteries) [27]	6 (90) 13 (90)	100	100	7	8	ns	33	22	ns	20 29	5 13	0.002 <0.001

ns = non-significant.

with stenting, means there is still room for improved outcomes with more advanced technologies.

Drug-eluting stents in CTO-PCI

There is limited data available on the impact that drug-eluting stents have had on the field of CTO-PCI. The majority of the data is with the Cypher® sirolimus-eluting stent (SES) (Cordis Johnson & Johnson, Miami Lakes, FL), which demonstrates a lower rate of restenosis compared to BMS.

In a retrospective analysis of 122 patients who underwent CTO-PCI between April 2002 and April 2004 and received a SES were compared to 259 patients who received a BMS for CTO lesions between April 2000 and April 2002. Angiographic follow-up was available in 80% of the BMS patients and 83% of the SES patients. At 6-month follow-up, restenosis was significantly lower in the SES group (9.2% versus 33.3%, $p < 0.001$), but there was no difference in death or MI [31]. This analysis is limited in that the groups of patients are not contemporaneous.

A retrospective analysis of 60 patients who received SES for CTO was performed compared to 120 patients who received BMS. At 6-month follow-up, the SES group (angiographic follow-up in 97%) had a lower incidence of binary restenosis (2% versus 32%, $p < 0.001$) and reocclusion (0% versus 6%, $p < 0.001$) than the BMS group (angiographic follow-up in 67%). There was no difference in the death, MI, or in-hospital

complication rate between groups, so the main difference was in revascularization (TVR 3% versus 30%, $p < 0.001$) [32]. The lack of angiographic follow-up in a significant number of the BMS patients limits the conclusions that can be drawn from this study.

There is very limited data on paclitaxel-eluting stent (PES) use in CTO. Binary restenosis rates in very small series appear to be 8–10%, which appears on par with SES [33,34]. There is no data available to aid in determining differences between SES and PES.

One randomized trial of DES in CTO-PCI has been reported, the PRISON II trial. Two centers enrolled 200 CTO patients and randomized them to receive either SES or the Bx Velocity™ (Cordis Johnson & Johnson, Miami Lakes, FL) BMS. Six-month angiographic follow-up was available on 94% of the patients. The remaining 12 patients were asymptomatic and had no clinical events. At 6 months, the SES group demonstrated a lower rate of restenosis (7% versus 36%, $p < 0.001$) and lower TLR (4% versus 19%, $p = 0.001$). There was no significant difference in recurrent angina CCS class III/IV, death, or MI between groups at 6-month and 12-month follow-up [35].

Long-term follow-up

A few registries of CTO-PCI patients have detailed long-term clinical outcomes (Table 3.3). In the PTCA era, a series of 257 CTO patients

Table 3.3 Long-term outcomes after CTO-PCI

CTO-PCI Registry	Follow-up (years)	n Success	Failure	Major finding in success group
Emory [8]	4	317	163	Higher death and MI-free survival 93% versus 89%, $p = 0.0044$
Thoraxcenter [37]	5	575	310	Higher survival 93.5% versus 88%, $p = 0.02$ Higher MI-free survival 89.6% versus 83.1%, $p = 0.02$
Mayo Clinic [5]	10	876	386	Higher survival % not reported, $p = 0.025$
Mid America Heart Institute [4]	10	1491	516	Higher survival 73.5% versus 65%, $p = 0.001$

at a single center demonstrated restenosis in 41% at 6 months, 66% at 1 year, and 77% at 2-year follow-up [36]. Piscione and colleagues' series of 83 patients with 26 CTO of <30-day duration and 59 CTO of >30-day duration found no difference in the composite of death, MI, and TVR between the two groups at 2-year follow-up [10]. 317 patients at Emory who had successful recanalization had higher death and MI-free survival at 4-year follow-up when compared to the 163 patients who had failed CTO-PCI (93% versus 89%, $p = 0.0044$) [8].

Three series of very long-term follow-up on CTO patients have been published in the literature: the experiences of the Mid America Heart Institute [4], the Thoraxcenter in Rotterdam [37], and the Mayo clinic registry [5]. Among 2007 patients who had CTO-PCI attempted between 1980 and 1999 and the Mid America Heart Institute, 1491 had successful procedures. These patients demonstrated a survival advantage at 10-year follow-up (73.5% versus 65%, $p = 0.001$). A propensity analysis matching these 2007 patients to 2007 patients who underwent non-CTO-PCI found no difference in death, MI, revascularization (composite of CABG and PCI), or stroke at 10-year follow-up [4].

A total of 874 patients with 885 CTO underwent attempted PCI at the Thoraxcenter between 1992 and 2002. Procedural success was 65%, of which 81% received bare metal stents. Patients with successful procedures had higher cumulative survival (93.5% versus 88%, $p = 0.02$) and higher survival free of acute MI (89.6% versus 83.1%, $p = 0.02$) at 5-year follow-up compared to patients with failed procedures [37].

The Mayo registry of 1262 patients who underwent CTO-PCI attempt between 1979 and 2005 had success rates that improved from 51% to 70% over time. Rates of TLR were significantly lower when comparing patients undergoing procedures after 1997 with those treated prior to that time. Mortality at 10-year follow-up was significantly greater in patients with a failed procedure ($p = 0.025$), although the separation of curves was not apparent until 6 years following PCI attempt. Multivariate analysis did not find technical failure to be an independent predictor of mortality, however [5].

Conclusions

Data is limited in the realm of CTO-PCI, but there is a reasonable amount of available evidence to draw certain conclusions. Successful CTO recanalization has been shown to be beneficial to patients, leading to reduced need for coronary artery bypass grafting (CABG), improved ejection fraction, and improved long-term mortality. Factors associated with procedural failure include multivessel disease, presence of bridging collaterals, moderate to severe calcification, longer CTO length, and longer CTO duration. Longer stented length and lower MLD following PCI have been shown to be associated with higher incidence of binary restenosis. Stent deployment is superior to PTCA at maintaining vessel patency following PCI. The limited data currently available on DES, specifically SES, demonstrate lower revascularization rates than following BMS deployment.

As technical success improves and long-term follow-up of patients verifies the benefits of CTO-PCI, interest in this procedure has been on the rise. Much of current evidence is retrospective and limited by small patient numbers, but the increasing enthusiasm is bound to lead to future well-designed trials that should solidify our knowledge of factors important to procedural success and sustained patency.

References

1 Christofferson RD, Lehmann KG, Martin GV, Every N, Caldwell JH, Kapadia SR. Effect of chronic total coronary occlusion on treatment strategy. *Am J Cardiol* 2005; **95**(9): 1088–1091.

2 Warren RJ, Black AJ, Valentine PA, Manolas EG, Hunt D. Coronary angioplasty for chronic total occlusion reduces the need for subsequent coronary bypass surgery. *Am Heart J* 1990; **120**(2): 270–274.

3 Noguchi T, Miyazaki MS, Morii I, Daikoku S, Goto Y, Nonogi H. Percutaneous transluminal coronary angioplasty of chronic total occlusions. Determinants of primary success and long-term clinical outcome. *Catheter Cardiovasc Interv* 2000; **49**(3): 258–264.

4 Suero JA, Marso SP, Jones PG *et al.* Procedural outcomes and long-term survival among patients undergoing percutaneous coronary intervention of a chronic total occlusion in native coronary arteries: a 20-year experience. *J Am Coll Cardiol* 2001; **38**(2): 409–414.

5 Prasad A, Rihal CS, Lennon RJ, Wiste HJ, Singh M, Holmes DR, Jr. Trends in outcomes after percutaneous coronary intervention for chronic total occlusions: a 25-year experience from the Mayo Clinic. *J Am Coll Cardiol* 2007; **49**(15): 1611–1618.

6 Kinoshita I, Katoh O, Nariyama J *et al.* Coronary angioplasty of chronic total occlusions with bridging collateral vessels: immediate and follow-up outcome from a large single-center experience. *J Am Coll Cardiol* 1995; **26**(2): 409–415.

7 Stewart JT, Denne L, Bowker TJ *et al.* Percutaneous transluminal coronary angioplasty in chronic coronary artery occlusion. *J Am Coll Cardiol* 1993; **21**(6): 1371–1376.

8 Ivanhoe RJ, Weintraub WS, Douglas JS, Jr *et al.* Percutaneous transluminal coronary angioplasty of chronic total occlusions. Primary success, restenosis, and long-term clinical follow-up. *Circulation* 1992; **85**(1): 106–115.

9 Tan KH, Sulke N, Taub NA, Watts E, Karani S, Sowton E. Determinants of success of coronary angioplasty in patients with a chronic total occlusion: a multiple logistic regression model to improve selection of patients. *Br Heart J* 1993; **70**(2): 126–131.

10 Piscione F, Galasso G, Maione AG *et al.* Immediate and long-term outcome of recanalization of chronic total coronary occlusions. *J Interv Cardiol* 2002; **15**(3): 173–179.

11 Dong S, Smorgick Y, Nahir M *et al.* Predictors for successful angioplasty of chronic totally occluded coronary arteries. *J Interv Cardiol* 2005; **18**(1): 1–7.

12 Olivari Z, Rubartelli P, Piscione F *et al.* Immediate results and one-year clinical outcome after percutaneous coronary interventions in chronic total occlusions: data from a multicenter, prospective, observational study (TOAST-GISE). *J Am Coll Cardiol* 2003; **41**(10): 1672–1678.

13 Sallam M, Spanos V, Briguori C *et al.* Predictors of re-occlusion after successful recanalization of chronic total occlusion. *J Invasive Cardiol* 2001; **13**(7): 511–515.

14 Choi SW, Lee CW, Hong MK *et al.* Clinical and angiographic follow-up after long versus short stenting in unselected chronic coronary occlusions. *Clin Cardiol* 2003; **26**(6): 265–268.

15 Sirnes PA, Myreng Y, Molstad P, Bonarjee V, Golf S. Improvement in left ventricular ejection fraction and wall motion after successful recanalization of chronic coronary occlusions. *Eur Heart J* 1998; **19**(2): 273–281.

16 Dzavik V, Carere RG, Mancini GB, *et al.* Predictors of improvement in left ventricular function after percutaneous revascularization of occluded coronary arteries: a report from the Total Occlusion Study of Canada (TOSCA). *Am Heart J* 2001; **142**(2): 301–308.

17 Chung CM, Nakamura S, Tanaka K *et al.* Effect of recanalization of chronic total occlusions on global and regional left ventricular function in patients with or without previous myocardial infarction. *Catheter Cardiovasc Interv* 2003; **60**(3): 368–374.

18 Sirnes PA, Golf S, Myreng Y *et al.* Stenting in Chronic Coronary Occlusion (SICCO): a randomized, controlled trial of adding stent implantation after successful angioplasty. *J Am Coll Cardiol* 1996; **28**(6): 1444–1451.

19 Sirnes PA, Golf S, Myreng Y *et al.* Sustained benefit of stenting chronic coronary occlusion: long-term clinical follow-up of the Stenting in Chronic Coronary Occlusion (SICCO) study. *J Am Coll Cardiol* 1998; **32**(2): 305–310.

20 Rubartelli P, Niccoli L, Verna E *et al.* Stent implantation versus balloon angioplasty in chronic coronary occlusions: results from the GISSOC trial. Gruppo Italiano di Studio sullo Stent nelle Occlusioni Coronariche. *J Am Coll Cardiol* 1998; **32**(1): 90–96.

21 Rubartelli P, Verna E, Niccoli L *et al.* Coronary stent implantation is superior to balloon angioplasty for chronic coronary occlusions: six-year clinical follow-up of the GISSOC trial. *J Am Coll Cardiol* 2003; **41**(9): 1488–1492.

22 Buller CE, Dzavik V, Carere RG *et al.* Primary stenting versus balloon angioplasty in occluded coronary arteries: the Total Occlusion Study of Canada (TOSCA). *Circulation* 1999; **100**(3): 236–242.

23 Sievert H, Rohde S, Utech A *et al.* Stent or angioplasty after recanalization of chronic coronary occlusions? (The SARECCO Trial). *Am J Cardiol* 1999; **84**(4): 386–390.

24 Hoher M, Wohrle J, Grebe OC *et al.* A randomized trial of elective stenting after balloon recanalization of chronic total occlusions. *J Am Coll Cardiol* 1999; **34**(3): 722–729.

25 Lotan C, Rozenman Y, Hendler A *et al.* Stents in total occlusion for restenosis prevention. The multicentre randomized STOP study. The Israeli Working Group for Interventional Cardiology. *Eur Heart J* 2000; **21**(23): 1960–1966.

26 Tamai H, Berger PB, Tsuchikane E *et al.* Frequency and time course of reocclusion and restenosis in coronary artery occlusions after balloon angioplasty versus Wiktor stent implantation: results from the Mayo-Japan Investigation for Chronic Total Occlusion (MAJIC) trial. *Am Heart J* 2004; **147**(3): E9.

27 Rahel BM, Suttorp MJ, Laarman GJ *et al.* Primary stenting of occluded native coronary arteries: final results of the Primary Stenting of Occluded Native Coronary Arteries (PRISON) study. *Am Heart J* 2004; **147**(5): e22.

28 Serruys PW, de Jaegere P, Kiemeneij F *et al.* A comparison of balloon-expandable-stent implantation with balloon angioplasty in patients with coronary artery

disease. Benestent Study Group. *N Engl J Med* 1994; **331**(8): 489–495.

29 Serruys PW, van Hout B, Bonnier H *et al.* Randomised comparison of implantation of heparin-coated stents with balloon angioplasty in selected patients with coronary artery disease (Benestent II). *Lancet* 1998; **352**(9129): 673–681.

30 Fischman DL, Leon MB, Baim DS *et al.* A randomized comparison of coronary-stent placement and balloon angioplasty in the treatment of coronary artery disease. Stent Restenosis Study Investigators. *N Engl J Med* 1994; **331**(8): 496–501.

31 Ge L, Iakovou I, Cosgrave J *et al.* Immediate and midterm outcomes of sirolimus-eluting stent implantation for chronic total occlusions. *Eur Heart J* 2005; **26**(11): 1056–1062.

32 Nakamura S, Muthusamy TS, Bae JH, Cahyadi YH, Udayachalerm W, Tresukosol D. Impact of sirolimus-eluting stent on the outcome of patients with chronic total occlusions. *Am J Cardiol* 2005; **95**(2): 161–166.

33 Werner GS, Krack A, Schwarz G, Prochnau D, Betge S, Figulla HR. Prevention of lesion recurrence in chronic total coronary occlusions by paclitaxel-eluting stents. *J Am Coll Cardiol* 2004; **44**(12): 2301–2306.

34 Werner GS, Schwarz G, Prochnau D *et al.* Paclitaxel-eluting stents for the treatment of chronic total coronary occlusions: a strategy of extensive lesion coverage with drug-eluting stents. *Catheter Cardiovasc Interv* 2006; **67**(1): 1–9.

35 Suttorp MJ, Laarman GJ, Rahel BM *et al.* Primary Stenting of Totally Occluded Native Coronary Arteries II (PRISON II): a randomized comparison of bare metal stent implantation with sirolimus-eluting stent implantation for the treatment of total coronary occlusions. *Circulation* 2006; **114**(9): 921–928.

36 Ellis SG, Shaw RE, Gershony G *et al.* Risk factors, time course and treatment effect for restenosis after successful percutaneous transluminal coronary angioplasty of chronic total occlusion. *Am J Cardiol* 1989; **63**(13): 897–901.

37 Hoye A, van Domburg RT, Sonnenschein K, Serruys PW. Percutaneous coronary intervention for chronic total occlusions: the Thoraxcenter experience 1992–2002. *Eur Heart J* 2005; **26**(24): 2630–2636.

PART II

PART II

Imaging

CHAPTER 4

CT Angiography: Application in Chronic Total Occlusions

Hidehiko Hara, MD, *John R. Lesser,* MD, *Nicholas Burke,* MD, *&*
Robert S. Schwartz, MD

Minneapolis Heart Institute and Foundation, Minneapolis, MN, USA

Introduction

Multislice computed tomography (MSCT) has demonstrated high qualitative and quantitative diagnostic accuracy among various patient populations [1,2]. It provides vessel wall plaque morphology and luminal stenosis quantitation from plaque measurements [3].

Percutaneous coronary intervention (PCI) of the chronic total occlusion (CTO) remains a significant interventional problem, but has shown very slow clinical progress. In recent series, procedural success rates range from 55% to 80%, with the variability reflecting differences in operator technique and experience, availability of advanced guidewires, CTO definition, and case selection [4]. The ability of CT angiography (CTA) to image plaque and three-dimensional vascular directions has given rise to the hope that advanced imaging by CTA may add incrementally to the success of PCI for CTOs. The present chapter discusses the present and future for CTA in CTO.

Overview of utility of CT scan to the coronary artery disease

Quantification of coronary artery calcification was first reported with electron beam CT (EBCT) [5]. This ability is the key since calcification

Chronic Total Occlusions, 1st edition. Edited by R. Waksman and S. Saito. © 2009 Blackwell Publishing, ISBN: 978-1-4051-5703-2.

plays a crucial role in difficulty of the coronary CTO. Histologic studies demonstrate an attenuation value of >130 HU as closely correlated with calcified plaque in the coronary arteries [6]. Additional studies provide evidence that EBCT underestimates the total coronary plaque burden. Modern cardiac CT scanners show the extent, distribution, and location of calcification [7,8].

Since the first generation of MSCT scanners were introduced in 2000, CT imaging has been made rapid advances. Modern scanners obtain 64 or more slices in one gantry rotation, and the temporal resolution has significantly decreased. Evidence for the utility of CT in coronary artery disease has accumulated over the years, and recent studies show its high quantitative and qualitative diagnostic accuracy when compared against quantitative coronary angiography [2]. It also has the potential for coronary plaque characterization in the proximal coronary system, perhaps comparable to intravascular ultrasound [9]. MSCT has now been applied to PCI for CTO [10,11].

Pathology

Pathological features of CTO vary, and depend on the mechanism of occlusion and its duration. Differential fibro-atheromatous plaque and thrombus content are frequent [12]. The acute event is likely plaque rupture, often causing thrombus formation and vessel occlusion [13]. Collagen and calcification replace the initial thrombus and cholesterol esters over time (Figure 4.1).

There may be a hard cap over the proximal and distal margins of the CTO which are comprised of fibrous tissue. Softer contents often occur between these caps (Figure 4.2). Proteoglycan is important for CTO lesions. Age-related changes in intimal plaque composition from cholesterol laden to fibrocalcific materials are seen in older CTOs and intimal plaque neovascular channels derived from the adventitia increase with age and are strongly associated with intimal cellular inflammation (Figure 4.3). Intimal plaque neovascularization formation is protective against the flow-limiting effects of intimal plaque growth [14].

How is pathology reflected by CTA imaging?

Previous investigations showed the importance of revascularizing CTO. Clinical improvements include symptoms, exercise tolerance, left ventricular function, and long-term survival [15–18]. While one of the most important reasons for procedural failure is the difficulty of the guidewire crossing occluded lesions, frequently creating difficulty due to the three dimensionality of its anatomical course visualized using only two-dimensional conventional coronary angiography (Figure 4.4).

The increased anatomic accuracy afforded by MSCT allows excellent resolution, and it may improve clinical success for PCI of CTO. Moreover,

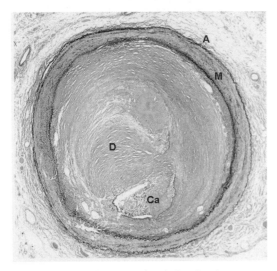

Figure 4.1 Human chronic total occlusion showing a "hard" plaque. Note regions of calcification (Ca, partially removed by histopathologic preparation process) and dense fibrous tissue (D). The media (M) and adventitia (A) are labeled, and the lumen is clearly occluded completely by the plaque (Elastin stain).

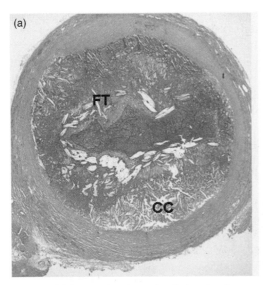

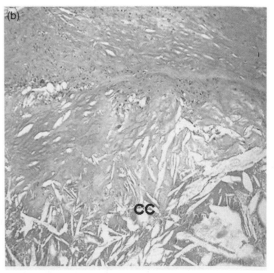

Figure 4.2 (a) Human chronic total occlusion showing a "soft' plaque." Note the cholesterol clefts (CC), where cholesterol was removed during the histolopathologic preparation. Loose fibrous tissue (FT) is also seen (Hematoxylin/Eosin stain). (b) Higher power magnification of (a).

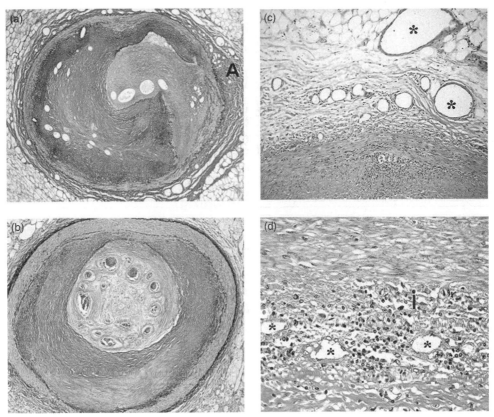

Figure 4.3 (a) Low-power view of a human chronic total occlusion with capillaries and neovascularization. (A indicates adventitia.) (b) Similar to (a), this photomicrograph shows an occluded central channel that has formed neovascular channels. The appearance of this occlusion suggests it is likely from a prior thrombotic episode. (c and d) Higher-power views of the microvascular channels, showing adventitial capillaries (*) and inflammation (I) around these channels.

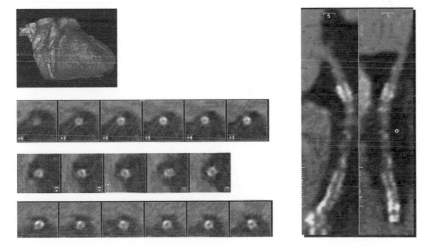

Figure 4.4 Cardiac CTA image of a chronic total occlusion of the right coronary artery. Cross-sections and longitudinal images are shown, with two regions of stenting. Plaque characterization consists of calcified and noncalcified plaque.

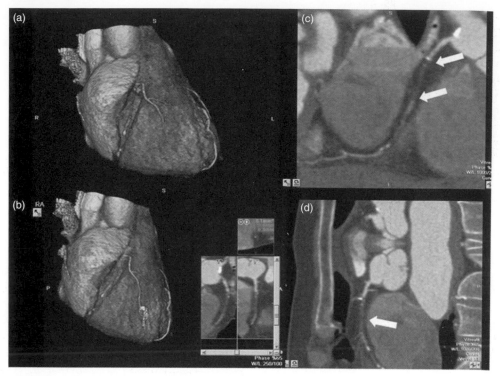

Figure 4.5 Similar to Figure 4.4, a cardiac CTA image of a chronic total occlusion showing calcified and noncalcified plaque. Arrows indicate the chronic total occlusion.

visualization and qualification of coronary atherosclerotic plaque is more difficult than assessing the coronary lumen narrowing. CTA shows not only the contrast enhanced lumen but also the vessel wall and atherosclerotic plaque (Figure 4.5). The potential for CTA lies in visualizing important predictors of the CTO lesion prior to PCI, and include spatial location and volume of calcification, and occluded lesion length from accumulation of cholesterol laden or fibrocalcific materials [19] (Figure 4.6).

What do we expect to see based on the CT density and spatial resolution?

CTA clearly identifies calcified lesions, and it may also be able to recognize lipid-rich plaque, fibrous plaque, and the degree of heavy calcification in CTO lesions according to various calcium scoring regimes. The most popular scoring was proposed by Agatston, with calcification defined at a threshold of >130 HU and an area threshold of >1 mm^2.

This score was calculated by multiplying the area of each calcified lesion by peak plaque density [5]. This score reveals incremental prognostic value in predicting sudden coronary death and nonfatal myocardial infarction in asymptomatic high-risk patients. Moreover, the calcification is an independent predictor of procedural failure for recanalization in CTO [20]. Identifying calcification is one of the most important predictors for clinical success. Extremely heavy calcification causes beam hardening and partial volume artifacts in the CTO image. Heavy calcification is associated with a high likelihood of adverse coronary events, not typically associated with plaque vulnerability. Moreover, the location of the calcified plaque within CTO is important for procedures and finding the true lumen within eccentrically calcified plaque. Recently, one study demonstrated the accuracy of 64-slice MSCT for classifying and quantifying plaque volumes in the proximal coronary arteries. The investigators detected not only calcified plaque but also hypodense spots (lipid pools) that were defined as structures larger than 2 mm^2 revealing a

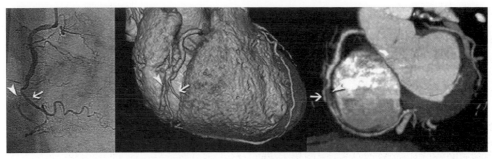

Figure 4.6 Conventional angiography image (left panel) showing a subtotal occlusion (arrowhead) of the mid part of the right coronary artery, distal to a right ventricular (RV) branch (arrow). Corresponding CT images using different image post-processing techniques: volume rendered (middle panel) and maximum intensity projection (right panel) images showing the subtotal occlusion (arrowhead) and RV branch (arrow) (Mollet et al. 2005).

density of at least 20 HU less than average value of surrounding noncalcified plaque tissue compared with intravascular ultrasound [9].

Most CT software creates three-dimensional volume rendered images of the coronary tree, multiplanar reconstruction, and maximal intensity projection images. Accurate roadmaps with good spatial resolution allow accurate guidewire placement in the occluded segment, while the lack of visualization of the course of an occluded artery and its distal lumen limits the effectiveness of various techniques.

Recent progress in MSCT spatial and temporal resolution uses decreased slice thickness and faster rotation times with reduced partial volume effects and motion artifacts for improved CTO visualization. One study revealed the complete visualization of coronary routes and plaque characterization in CTO segments with 16-slice MSCT, providing higher resolution. The investigators conclude that an excellent PCI success rate for CTO lesions is achieved using MSCT guidance [11].

Clinical results to date and impact on the interventional procedure

Several small studies demonstrate favorable results using MSCT for PCI in patients with CTO. Yokoyama and coworkers found an overall procedural success of 91.3% among 23 CTO lesions using MSCT guidance [11]. The investigators treated 23 angiographic CTO in 22 patients (average age 69 ± 5 years, 17 male), and 16-slice

MSCT was performed prior to PCI. All coronary routes of the CTO segment were accurately visualized including markedly angulated CTO lesions (13.0%) which could not be detected. Most lesions were occluded for longer than 3 months (95.7%), and 87.0% of those cases received grade 3 collaterals from other coronary arteries. The lesion length was 15.8 ± 10 mm and vessel diameter was 2.2 ± 0.4 mm. Calcification were divided into three groups comprising noncalcified, moderately calcified, and exclusively calcified. The majority of calcified plaque was located in the proximal, or both proximal and distal segments. MSCT revealed exclusively calcified plaque in 50.0% of those lesions. The authors conclude that MSCT should become a useful tool in PCI of CTO. They achieved excellent procedural results even with complicated and/or calcified lesions.

Mollet and de Feyter recently demonstrated independent predictors of procedural failure of PCI to the 45 patients with CTO by using 16-slice MSCT variables [3]. They found that long occlusions and severe calcification on MSCT coronary angiogram are important predictors of procedural failure, while neither variable was identified as an independent predictor on conventional CAG. Also, they pointed out the issue of relatively high radiation exposure during MSCT previously reported between 6.7 mSv and 13.0 mSv [21,22]. MSCT coronary angiography may reduce the procedural time for PCI of the CTO, because it may suggest a therapeutic strategy and the total radiation exposure dose may be decreased.

A recent 64-slice MSCT study, Kaneda and Saito and others demonstrated that technical success was higher in patients with MSCT imaging than without imaging (87% versus 80%, respectively) among patients with scheduled PCI for CTO lesions. They suggested a difference in procedural success among vessels, where 91% (20/22 cases) success was achieved in the left anterior descending and circumflex arteries with MSCT imaging, whereas motion artifacts limited use in the right coronary artery. They concluded that 64-slice CT facilitated PCI was a promising adjunctive modality to the CTO lesions [10].

Future perspectives

MSCT has progressed remarkably within the past decade. Better temporal and spatial resolution is still needed. 256-slice CT images are under investigation [23], and improved new models will likely improve these numbers.

Conclusions

MSCT coronary angiography prior to scheduled PCI of CTO lesions is promising, since this technology allows not only seeing the true three-dimensional course of occluded coronary arteries, but also reveals the characteristics of the occluded segment such as bending and severe calcification which are independent predictors of procedural failure. This modality is still developing and may ease some procedural difficulties, but needs to be further explored especially to the complex coronary intervention such as CTO lesions.

See Plates 3 and 4 in the color plate section.

References

1 Leber AW, Knez A, von Ziegler F et al. Quantification of obstructive and nonobstructive coronary lesions by 64-slice computed tomography: a comparative study with quantitative coronary angiography and intravascular ultrasound. J Am Coll Cardiol 2005; 46(1): 147–154.

2 Raff GL, Gallagher MJ, O'Neill WW, Goldstein JA. Diagnostic accuracy of noninvasive coronary angiography using 64-slice spiral computed tomography. J Am Coll Cardiol 2005; 46(3): 552–557.

3 Mollet NR, Hoye A, Lemos PA et al. Value of preprocedure multislice computed tomographic coronary angiography to predict the outcome of percutaneous recanalization of chronic total occlusions. Am J Cardiol 2005; 95(2): 240–243.

4 Stone GW, Reifart NJ, Moussa I et al. Percutaneous recanalization of chronically occluded coronary arteries: a consensus document: Part II. Circulation 2005; 112(16): 2530–2537.

5 Agatston AS, Janowitz WR, Hildner FJ, Zusmer NR, Viamonte M, Jr., Detrano R. Quantification of coronary artery calcium using ultrafast computed tomography. J Am Coll Cardiol 1990; 15(4): 827–832.

6 Rumberger JA, Simons DB, Fitzpatrick LA, Sheedy PF, Schwartz RS. Coronary artery calcium area by electron-beam computed tomography and coronary atherosclerotic plaque area. A histopathologic correlative study. Circulation 1995; 92(8): 2157–2162.

7 Rumberger JA, Sheedy PF, Breen JF, Schwartz RS. Electron beam computed tomographic coronary calcium score cutpoints and severity of associated angiographic lumen stenosis. J Am Coll Cardiol 1997; 29(7): 1542–1548.

8 Rumberger JA, Sheedy PF, 3rd, Breen JF, Schwartz RS. Coronary calcium, as determined by electron beam computed tomography, and coronary disease on arteriogram. Effect of patient's sex on diagnosis. Circulation 1995; 91(5): 1363–1367.

9 Leber AW, Becker A, Knez A et al. Accuracy of 64-slice computed tomography to classify and quantify plaque volumes in the proximal coronary system: a comparative study using intravascular ultrasound. J Am Coll Cardiol 2006; 47(3): 672–677.

10 Kaneda H, Saito S, Shiono T, Miyahita Y, Takahashi S, Domae H. Sixty-four-slice computed tomography-facilitated percutaneous coronary intervention for chronic total occlusion. Int J Cardiol 2007; 115(1): 130–132.

11 Yokoyama N, Yamamoto Y, Suzuki S et al. Impact of 16-slice computed tomography in percutaneous coronary intervention of chronic total occlusions. Catheter Cardiovasc Interv 2006; 68(1): 1–7.

12 Aziz S, Ramsdale DR. Chronic total occlusions–a stiff challenge requiring a major breakthrough: is there light at the end of the tunnel? Heart 2005; 91(Suppl 3): iii42–iii48.

13 Strauss BH, Segev A, Wright GA et al. Microvessels in chronic total occlusions: pathways for successful guidewire crossing? J Interv Cardiol 2005; 18(6): 425–436.

14 Srivatsa SS, Edwards WD, Boos CM et al. Histologic correlates of angiographic chronic total coronary artery occlusions: influence of occlusion duration on neovascular channel patterns and intimal plaque composition. J Am Coll Cardiol 1997; 29(5): 955–963.

15 Finci L, Meier B, Favre J, Righetti A, Rutishauser W. Long-term results of successful and failed angioplasty

for chronic total coronary arterial occlusion. *Am J Cardiol* 1990; **66**(7): 660–662.

16 Puma JA, Sketch MH, Jr., Tcheng JE *et al.* Percutaneous revascularization of chronic coronary occlusions: an overview. *J Am Coll Cardiol* 1995; **26**(1): 1–11.

17 Rambaldi R, Hamburger JN, Geleijnse ML *et al.* Early recovery of wall motion abnormalities after recanalization of chronic totally occluded coronary arteries: a dobutamine echocardiographic, prospective, single-center experience. *Am Heart J* 1998; **136**(5): 831–836.

18 Suero JA, Marso SP, Jones PG *et al.* Procedural outcomes and long-term survival among patients undergoing percutaneous coronary intervention of a chronic total occlusion in native coronary arteries: a 20-year experience. *J Am Coll Cardiol* 2001; **38**(2): 409–414.

19 Mollet NR, Cademartiri F, de Feyter PJ. Non-invasive multislice CT coronary imaging. *Heart* 2005; **91**(3): 401–407.

20 Noguchi T, Miyazaki MS, Morii I, Daikoku S, Goto Y, Nonogi H. Percutaneous transluminal coronary angioplasty of chronic total occlusions. Determinants of primary success and long-term clinical outcome. *Catheter Cardiovasc Interv* 2000; **49**(3): 258–264.

21 Hunold P, Vogt FM, Schmermund A *et al.* Radiation exposure during cardiac CT: effective doses at multidetector row CT and electron-beam CT. *Radiology* 2003; **226**(1): 145–152.

22 Morin RL, Gerber TC, McCollough CH. Radiation dose in computed tomography of the heart. *Circulation* 2003; **107**(6): 917–922.

23 Mizuno N, Funabashi N, Imada M, Tsunoo T, Endo M, Komuro I. Utility of 256-slice cone beam tomography for real four-dimensional volumetric analysis without electrocardiogram gated acquisition. *Int J Cardiol* 2007; **120**(2): 262–267.

CHAPTER 5

Magnetic Navigation Wire

Steve Ramcharitar, BMBCh, DPhil & *Patrick Serruys*, MD, PhD

The Thoraxcenter, Erasmus Medical Center, The Netherlands

Introduction

Magnetic Navigation System (MNS) is a rapidly growing technology with nearly 100 systems globally installed [1]. It was first utilized in the field of neurosurgery and cardiac electrophysiology [2] and is now being extended to percutaneous coronary interventions (PCI). In PCI, the Niobe®, MNS (Stereotaxis, St Louis, MO, USA) offers a novel approach to cross a lesion by precisely controlling of the tip of a magnetically enabled wire *in vivo* [3,4]. The system comprises of four key components: (i) two permanent adjustable magnets mounted on mechanical positioners situated at either side of the fluoroscopy table, (ii) a navigation software (Navigant®) that creates a virtual roadmap and vectors after inputting imaging data, (iii) a real time fluoroscopy system to display a virtual roadmap on the live image, and (iv) a sterile touch screen monitor ideally placed at the operating table for the operator to control the system. The magnetic guide wire used together with this system has a nominal diameter of 0.014 inch/0.36 mm and a nominal length of 185 cm or 300 cm [5]. The wire is configured with a 2 or 3 mm embedded gold encapsulate neodynium iron boron magnet at the distal tip. The first generation wires called the Cronus™ was hydrophilically coated with a tapering end that led to a 2 cm floppy or 3 mm intermediate coiled segment to which the magnet was attached (Figure 5.1) [6]. These tiny magnets when placed

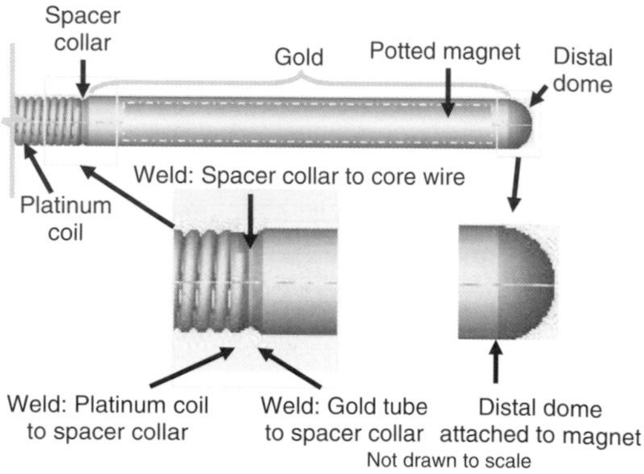

Figure 5.1 The basic design at the tip of a magnetically enabled wire.

in the magnetic field generated by the MNS aligned themselves in the direction of the applied field [7]. Once the tip direction is aligned in the desired direction then the wire can be manually advanced until another change of direction is required [8]. This basic principle of wire guidance is retained in the newer generation wires and towards the development of a radiofrequency enabled magnetic wire aimed at coronary and peripheral occlusion.

The current and future magnetic navigation wires

The newest family of magnetic wires that is currently commercially available is the Titan™ range. Like the Cronus™ wires they are available in either angled or straight 2 or 3 mm magnetic tips. Although the basic design of the wires is the same as the Cronus™ these wires are superior in their ability to deliver a device. Three-point deflection

Chronic Total Occlusions, 1st edition. Edited by R. Waksman and S. Saito. © 2009 Blackwell Publishing, ISBN: 978-1-4051-5703-2.

testing performed by supporting the wires at two points and measuring the force required to deflect the mid-point to 4 mm showed that they stiffen quicker in order to improve device delivery (Figure 5.2).

It gives the Titan™ wires a profile more similar to that of a Balance Medium Weight (BMW, Abbott Vascular Devices, Redwood, CA, USA) moderate support wire. At present the Titan™ wires are used in the majority of magnetic assisted PCI and these can include chronic total occlusions (CTOs) provided that the occlusion is short and not very old. However, when a stiffer wire that has greater pushability is desirable then the Titan™ Assert wire can be used as the shaft and tip load has similar characteristics to a Miracle 3 g (Asahi Intccc., Nagoya,

Japan). The tip-load measures the force to buckle the guidewire with 1 cm of extension (Figure 5.3).

The new Pegasus™ wires will soon supersede the Titan™ range. These wires are different as they are manufactured using nitinol in the distal shaft allowing a greater retention in the shape during the magnetic-assisted PCI. The proximal shaft is stainless steel to provide pushability. As with other magnetic wires they are hydrophilically coated to facilitate a smooth wire transit. At the tip of the wire is attached the 2 or 3 mm magnet. Various degrees of wire stiffness (moderate or intermediate) are possible by varying the diameter of the nitinol shaft under the coil. The three-point deflection test pattern shows that the Pegasus™ Moderate and Assert have similar support profiles. However, the very distal 2 cm of the Assert is stiffer to transmit more force when crossing tight or total occlusions (Table 5.1).

There are a number of improvements scheduled in the near future to the magnetic wires beyond Pegasus™. These include having smaller, but more, magnets embedded in a polymer tipped wire so as to have smoother transitions and larger, sharper magnetic deflections.

Navigational modes to orientate the magnetic tip

The magnets when correctly positioned and iso-centered interact to produce a uniformly spherical 15 cm magnetic field of 0.08 T called

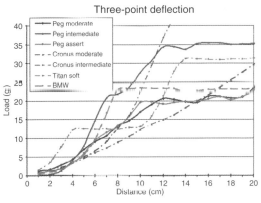

Figure 5.2 The lateral stiffness of magnetically enabled wire as determined by three-point testing.

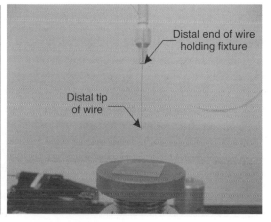

Tip load @ 1 cm extension	
Guidewire	Tip load (gf)
Cronus Soft	1.0
Cronus Moderate	1.8
Cronus Assert	3.5
Titan Soft	1.3
Titan Super Support	1.8
Titan Assert	3.5
BMW	0.6
Asahi Miracle 3	3.3

Figure 5.3 The tip-load comparison of magnetically enabled and conventional wires.

Table 5.1 Characteristics of the stereotaxis guidewire family

		Stereotaxis guidewire family comparison		
Guidewire	Distal core	Proximal core	Magnet tip length	Distal hydrophilic coating
Cronus	Nitinol	Nitinol	2 and 3 mm	25 cm
Titan	Stainless Steel	Stainless Steel	2 and 3 mm	10–34 cm
Pegasus	Nitinol	Stainless Steel	2 and 3 mm	40 cm

the magnetic volume. Within this volume any applied magnetic field vector precisely directs the tiny magnet mounted on the tip of a wire. Preset vectors of major vessels can be selected by the operator and advanced via the touch screen monitor. In doing so the magnets rotate, tilt, or translate to align the magnetic field to the orientation of the vector. The desired vector is displayed on the live fluoroscopy image and as the magnets move a second vector is displayed that eventually assumes the same orientation of the desired vector confirming the desired magnetic orientation is reached. In addition to the preset, vectors can also be created from two-dimensional maps of angiographic images or by using dedicated three-dimensional reconstruction software to generate a virtual road map of the vessel lumen. This virtual road map is displayed as a static centre white line on the live fluoroscopy image. The latter programme has the ability to create an endoluminal view of the coronary artery that can accentuate subtle changes in the direction of the vectors [9]. In the initial experience to extend MNS to CTOs it was described that the 'bull's eye view' that allows navigation around a central axis was a particularly useful technique [6]. In this approach the tip of the guidewire can be automatically or manually orientated to follow points that mimic a bull's eye used for target shooting. In doing so microchannels within the CTO can be locate through which the magnetic wire can enter (Figure 5.4).

The theory of radio frequency (RF) ablation in CTO

An attractive strategy for CTOs using the following concepts has been postulated by Serruys [10]: first, using magnetic navigation to steer a guidewire towards the occlusion; second, a technology to

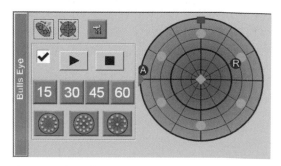

Figure 5.4 The Bull's Eye Navigational mode depicting the various interrogation patterns and tip angulations that can be utilized in searching for a microchannel in a CTO.

look forward within the vessel, either through the use of an optical coherence tomography or an intravascular ultrasound (IVUS) system or multislice computer tomography (MSCT) cross-sections to ensure ideal positioning of the wire in the true lumen; finally, some ablative power is needed at the tip of the wire to recanalize the CTO. Radiofrequency ablation has previously been reported with the Safe-Cross RF wire (Intraluminal Therapeutics, Carlsbad, CA, USA) uses optical reflectometry to verify the intraluminal position of the wire prior to radiofrequency ablation [11]. In the treatment of CTOs using RF ablation the first step required is energy delivered through mono or bipolar electrodes in order to generate a current that travels between the active electrode and the ground electrode (or dispersive electrode). In addition, continuous RF energy of frequencies greater than 100 kHz is desirable as this avoids neuromuscular stimulation without compromising the ablating potential. The distribution of this current is dictated by the size of the ablating active electrodes and the characteristics of the tissues surrounding the electrodes. The potential difference between the active electrode and the ground electrode determines the impedance and when low is the preferred pathway for current flow. When an RF voltage is applied to the electrodes, the polarity of the electrodes alternates at a given frequency. Polar molecules are alternatively attracted to the active electrode and then to the ground electrodes during each cycle of RF current, resulting in the generation of heat. The bioheat equation is used to describe how the temperature changes as a result of RF current delivery [12]:

$$T = \frac{1}{\sigma \rho c} J^2 t + T_0$$

where
T = final temperature (K)
σ = electrical conductivity (S/m)
ρ = tissue density (kg/m^3)
J = magnitude of the current density (A m^2)
t = duration of activation (s)
T_0 = initial temperature (K)

Furthermore, if the electric field between the tissue and electrode is large enough, arcing can occur. Electrical arcs are focused very high-energy sparks that are thought to vaporized cells in front of the active electrode and in so doing disrupt the tissue layer for effective ablating/cutting. Theoretical calculations show arcs can heat tissue from 37°C to 100°C in microseconds. Studies of electrical characteristics along with observation of the tip during cutting with the RF guidewire indicate two distinct phases in the cutting/ablation process [13]:

Phase 1: Water around the active electrode heats up and vaporizes. A capacitive vapor layer (dielectric layer) separates the electrode and the tissue.

Phase 2: Along the points on the electrode where the voltage potential is sufficient to break down the dielectric layer, an arc jumps from the electrode to the tissue.

Each arc quickly vaporizes water within the occlusion on contact, disrupting the tissue to allow easy passage of the electrode. If the vapor layer is maintained, then continuous arcing and steady cutting occurs.

The magnetically enabled RF wire

At present this wire is still being developed by Stereotaxis with the final testing due to be completed

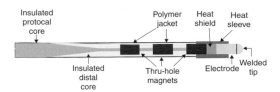

Figure 5.5 The magnetically enabled RF wire.

later this year. The latest prototype (Figure 5.5) consists of an insulated core wire, three spaced magnets in a polymer jacket and a heat shield surrounded by a heat sleeve attaching the RF electrode.

Its electrically conductive nitinol core wire is supportive on the proximal end whilst being flexible and durable on the distal end. For safe delivery of the RF energy to the electrode tip of the wire, the length of the core is electrically insulated with a PTFE (polytetrafluoroethylene) coating. The degree of insulation of the distal and the proximal section takes into account the wires function. In the distal section only very thin insulation is used so as to provide adequate dielectric strength without affecting the wire's flexibility. In the proximal section the insulation has a higher dielectric strength than the distal section since it is to be handled by the operator. As PTFE is naturally lubricious it avoids the need for an additional coating. Different designed magnets ('thru-hole magnets') having hollow central cores are placed proximally along the distal tip of the wire and are specially treated to prevent corrosion. A heat shield and sleeve protects them as since the intense heat generated can result in their demagnetization. The RF electrode is manufactured from the composite metal alloy and the entire wire is encased in a polyurethane polymer jacket for smooth transitions between the different components. In house *in vivo* studies were performed in porcine models having artificially created occlusions of the femoral arteries. The occlusions were typically 5–8 cm in length and aged 6–8 weeks to form the tough end caps and induce collateral formation. The device proved capable of engaging and perforating the proximal cap and entering the occlusion. It also proved capable of progressing within the occlusion, traversing the entire occlusion and exiting the distal cap into the distal patent section of artery.

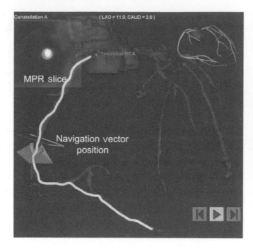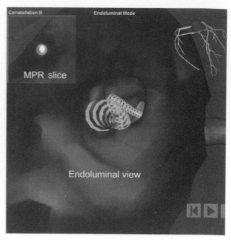

Figure 5.6 Navigation through MSCT co-integration demonstrating the MPR cross-section slice (left upper quadrant at the site of the navigational vector and the corresponding endoluminal view in the right panel).

Magnetic navigation and MSCT co-integration in CTOs

In a CTO the inability to image the artery with contrast media means that an alternative imaging modality is require to create the three-dimensional roadmap. MSCT offers the ability to visualize the occluded coronary artery and can provide a full three-dimensional roadmap of the coronary tree in Navigant® [14]. In the newest version (Navigant® 2.11) a segmented MSCT volume that only shows the coronary tree (Siemens Medical Solutions, Forchheim, Germany) can be imported into the software. In addition, the operator has access to the endoluminal view that simulates looking through the vessel lumen and simultaneously to the corresponding Multiplanar reconstruction (MPR) slice, as well as an automated update of the magnetic vector as the wire is advanced. The latter means that the operator can fully concentrate on the wire advancement guided by the moving vectors on the live fluoroscopy image. Moreover, as the vector is sequentially updated so too are the MPR slices together with the endoluminal views so that the operator can always have prior knowledge of the lesion in front of the wire (Figure 5.6). Clinical evaluation of the magnetically enabled RF wire with MSCT co-integration of chronically occluded stents is in the final stages of preparation.

Limitations

One major limitation with current wire designs is that the magnet is stuck on to the tip of the wire and this can influence the wire's ability to transit smoothly across a lesion. In the future generation wires the multimagnet design as used in the RF wire will try to accommodate this limitation. Another limitation with the current technology in that the uploaded MSCT dataset for managing CTO creates a static roadmap of the vessel, while the heart is a beating dynamic organ. In the future a dynamic roadmap created from the MSCT will be needed so that the wire advancement can be appropriately gated to the image to maximize the probability that it will be within the true lumen.

Conclusion

Magnetic Navigation is a promising technology in the management of CTOs. Over the past 5 years the improvement in magnetic guide wire designs has led to wires with comparable characteristics to conventional wires. The development of the magnetically enabled RF ablating wire together with the recent upgrades in MSCT co-integration software has brought the MNS closer to realizing its full potential to the CTO field.

See Plates 5 and 6 in the color plate section.

References

1 Patterson MS, Schotten J, van Mieghem C, Kiemeneij F, Serruys PW. Magnetic navigation in percutaneous coronary intervention. *J Interv Cardiol* 2006; **19**: 558–565.

2 Ernst S, Ouyang F, Linder C *et al.* Initial experience with remote catheter ablation using a novel magnetic navigation system: magnetic remote catheter ablation. *Circulation* 2004; **109**: 1472–1475.

3 Faddis MN, Chen J, Osborn J, Talcott M, Cain ME, Lindsay BD. Magnetic guidance system for cardiac electrophysiology: a prospective trial of safety and efficacy in humans. *J Am Coll Cardiol* 2003; **42**: 1952–1958.

4 Hertting K, Ernst S, Stahl F *et al.* Use of the novel magnetic navigation system Niobe™ in percutaneous coronary interventions; the Hamburg experience *Eurointervention* 2005; **1**: 336–339.

5 Atmakuri SR, Lev EI, Alviar C *et al.* Initial experience with a magnetic navigation system for percutaneous coronary intervention in complex coronary artery lesions. *J Am Coll Cardiol* 2006; **47**: 515–521.

6 Tsuchida K, Garcia Garcia HM, van der Giessen WJ *et al.* Guidewire navigation in coronary artery stenoses using a novel magnetic navigation system: first clinical experience. *Catheter Cardiovasc Interv* 2006; **67**: 356–363.

7 Ramcharitar S, Patterson MS, van Geuns RJ *et al.* A randomised controlled study comparing conventional and magnetic guidewires in a two-dimensional branching tortuous phantom simulating angulated coronary vessels. *Catheter Cardiovasc Interv* 2007; **70**: 662–668.

8 Ramcharitar S, Patterson MS, van Geuns RJ, Serruys PW. Magnetic navigation system used successfully to cross a crushed stent in a bifurcation that failed with conventional wires. *Catheter Cardiovasc Interv* 2007; **69**: 852–855.

9 Patterson M, Tanimoto S, Tsuchida K, Serruys PW. Magnetic navigation with the endo-luminal view and the X-ray overlay – Major advances in novel technology. *Eurointervention* 2008; in press.

10 Serruys PW. Fourth annual American College of Cardiology international lecture: a journey in the interventional field. *J Am Coll Cardiol* 2006; **47**: 1754–1768.

11 Werner GS, Fritzenwanger M, Prochnau D *et al.* Improvement of the primary success rate of recanalization of chronic total coronary occlusions with the Safe-Cross system after failed conventional wire attempts. *Clin Res Cardiol* 2007; **96**: 489–496.

12 Pearce JA. *Electrosurgery*, 1986. London: Chapman and Hall.

13 Honig WM. The mechanism of cutting in electrosurgery. *IEEE Trans Biomed Eng* 1975; January: 58–62.

14 Garcia-Garcia HM, Tsuchida K, van Mieghem C *et al.* Multi-slice computed tomography and magnetic navigation-initial experience of cutting edge new technology in the treatment of chronic total occlusions. *Eurointervention* 2008; in press.

CHAPTER 6

IVUS-Guided Recanalization of CTO

Etsuo Tsuchikane, MD, PhD

Department of Cardiology, Toyohashi Heart Center, Aichi, Japan

Intravascular ultrasound (IVUS) is one of the imaging modalities for vascular assessment and intervention which provides cross-sectional information of the vessel and area surrounding the vessel. Therefore, it can provide some useful information which can not be evaluated only by angiography. Currently, during the percutaneous coronary intervention of chronic coronary total occlusion (CTO-PCI), IVUS is sometimes used for assessment of plaque morphology and lesion length as well as vessel caliper after successful wiring followed by small balloon (usually 1.5 mm) so that ideal stent implantation can be performed. Of course, this procedure is not mandatory in CTO-PCI; however, for example, it is effective to avoid the vessel rupture by oversized stenting for shrunk vessel. Besides these evaluations after successful wiring of the occlusion, IVUS can be used to improve the success rate of wiring during CTO-PCI. In this chapter, we describe the effectiveness of IVUS on wiring procedure in CTO-PCI. There are mainly two types of IVUS-guided wiring techniques: IVUS-guided wiring at CTO entrance and IVUS-guided penetration from subintimal space.

Chronic Total Occlusions, 1st edition. Edited by R. Waksman and S. Saito. © 2009 Blackwell Publishing, ISBN: 978-1-4051-5703-2.

IVUS-guided wiring at CTO entrance

Confirmation of the entrance of CTO

In general, contralateral angiography precisely helps to identify an entry of a CTO despite the absence of stamp in the total occlusion of a bifurcation lesion. It is not so difficult to detect a dimple in the entry by wiring around the CTO if the operator can presume a route and a location of the passage. However, the use of angiography sometimes fails to identify the entry point. In this situation, IVUS is useful to detect the entry point of the CTO if the branch is large enough to advance an IVUS catheter (Figure 6.1). To perform this technique, the IVUS catheter is initially advanced into the branch at the occlusion. Based on a series of IVUS images, the catheter is positioned at the occlusion in the main vessel and angiography is performed subsequently. The entry exists at the location of IVUS transducer on angiography. Then, the operator seeks a dimple at the entry with careful wire manipulation. This technique also helps to examine the plaque hardness at the entrance.

Examination of the wire entry point into CTO

When the proximal vessel caliper is big enough to advance both IVUS catheter and support catheter for wiring, we can check the entry point of the wire into CTO by IVUS. This examination sometimes plays a very important role when the first wire goes into the subintimal space (Figure 6.2). In CTO-PCI, unfortunately,

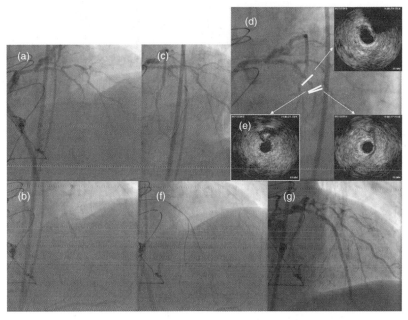

Figure 6.1 (a) Mid-LAD-CTO. (b) Although the LAD was completely blocked around mid-portion, it was hard to identify the entrance of a CTO despite the contra-lateral injection was performed. (c) Then an IVUS catheter was inserted into the distal septal branch. (d and e) IVUS image was then easily identified the CTO entrance. (f) This confirmation was also effective to choose a stiff wire to penetrate the tight proximal fibrous cap. (g) Final angiographic result after stenting.

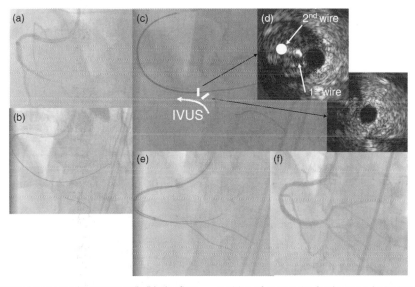

Figure 6.2 (a) Distal RCA-CTO (re-attempted). (b) The first attempt to cross the CTO by wiring was failed. In the second attempt, the first wire (intermediate) easily went out of the true channel. (c) This first wire was left and then an IVUS catheter was inserted into the small branch at CTO entrance. The images clearly showed that the entry point of the first wire was too close to the branch (d) so that it easily advanced into the subintimal space. The correct position of entry point for the second wire is in the center of the obstructed true channel which indicated the opposite direction to the branch. (e) Therefore, the course of the second wire was intentionally changed from the CTO entrance towards the opposite direction to the branch angiographically. Then this wire easily got into the distal small branch. (f) Final angiographic result after stenting.

the first wire often goes into the subintimal space, sometimes from the entrance of CTO. In these situations, the first wire should be left there and IVUS examination should be conducted if possible to check the entry point of the first wire. When the entry point is located around the center of the entrance circle detected by IVUS, the second wire should be advanced into the occlusion along the first wire to seek another channel inside the occlusion. When the entry point of the first wire is located on the marginal position of the circle, this wire must go into subintimal space from the entrance of CTO. In other words, the second wire should be advanced from the center of circle to another direction. Correct direction can be determined by side branch as shown in Figure 6.2. Also the correct entry point of the second wire can be identified by simultaneous wiring with IVUS catheter. Of course, an 8 Fr guiding catheter is indispensable for this procedure. This wiring technique should be called "IVUS-guided parallel wiring technique."

IVUS-guided penetration from subintimal space

Even when using the standard parallel wiring technique, the wires occasionally enlarge the subintimal space in difficult CTO procedures. Once the subintimal space expands beyond the distal end of CTO, the distal true lumen can be hardly seen in fluoroscopy. In these situations we often have to abandon the subsequent procedure when only the angiographical guidance is used. However, IVUS has a potential to make a breakthrough in these situations. IVUS can differentiate a true lumen from a false lumen by identifying the presence of side branches (which arise only from the true lumen) and intima and media (which surround the true lumen, but not the false lumen). Similarly, IVUS can confirm when the guidewire has reentered the true lumen from the false lumen [1]. This concept was first described by Werner *et al.* in 1997 [2]. With IVUS-guided wiring in subintimal space, the IVUS catheter is advanced through the first wire in the subintimal space. Enlargement of the subintimal space by wiring often collapses the distal true lumen; therefore, it would be failed to observe on angiography. However, the IVUS image clearly shows the cross sectional information which is useful to guide the second wire into the true lumen. Stiff wires (Confianza or Miraclebros 12, Asahi Intecc, Japan) should be used as the second wire to penetrate the true channel. Figure 6.3 illustrates IVUS-guided penetration technique from

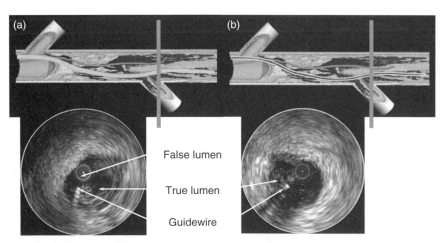

False lumen

True lumen

Guidewire

Figure 6.3 Concept of IVUS-guided penetration technique from subintimal space: (a) The distal true channel is completely collapsed by the enlargement of subintimal space. The IVUS catheter is intentionally inserted into space to examine the cross-sectional information. The IVUS image clearly indicates the collapsed true channel and the wire in expanded subintimal lumen. (b) Under this IVUS guidance, it can be performed to lead the wire into the collapsed true channel.

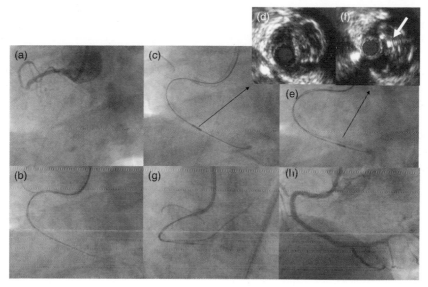

Figure 6.4 (a) Long RCA-CTO. (b) Parallel-wiring technique using stiff wires could not provide successful wire crossing. (c) An IVUS catheter was advanced through the wire in the false channel. (d) The image clearly showed an expanded subintimal space and a collapsed true channel. (e and f) Then a tapered stiff wire (Confianza, Asahi Intecc, Japan) was delivered under the IVUS guidance to penetrate the true channel from subintimal space and finally this procedure was succeeded. (g) The wire was carefully advanced to the distal true lumen. (h) Final angiographic result after multiple stenting.

subintimal space. This technique sometimes requires balloon dilatation in the subintimal space to deliver the IVUS catheter, and so it should never be performed when wire perforation from the subintimal space is already detected. Also an 8 Fr guiding catheter is indispensable to conduct the simultaneous wiring under IVUS guidance. After successful wire crossing, multiple stenting is mandatory to fully cover the enlarged subintimal space. However, by using this technique, we can retrieve some of unsuccessful CTOs initially performed by angiographical guidance [3,4]. Thus, this technique could be one of the last alternatives in the antegrade approach when standard wiring procedures fail in cases without a chance of retrograde approach. A representative case is shown in Figure 6.4.

See Plates 7 through 11 in the color plate section.

References

1 Stone GW, Colombo A, Teirstein PS *et al.* Percutaneous recanalization of chronically occluded coronary arteries : procedural techniques, device, and results. *Cathet Cardiovasc Interv* 2005; **66**(2): 217–236.

2 Werner GS, Diedrich J, Schlz KH, Knies A, Kreuzer H. Vessel reconstruction in total coronary occlusions with a long subintimal wire pathway: use of multiple stents under guidance of intravascular ultrasound. *Cathet Cardiovasc Diagn* 1997; **40**(1): 46–51.

3 Ito S, Suzuki T, Ito T *et al.* Novel technique using intravascular ultrasound-guided guidewire cross in coronary intervention for uncrossable chronic total occlusions. *Circ J* 2004; **68**(11): 1088–1092.

4 Matsubara T, Murata A, Kanyama H *et al.* IVUS-guided wiring technique: promising approach for the chronic total occlusion. *Catheter Cardiovasc Interv* 2004; **61**(3): 381–386.

PART III

Wires Technology

CHAPTER 7

Deflecting Tip Wires

Mirko Schiemann, MD

University Hospital Frankfurt, Frankfurt, Germany

Chronic total occlusion (CTO) remains a relative contraindication and the main cause of failure of coronary angioplasty. Approximately 30% of all coronary angiograms in patients with coronary artery disease will show a CTO and its presence often excludes patients from treatment by percutaneous coronary intervention (PCI) [1].

Coronary vessels that are excessively tortuous, clacified, and have angulated branches can lead to technical limitations in reaching and crossing distal, eccentric, and long coronary stenoses resulting in PCI failure [2]. In a large series by Kinoshita *et al.* [3], reasons for procedural failure included inability to cross the lesion with a guidewire (63% of cases), long intimal dissection with creation of a false lumen (24%), dye extravasation (11%), failure to cross the lesion with the balloon or dilate adequately (2%), and thrombus (1.2%). Effective therapy can therefore be limited by the occasional inability of the interventionalist to navigate the standard available guide wires through anatomically challenging regions of coronary vasculature and atherosclerotic disease accompanied with high radiation dose and extensive use of contrast, which may result in contrast nephropathy [4] and/or dermatologic x-ray toxicity [5–9]. Despite advances in experience and equipment, CTO recanalization with the use of contemporary guidewires and techniques may still be unsuccessful in ≥25% of cases. Numerous devices have been developed to approach such refractory and complex cases.

Many of these devices never progressed beyond the investigational phase because their use in small numbers of patients demonstrated either excessively high rates of complications (typically either dissection and/or perforation) or success rates not clearly greater than those achieved by standard equipment. Examples of failed CTO devices include the Magnum/Magnarail system [10,11], the Kensey Catheter [12], the ROTACS Low Speed Rotational Atherectomy Catheter [13], and the Excimer Laser Wire [14].

Most guidewire tips can be shaped by the physician during use or are supplied preshaped by the vendors. These conventional guidewires generally must be removed for reshaping and reinserted thereafter. During long and complex anatomic circumstances the shape of the wire tip can get lost. Limitations for these conventional wire systems are besides CTO, tortous vessel anatomy, through deployed stents, side-branch conditions, bifurcation/trifurcation, and acute take-offs. Routine guidewires used to cross non-occlusive lesions do not have the tip stiffness or push sufficient to traverse the tough fibrous cap of CTOs. Specialized guidewires have a thicker core that gradually tapers towards the tip, increasing tip stiffness and support.

The success rates for percutaneous CTO recanalization have undoubtedly improved over the last 5 years; a major reason is the introduction of stiffer, more powerful, and more supportive wires with greater torque response (e.g., Asahi Intec Miracle Brothers 3 to 12 g wires), tapered tip wires (e.g., Asahi Intec Confianza and Confianza Pro 9-g and Guidant Cross-It 100 to 400 wires), and wires with hydrophilic coatings (e.g., Guidant Whisper

Chronic Total Occlusions, 1st edition. Edited by R. Waksman and S. Saito. © 2009 Blackwell Publishing, ISBN: 978-1-4051-5703-2.

and Pilot, Boston Scientific Choice PT and PT Graphics, Terumo Crosswire and Confianza Pro). Hydrophilic wires, however, have the tendency for subintimal passage and perforation of end capillaries resulting in vessel occlusion or perforation and may also prohibit future surgical grafting of the coronary artery. These wires also may easily enter the thin-walled vasa vasorum, which are prone to perforation either directly from the wire or from subsequent dilatation.

Routine incorporation of novel or advanced procedural techniques, including contralateral injections to visualize the distal vessel via collaterals, and the parallel wire technique have also contributed to the improving success rates in catheter-based CTO revascularization. The Shinobi guidewire (Cordis, Johnston & Johnston) is specifically designed to cross CTOs and has a one piece core with a broad transition and increased stiffness, with a tip diameter of 0.014 inch. The distal 25 cm of the guidewire has a Teflon coating. The Miracle guidewires (Asahi Intecc, Japan) have 0.014 inch tips and are available in several degrees of stiffness (3 g/4.5 g/6 g/12 g). The Conquest guidewire (Asahi Intecc) has a tip stiffness of 9 g and a distal diameter of 0.009 inch. Extreme care must be taken when using these stiff guidewires to cross CTOs, as they are more likely to create false channels, dissection and perforation. Two devices specifically designed for refractory CTO recanalization have demonstrated sufficient safety and efficacy to have received approval by the Food and Drug Administration for sale in the US: the Safe Cross-RF guidewire and the Frontrunner catheter [15].

The first *in vivo* deflecting tip wire was from Medtronic Corp. (1986) with a unidirectional deflecting tip. In 1992 Pilot Cardiovascular Systems Inc. presented a 0.014-inch stainless-steel wire with a 5 mm deflecting tip and a 165 cm length. At this time the tip deflection was not durable *in vivo* – the transition from deflection joint to support zone was too abrupt and the ergonomics of handle design less comfortable.

The Safe Cross-RF guidewire (Intraluminal Therapeutics) is a steerable 0.014-inch intermediate-stiffness guidewire incorporating optical coherence reflectometry, which measures the reflection of near-infrared light (10–30 μm resolution) ahead of the wire tip [16]. Optical coherence reflectometry (OCR) uses the low coherence light transmitted from the 0.007 inch optical fibre incorporated into the tip of the guidewire to reflect from the tissue ahead. Depending on the absorption and scatter pattern present in the reflected signal, the detector can differentiate between plaque and normal artery wall. This information is displayed as a waveform on a screen, which enables the operator to determine the location of the guidewire within the occlusion. A visible and audible signal warns the operator when the wire tip approaches within 1 mm of the outer vessel wall, allowing the wire to be redirected before dissecting or perforating. Radiofrequency energy (100 ms pulses; 250–500 kHz) is emitted from the tip of the wire that enables it to traverse the tough fibrous cap of refractory CTOs [17]. Early pilot experiences [16,17] and a subsequent controlled multicenter registry [18] demonstrated that this active guidewire is able to cross 50% to 60% of lesions refractory to a 10 min attempt with a standard guidewire. Perforations related to the device have occurred in <1% of patients. In a registry of 32 patients whose CTO could not be crossed with a conventional guidewire, the device achieved recanalization in 81% of cases without device complication [19]. However, two further small studies report success in only 52–60% of such cases [20,21] following limited steerability within the lesion. Interchange between conventional guidewires and SafeCross was necessary in hard lesions.

The Frontrunner Catheter (LuMend Inc, Redwood City, California) is a manually operated device incorporating a bilaterally hinged distal tip that can be angled to 25° and 36°, and spreads tissue planes via the principle of blunt microdissection [22]. The device is supported by a probing and recanalization catheter (4.5 F Micro Guide Catheter) as it is passed across the occlusion. The current X-39 Frontrunner has an outer diameter of 0.03 to 0.04 inches, with a 2.8 F distal tip. Lesion success rates with the Frontrunner have been achieved in 50–60% of refractory occlusions, although rates are slightly lower in tortuous right coronary arteries [22]. Perforations have occurred in 0.9% of cases. This device may have a special role in refractory in-stent CTOs, wherein the stent serves to confine the device as it passes through the

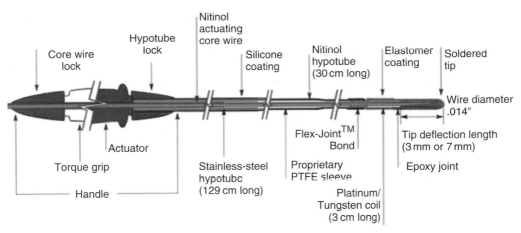

Figure 7.1 Wire Construction of the Cordis STEER-IT® Deflecting Tip Guidewire. A nitinol core wire runs the entire length of the wire. Proprietary Teflon (PTFE) sleeve over the nitinol hypotube to create a lubricious surface on the distal 30 cm of the wire (excluding the tip). FLEX-JOINT™ Bond attaches the platinum/tungsten coils to the nitinol hypotube (www.cordis.com).

occlusion [23]. The dissection planes are limited to the fibrocalcific plaque, which is more rigid and less stretchable than the vessel adventitia – reducing the risk of vessel perforation [24,25]. After 342 cases, reported complications were infrequent with a 2% perforation rate and no device related deaths [26].

The Cordis STEER-IT wire (Figure 7.1) is a new 0.014-inch movable core guidewire with a flexible, radiopaque platinum alloy on the distal tip coated with an elastomer to achieve longevity. In contrast to the Cordis Wizdom Steerable Guidewire the longitudinal distal/proximal movement of the handle mechanism, located at the proximal end of the guidewire, enables to deflect the distal tip in two directions with a minimum of 45°. This allows changing of the wire orientation without much torque. The handle mechanism is butted in a stainless-steel hypotube, which is soldered to a nitinol hypotube. The handle mechanism is similar to the USCI Commander™ Deflectable Guide Wire. The guidewire has a nitinol core covered with a proprietary nonstick coating sleeve to assist advancing the device providing an adequate lateral support. Potential limitations of the STEER-IT WIRE may include: the transition point around the flex joint is less then ideal for a smooth negotiation around extreme bends, the torque ability is not equal to best in class conventional wires, there is only a single wire stiffness

available and at the moment there is no possibility of coupling with other energy source or guidance system to facilitate crossing CTOs. The Cordis STEER-IT WIRE is not FDA-cleared for the use in CTO.

The Venture Catheter (St. Jude Medical; Velocimed, Minnesota) is a 6French compatible, single-use, over-the-wire support tip-deflecting catheter deflecting all commercially available 0.014-inch-long guidewire tips up to 90°. It enables to change the direction of current fixed-shaped guidewire tip angles which provides more precise wire control in the engagement of target vessels/lesions with difficult take-off angles and it helps the wire advancement around bends and in steering wire away from dissection planes. Patient study observations from Naidu *et al.* (1 patient) [27], McNulty *et al.* (2 patients) [28], and McClure *et al.* (20 patients) [29] described the successful use of the Venture Catheter involving left circumflex artery, as well as for diagonal branches and saphenous vein graft anastomotic lesions. The Venture Catheter also provides more effective back up support for guidewires to pass complex lesions. However, the 0.0175-inch catheter offers a rather low clearance for friction free 0.014-inch wire manipulation. The exchange from the soft to the stiff part is not smooth when the catheter tip is in a deflected position. Moreover the ability to change the guidewire tip angle is

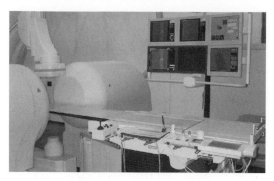

Figure 7.2 Setup of the Stereotaxis Inc. Magnetic Guidance System integrated with a modified Siemens C-arm single-plane digital angiography system (AXIOM Artis *d*FC, Siemens, Forchheim, Germany) (Schiemann M, *et al.* [33]).

diminished with stiffer CTO wires like Confienzy™ and SafeCross™.

Further novel guidance modalities are under development, including forward-looking ultrasound [30,31] and magnetically enabled three-dimensional wire guidance [32,33]. The magnetic guidance system (Stereotaxis Inc., St. Louis, MO) (Figure 7.2) is comprised of two focus-field permanent 0.08 T magnets, encased within fiberglass housings and normally kept in a stowed position laterally opposed to the walls of the angiography lab. When activated, the magnets rotate into the navigation position on either side of the patient table and become computer-integrated with the digital angiography system. In this position the maximum x-ray imaging angle is limited to 30° LAO/RAO (left anterior oblique/right anterior oblique). Using a table-sided interface system the interventionalist may direct the resultant magnetic vector to any orientation in three-dimensional space. Magnetic navigation results from placing a magnetically tipped guidewire within the magnetic field and allowing the magnetically driven deflection of the distal tip to guide the wire through angulated segments while manually advancing the wire. Although the magnetic field strength is considerably low, patients should be routinely screened for magnetic exclusions like before an MRI procedure. The length and rigidity of the distal segment of the magnetic wire might be a risk for dissection and inhibit effective magnetic navigation. As the curve of the wire is not preshaped, control of the wire tip without

the magnetic field is very limited. Experimental [33] and clinical studies with the use of magnetic ablation catheters in EP labs [32] already show the technical feasibility of magnetic navigation but here especially the cost-effectiveness must be considered and evaluated.

Although manually reshaping wires, use of alternate wires, and support with over the wire balloons may facilitate interventions in excessively angulated vessels tip-deflecting devices might provide an alternative strategy improving procedure success and decreasing procedure time. Prospective randomized trials are required comparing these novel approaches and devices with contemporary angioplasty equipment and techniques.

See Plate 12 in the color plate section.

References

1 Bourassa MGRG, Detre KM. Bypass angioplasty revascularization investigation: patient screening, selection, and recruitment. *Am J Cardiol* 1995; **75**: 3C–8C.

2 Safian RD, McCabe CH, Sipperly ME, McKay RG, Baim DS. Initial success and long-term follow-up of percutaneous transluminal coronary angioplasty in chronic total occlusions versus conventional stenoses. *Am J Cardiol* 1988; **61**: 23G–28G.

3 Kinoshita I, Katoh O, Nariyama J, *et al.* Coronary angioplasty of chronic total occlusions with bridging collateral vessels: immediate and follow-up outcome from a large single-center experience. *J Am Coll Cardiol* 1995; **26**: 409–415.

4 Lindsay J, Apple S, Pinnow EE, *et al.* Percutaneous coronary intervention-associated nephropathy foreshadows increased risk of late adverse events in patients with normal baseline serum creatinine. *Catheter Cardiovasc Interv* 2003; **59**: 338–343.

5 Wagner LK, McNeese MD, Marx MV, Siegel EL. Severe skin reactions from interventional fluoroscopy: case report and review of the literature. *Radiology* 1999; **213**: 773–776.

6 Koenig TR, Wolff D, Mettler FA, Wagner LK. Skin injuries from fluoroscopically guided procedures: Part 1, characteristics of radiation injury. *Am J Roentgenol* 2001; **177**: 3–11.

7 Nikolic B, Spies JB, Lundsten MJ, Abbara S. Patient radiation dose associated with uterine artery embolization. *Radiology* 2000; **214**: 121–125.

8 Nahass GT, Cornelius L. Fluoroscopy-induced radiodermatitis after transjugular intrahepatic portosystemic shunt. *Am J Gastroenterol* 1998; **93**: 1546–1549.

9 Shope TB. Radiation-induced skin injuries from fluoroscopy. *Radiographics* 1996; **16**: 1195–1199.

10 Allemann Y, Kaufmann UP, Meyer BJ, *et al.* Magnum wire for percutaneous coronary balloon angioplasty in 800 total chronic occlusions. *Am J Cardiol* 1997; **80**: 634–637.

11 Pande AK, Meier B, Urban P, *et al.* Magnum/Magnarail versus conventional systems for recanalization of chronic total coronary occlusions: a randomized comparison. *Am Heart J* 1992; **123**: 1182–1186.

12 Lukes P, Wihed A, Tidebrant G, Risberg B, Ortenwall P, Seeman T. Combined angioplasty with the Kensey catheter and balloon angioplasty in occlusive arterial disease. A preliminary report. *Acta Radiol* 1992; **33**: 230–233.

13 Kaltenbach M, Hartmann A, Vallbracht C. Procedural results and patient selection in recanalization of chronic coronary occlusions by low speed rotational angioplasty. *Eur Heart J* 1993; **14**: 826–830.

14 Serruys PW, Hamburger JN, Koolen JJ, *et al.* Total occlusion trial with angioplasty by using laser guidewire. The TOTAL trial. *Eur Heart J* 2000; **21**: 1797–1805.

15 Stone GW, Reifart N, Moussa I, *et al.* Percutaneous recanalization of chronically occluded coronary arteries. *Circulation* 2005; **112**: 2530–2537.

16 Cordero H, Warburton KD, Underwood PL, Heuser RR. Initial experience and safety in the treatment of chronic total occlusions with fiberoptic guidance technology: optical coherent reflectometry. *Catheter Cardiovasc Interv* 2001; **54**: 180–187.

17 Shammas NW. Treatment of chronic total occlusions using optical coherent reflectometry and radiofrequency ablative energy: incremental success over conventional techniques. *J Invasive Cardiol* 2004; **16**: 58–59.

18 Baim DS, Braden G, Heuser R, *et al.* Utility of the safe-cross-guided radiofrequency total occlusion crossing system in chronic coronary total occlusions (results from the Guided Radio Frequency Energy Ablation of Total Occlusions Registry Study). *Am J Cardiol* 2004; **94**: 853–858.

19 Braden G. Clinical experience in crossing total occlusions with the safe-cross system. *Am J Cardiol* 2003; **92** (Suppl 6A): 66L.

20 Hoye A, Onderwater E, Cummins P, Sianos G, Serruys PW. Improved recanalization of chronic total coronary occlusions using an optical coherence reflectometry-guided guidewire. *Catheter Cardiovasc Interv* 2004; **63**: 158–163.

21 Ng W, Chen W, Lee P. Initial experience and safety in the treatment of chronic total coronary occlusions with a new optical coherent reflectometry-guided radiofrequency ablation guidewire. *Am J Cardiol* 2003; **92**: 732–734.

22 Whitbourn RJ, Cincotta M, Mossop P, Selmon M. Intraluminal blunt microdissection for angioplasty of coronary chronic total occlusions. *Catheter Cardiovasc Interv* 2003; **58**: 194–198.

23 Yang YM, Mehran R, Dangas G, *et al.* Successful use of the frontrunner catheter in the treatment of in-stent coronary chronic total occlusions. *Catheter Cardiovasc Interv* 2004; **63**: 462–468.

24 Tadros P. Successful revascularization of a long chronic total occlusion of the right coronary artery utilizing the frontrunner X39 CTO catheter system. *J Invasive Cardiol* 2003; **15**(11): 3 p.

25 Simonton SA. Chronic total occlusions: a new frontier. *J Invasive Cardiol* 2004; **16**(Suppl B): 1–2.

26 Selmon M, Daniel M. Catheter assisted recanalization of chronic total occlusions in the coronary vasculature. *Cardiol Int* 2003; **4**: 79–82.

27 Naidu SS, Wong SC. Novel intracoronary steerable support catheter for complex coronary intervention. *J Invasive Cardiol* 2006; **18**: 80–81.

28 McNulty E, Cohen J, Chou T, Shunk K. A "grapple hook" technique using a deflectable tip catheter to facilitate complex proximal circumflex interventions. *Catheter Cardiovasc Interv* 2006; **67**: 46–48.

29 Mc Clure S, Wahr D, Webb J. Venture wire control catheter. *Catheter Cardiovasc Interv* 2005; **66**: 346–350.

30 Demirci U, Ergun AS, Oralkan O, Karaman M, Khuri-Yakub BT. Forward-viewing CMUT arrays for medical imaging. *IEEE Trans Ultrason Ferroelectr Freq Control* 2004; **51**: 887–895.

31 Wang Y, Stephens DN, O'Donnell M. Optimizing the beam pattern of a forward-viewing ring-annular ultrasound array for intravascular imaging. *IEEE Trans Ultrason Ferroelectr Freq Control* 2002; **49**: 1652–1664.

32 Ernst S, Hachiya H, Chun JK, Ouyang F. Remote catheter ablation of parahisian accessory pathways using a novel magnetic navigation system – a report of two cases. *J Cardiovasc Electrophysiol* 2005; **16**: 659–662.

33 Schiemann M, Killmann R, Kleen M, Abolmaali N, Finney J, Vogl TJ. Vascular guide wire navigation with a magnetic guidance system: experimental results in a phantom. *Radiology* 2004; **232**: 475–481.

CHAPTER 8

ASAHI Wires

Shigeru Saito, MD, FACC, FSCAI, FJCC

Shonan Kamakura General Hospital, Kamakura, Japan

Introduction

The conventional guidewire techniques for chronic total occlusion (CTO) lesions might have not been developed without the presence of various guidewires manufactured by ASAHI INTECC Company, Japan. The conventional guidewire techniques are classified into "drilling" and "penetrating" techniques. In the "drilling" technique, the guidewire is rotated clockwise and counterclockwise while the tip is pushed modestly against the CTO lesion. The guidewire can be advanced such as a drill is going into an objective. In the "penetrating" technique, the operator aims at the target by the tip of the guidewire without clockwise and counterclockwise rotation. Generally, the first technique is better, since the chance of guidewire perforation is less and work for most of the lesions, Miracle series guidewires are best for this technique. However, if the proximal cap of the CTO lesion is very hard, we need to penetrate it. In this purpose, the tapered-tip guidewires are adequate, since the penetration ability is dependent on the tip stiffness, tip cross sectional area and the slippery coating. The majority of CTO lesions can be passed through by using Miracle 3 guidewire. However, some lesions need very stiff guidewires like Conquest-Pro 12, in which penetration technique is necessary.

Chronic Total Occlusions, 1st edition. Edited by R. Waksman and S. Saito. © 2009 Blackwell Publishing, ISBN: 978-1-4051-5703-2.

Important parameters for PCI guidewires

In order to develop the guidewires for CTO lesions, ASAHI INTECC Company has developed several concepts which can define the performance of each guidewire. These include "tip load," "shaping ability and memory," "tip flexibility," "shaft support," "torque transmission," "slipping ability," "trackability," and "trap resistance."

Tip load (tip stiffness)

We are very frequently using the terminology of "tip stiffness." How we can define the tip stiffness? The simplest way of its definition is the load, when the tip of the guidewire starts to buckle. In ASAHI INTECC Company, the load in grams against the electronic balance, when the tip of the guidewire starts to buckle, is defined as tip stiffness. The distance from the lower end of the pipe to the upper side of the electronic balance is fixed at 10 mm (Figure 8.1a).

Normally, the guidewires for CTO lesions have tip stiffness of 3 g or greater. Regular floppy guidewires have tip stiffness of less than 1 g.

Shaping ability and memory

Tip shaping ability and memory are very important especially for CTO lesions. Shape memory ability can be tested by the test system as Figure 8.1b. After inserting a shaped test guidewire into the tube and rotating it clockwise and counterclockwise several fixed times and then pulling out it, how much completely the original shape

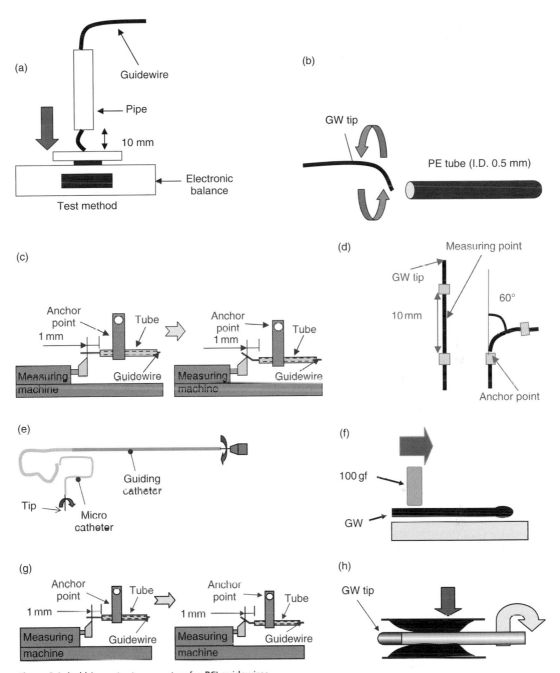

Figure 8.1 (a–h) Important parameters for PCI guidewires.

has recovered is measured. ASAHI wires have a flat shaping core ribbon, which provides good shaping ability and memory.

Tip flexibility

Tip flexibility is the concept contrary to tip stiffness. If tip flexibility is not enough, the guidewire creates intimal dissection very easily. Tip flexibility is a function of the distance from the tip of the guidewire. Thus, it is measured by using the test system as Figure 8.1c. The testing guidewire is extended by the index distance from the tip plus 1 mm from a microtube. Then, the bending load is applied to the guidewire at the index distance from the tip (1 mm from the tip of the microtube). This load is a function of the distance from the tip of the guidewire and characterizes the tip flexibility of the wire.

Shaft support

Shaft support is defined as the force which is required to bend the wire shaft for 60° at the anchor point of the index distance from the tip of the wire by applying the bending force to the point 10 mm distal to the anchor point (Figure 8.1d). This force is measured every 10 mm point starting at 30 mm from the tip of the wire and going up to 150 mm.

This parameter is very important in transporting such stiff devices as balloon catheters or stents over the guidewire through the tortuous or bending arterial anatomy.

Torque transmission

Torque transmission is the most important parameter in steering the tip of the guidewire. Placing the guidewire in a tortuous catheter, the proximal end of it is rotated by index angles, and the rotational response of the distal end of the guide-wire is measured (Figure 8.1e).

Slipping ability

Lubrication of the outer surface of each guidewire is important in transmitting torque to the tip of the guidewire as well as in navigating the tip through the tortuous arteries. Slipping ability is measured by estimating the minimum pulling force while clipping the guidewire under 100 g load (Figure 8.1f).

Trackability

Trackability is decided by several physical properties including slipping ability, tip flexibility, shaft support, as well as tip load. If the trackability is good, the guidewire can reach far in a tortuous artery. By inserting a test guidewire into tortuous vessel model with adding certain torque power, how far the guidewire has reached is measured (Figure 8.1g).

Trap resistance

Because the CTO lesions consist of mixed plaques, the tip of the guidewire is often trapped within the lesions. This entrapment of the guidewire is sometimes dangerous, since it is associated with the risk of the wire separation. The trap resistance can be tested by gripping the tip of the guidewire with index gripping power while rotating the proximal shaft of the guidewire. If the trap resistance is higher, the tip of the guidewire can be rotated with the rotation of the proximal shaft even under higher gripping power. The maximum gripping power, under which the test guidewire can be freely rotated, is defined as trap resistance (Figure 8.1h).

Line-up of ASAHI guidewires

ASAHI INTECC has full line-up of PCI guidewires, which can be used in different situations or anatomies. These are listed in Table 8.1.

The guidewires specific for CTO lesions or retrograde approach need to be described further.

CTO guidewires

Miracle series

Miracle series guidewires consist of Miracle 3, 4.5, 6, and 12 g. Their structure is characterized by the combination of "one-piece core wire" design and "joint-less spring coil" (Figure 8.2). In the one-piece core wire design, the shaping ribbon is directly attached to the center of the distal core wire tip. This design enables direct transmission of pushing power from the proximal shaft to the tip of the guidewire. In the joint-less spring coil design, the distal platinum spring coil is directly welded to the proximal stainless spring coil. This design improves the torque transmission (Figure 8.3).

Table 8.1 ASAHI PTCA GW

Category	Product name	O.D. (inch)	Length (cm)	Radiopaque length (cm)	Tip load (g)	Spring coil length (cm)
Frontline cases	Light	0.014	180	3	0.5	20
	Soft	0.014	180	3	0.7	30
	Route/PROWATERflex	0.014	180	3	0.8	20
	Rinato/Prowater	0.014	180	3	0.8	20
	Marker Wire	0.014	180	3	0.7	30
	Zeroclear	0.014/0.020	180	2.5	0.7	30
Frontline cases & chronic occlusion cases	Fielder	0.014	180	3	1	12
	Fielder FC	0.014	180	3	0.8	11
Chronic occlusion cases	Intermediate/Medium	0.014	180	3	3.0	30
	Miracle Primo	0.014	180	3	2.5	30
	Miracle 3/Miraclebros 3	0.014	180	11	3.0	11
	Miracle 4.5/Miraclebros 4.5	0.014	180	11	4.5	11
	Miracle 6/Miraclebros 6	0.014	180	11	6.0	11
	Miracle 12/Miraclebros 12	0.014	180	11	12.0	11
	Conquest/Confianza 9	0.014/0.009	180	20	9.0	20
	Conquest 12	0.014/0.009	180	20	12.0	20
	Conquest Pro/Confianza Pro 9	0.014/0.009	180	20	9.0	20
	Conquest Pro 12/Confianza Pro 12	0.014/0.009	180	20	12.0	20
	Conquest Pro 8-20/Confianza Pro 8-20	0.014/0.009	180	20	20.0	20
Extra support cases	Grand Slam	0.014	180	4	0.7	4
Decillion series						
Frontline cases	Decillion FL	0.010	180	3	0.8	8
Chronic occlusion cases	Decillion MD	0.010	180	3	3.0	8
X-treme						
Frontline cases & chronic occlusion cases	X-treme	0.014/0.009	190	16	0.8	16

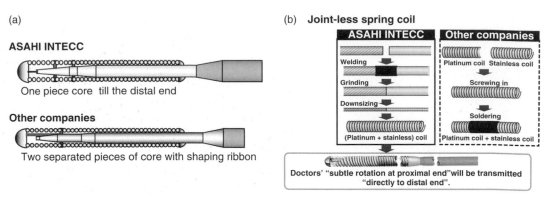

Figure 8.2 (a,b) Structure of ASAHI guidewires.

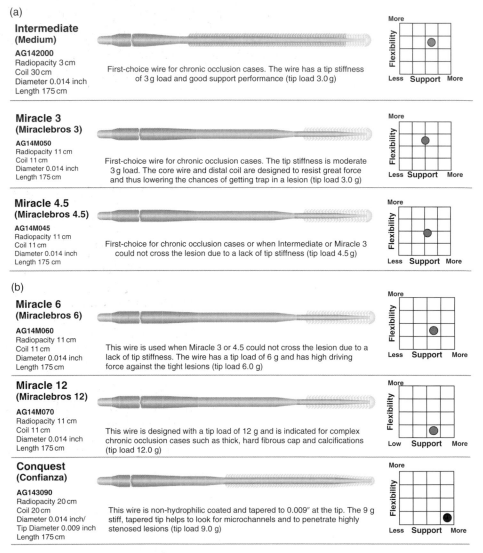

Figure 8.3 (a–c) Characteristics of each ASAHI guidewire.

(c)

Conquest Pro
(Confianza Pro)

AGH143090
Radiopacity 20 cm
Coil 20 cm
Diameter 0.014 inch/
Tip diameter 0.009 inch
Length 175 cm

Similar structure and tip stiffness as Conquest except that the coil area is hydrophilic coated which provides greater lubricity while crossing a lesion. The distal ball tip is not hydrophilic coated to allow it to catch on to the entry point of the lesions (tip load 9.0 g)

Conquest Pro 12
(Confianza Pro 12)

AGH143091
Radiopacity 20 cm
Coil 20 cm
Diameter 0.014 inch/
Tip diameter 0.009 inch
Length 175 cm

This wire is designed with a tip load of 12 g and is indicated for complex chronic occlusion cases such as thick, hard fibrous cap and calcifications (tip load 12.0 g)

Conquest Pro 8-20
(Confianza Pro 8-20)

AGH143091
Radiopacity 20 cm
Coil 20 cm
Diameter 0.014 inch/
Tip diameter 0.008 inch
Length 175 cm

This wire is designed to be used for complex lesions, specifically those with heavy calcifications and tough fibrous tissues. It possesses a tip load of 20 g and 0.008 inch tapered tip which makes it the stiffest and finest of the current NEO'S PTCA guidewire series (tip load 20.0 g)

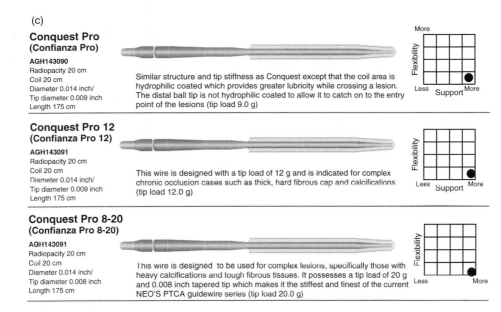

Figure 8.3 (Continued)

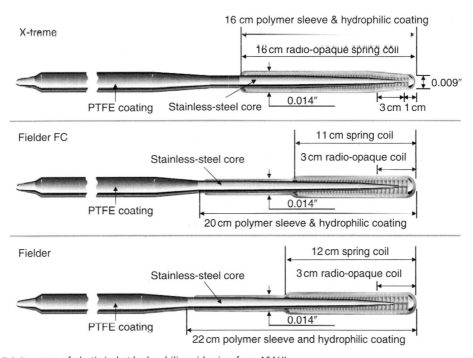

Figure 8.4 Structure of plastic-jacket hydrophilic guidewires from ASAHI.

Conquest (Confianza) series

The structure of Conquest series is essentially not different from other ASAHI INTECC guidewires except their tip diameter tapered to 0.009 or 0.008 inches. The sprint coil is coated by hydrophilic coating in Conquest Pro guidewires.

Special guidewires for retrograde approach

The retrograde approach needs very lubricant and high torque-controllable guidewires. These include Fielder, Fielder FC, and Fielder X-treme (Figure 8.4).

Conclusion

ASAHI INTECC developed PCI guidewires studied several important characteristics of PCI guidewires and established the test methods for these parameters. Based on the tests, different kinds of PCI guidewires have been developed for different subsets of lesions and situations. Each operator has to be familiarize *himself or herself* with the different characteristics of these guidewires.

See Plate 12 in the color plate section.

CHAPTER 9

Tornus Catheter

Hideaki Kaneda, MD, PhD

Cardiology and Catheterization Laboratories, Shonan Kamakura General Hospital, Kanagawa, Japan

Introduction

Despite the marked reduction in restenosis realized with drug-eluting stents, clinical efficacy is hampered by procedural failure (inability to perform stent implantation) in subsets of patients. Although procedural failure arises mainly from inability to cross the lesion (mainly occluded segment) with a guidewire, severe coronary artery stenosis, such as severe calcification or chronic total occlusions (CTO), sometimes hinders the crossing of a conventional balloon or a microcatheter afterward. Several techniques have been proposed to create a better backup support. Deep engagement of the guiding catheter into the coronary artery [1,2] and a buddy wire technique [3] are already well known for increasing backup support. A new technique, the anchor balloon technique, was recently reported [4,5].

Ablation of the (calcified) plaque is another option. Although ablation with high-speed rotational atherectomy is efficacious for these lesions [6], atherectomy requires the RotaWire (Boston Scientific, Miami, FL) crossing the lesion (or exchanging of a guidewire to the RotaWire), which is not always successful. Although the excimer laser catheter may be of help in these situations,

the use of this technology is still limited in practice because of its low-cost performance [7,8].

Recently, a new penetration catheter (Tornus, Asahi Intecc, Japan; Abbott Vascular, Redwood City, CA) was developed to enable balloon crossing (and subsequent dilatation of the lesion) when any balloon catheter or microcatheter has failed to cross through the lesion after successful wire crossing [9]. The Tornus catheter has a unique function of enlarging the vessel channel in a tight lesion through its screwing effect.

Device description

The Tornus catheter consists of three parts: the main shaft with surface coating, the polymer sleeve, and the hub connector (Figure 9.1). The catheter has hydrophobic coating in the inner lumen to provide greater lubricity. The main shaft is a coreless stainless coil that is right-handed lay (clockwise). Eight stainless wires are stranded in the coil. The outside diameter is 0.70 mm (2.1 Fr), and the inside diameter (0.41–0.46 mm) is compatible for a 0.014-inch guidewire. A platinum marker at the very end of distal tip (1 mm) facilitates fluoroscopic identification of the catheter tip (0.62 mm [1.9 Fr] in diameter). The sleeve prevents back-bleeding from the clearance gap of the shaft, prevents crushing of the shaft caused by clamping of the Y-connector valve, and acts as a safety indicator for catheter shaft breakage due to excessive catheter rotation (see below).

Chronic Total Occlusions, 1st edition. Edited by R. Waksman and S. Saito. © 2009 Blackwell Publishing, ISBN: 978-1-4051-5703-2.

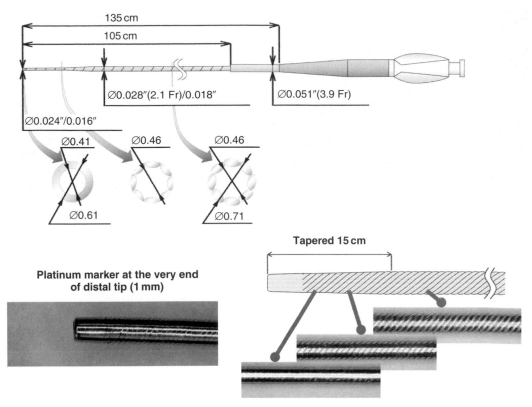

Figure 9.1 Whole picture of the Tornus catheter and cropped image of the catheter tip.

Recently, a larger size catheter (TORNUS 88 FLEX; 2.6 Fr) was introduced to improve backup support and pushability despite less flexibility for tortuous anatomy.

Penetration and removing

To penetrate the severe stenosis (advance the catheter), the Tornus catheter should be rotated in a counterclockwise direction (screwing). A torque control device should be held at all times to avoid the Tornus catheter and guidewire to be rotated together. To avoid overtorquing, it is recommended to use only one hand to rotate the Tornus catheter. Maximal rotation is recommended not to exceed 20 times in one direction. Torque transmission delay may sometimes occur, manifested by the distal part continuing to rotate even after the proximal part stops rotating. If the Tornus catheter does not advance despite counter-clockwise rotation, the Tornus catheter should be released,

to allow it to rewind to avoid breakage of the shaft (see below). Care should be taken to assure that the guidewire is secure while the Tornus catheter is rewinding.

To remove the Tornus catheter, it should be carefully rotated, in a clockwise direction, until the catheter enters into the guiding catheter. An extension wire or 300-cm exchange guidewire is needed, to make sure that the guidewire is not removed along with the Tornus catheter. The so-called "Nanto-Method" should not be used (applying pressure to the central guidewire lumen of the catheter with the inflation device) [10].

Breakage of the shaft

When the tip of the shaft is stuck, excessive rotational force may cause breakage of the shaft at the distal part as shown in Figure 9.2c. In order to avoid this breakage, the shaft at the proximal end in the sleeve is tapered to make it weakest

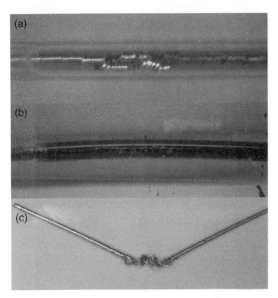

Figure 9.2 Examples of shaft breakage: (a) Breakage of shaft is first observed at the sleeve (the weakest segment), (b) Visibility of shaft structure may be affected by blood, and (c) distal shaft breaks if rotations continue after breakage of proximal shaft.

dynamically. This weakest segment at the proximal end will be damaged first (Figure 9.2a). The part of the sleeve that covers the weakest part of the shaft is thickened. Visibility of the shaft structure may be affected by blood (Figure 9.2b). If any breakage is observed in the safety sleeve, stop the screwing rotation and exchange the Tornus catheter carefully.

Another use of Tornus

Indicated not only for penetrating the lesion (after successful wire crossing), the Tornus catheter is useful before wire crossing. Because the Tornus catheter could provide stronger backup support for guidewire manipulations than a conventional over-the-wire balloon, the Tornus catheter is useful when strong backup support is needed for wire crossing, such as in the treatment for CTO lesions [11]. However, the handling time should be limited to avoid thrombosis in the wire lumen. Special care (wiping the guidewire surface at every exchange) should be taken because thrombus may affect the performance of the Tornus catheter.

Possible complication

It is important to make sure a guidewire is in the true lumen before advancing the Tornus catheter. With device improvements, more total occlusions have been crossed with a guidewire, though true intraluminal access is not always achieved, which is not easily apparent on coronary angiography. The Tornus catheter could enlarge the false lumen, resulting in coronary perforation, or stent implantation in the false lumen, leading to distal dissection or branch occlusion. To avoid such complications, careful examination with intravascular ultrasound might be required to ensure true intraluminal passage before advancing the Tornus catheter.

There is risk of vessel damage due to shaft breakage, if it occurs in the coronary artery. However, this may be avoided if special care is taken to monitor the safety system at the proximal end (see above), as well as the catheter tip under fluoroscopy during rotation.

Transradial approach

Although transradial access has gained popularity over the past decade due to its benefits, such as improved patient comfort and decrease in access site bleeding complications [12,13], inadequate catheter support due to the small guiding catheter size may limit its effectiveness in some complex lesions, including CTO lesions [14]. The Tornus catheter, which enables the crossing of the lesion, even with inadequate catheter support, may improve procedural outcomes in the treatment for CTO lesions through the radial approach.

Case presentation

A 79-year-old man with a history of myocardial infarction presented with angina in September 2005. His coronary risk factors included hyperlipidemia and diabetes (oral drug therapy). Coronary angiography revealed a total occlusion in the proximal segment of his right coronary artery (RCA; Figure 9.3a). Angioplasty for the CTO in the RCA was attempted in September 2005. After 10,000 units of heparin was administered, the RCA was engaged with a 7 Fr SAL (short amplatz left) 1.5 catheter with side holes via the right radial

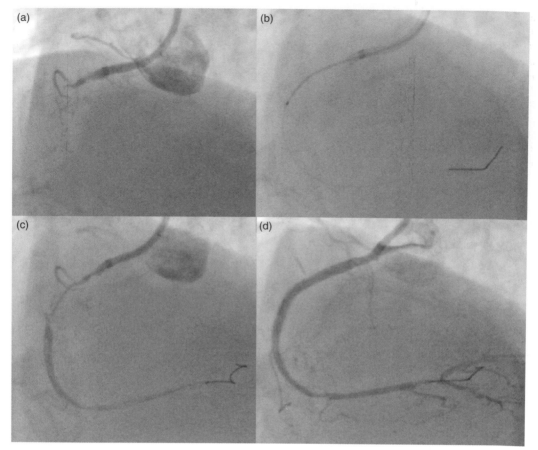

Figure 9.3 Case presentation: coronary angiogram showing a total occlusion in the proximal segment of his right coronary artery (a). After penetration with the Tornus catheter (b), the balloon catheter could pass through the CTO lesion (c), resulting in successful sirolimus-eluting stent implantation (d).

artery. With a 1.5 mm × 20 mm balloon (Ryujin-OTW, Terumo, Japan), a guidewire (Runthrough-intermediate, Terumo, Japan) successfully crossed the lesion. However, due to inadequate catheter support, the balloon catheter could not pass through the CTO lesion. After penetration with the Tornus catheter (Figure 9.3b), the balloon catheter could pass through the CTO lesion (Figure 9.3c), resulting in successful sirolimus-eluting stent implantation (Figure 9.3d, Cypher, 3.0 mm × 33 mm, Cordis, Johnson and Johnson Interventional Systems, Warren, NJ).

In conclusion, the Tornus catheter has the unique function of enlarging the vessel channel in a tight lesion through its screwing effect and enables balloon crossing (and subsequent dilatation of the lesion) when any balloon catheter or microcatheter failed to cross through the lesion after successful wire crossing. The Tornus catheter could improve treatment outcome, for complex lesion subsets including CTO lesions. See Plate 13 in the color plate section.

Acknowledgment

The author thanks Heidi N. Bonneau, RN, MS, for her expert review of the manuscript.

References

1 Peels HO, van Boven AJ, den Heijer P, Tio RA, Lie KI, Crijns HJ. Deep seating of six French guiding catheters for

delivery of new Palmaz-Schatz stents. *Cathet Cardiovasc Diagn* 1996; **38**: 210–213.

2 Bartorelli AL, Lavarra F, Trabattoni D *et al.* Successful stent delivery with deep seating of 6 French guiding catheters in difficult coronary anatomy. *Catheter Cardiovasc Interv* 1999; **48**: 279–284.

3 Saucedo JF, Muller DW, Moscucci M. Facilitated advancement of the Palmaz-Schatz stent delivery system with the use of an adjacent 0.018″ stiff wire. *Cathet Cardiovasc Diagn* 1996; **39**: 106–110.

4 Fujita S, Tamai H, Kyo E *et al.* New technique for superior guiding catheter support during advancement of a balloon in coronary angioplasty: the anchor technique. *Catheter Cardiovasc Interv.* 2003; **59**: 482–488.

5 Hirokami M, Saito S, Muto H. Anchoring technique to improve guiding catheter support in coronary angioplasty of chronic total occlusions. *Catheter Cardiovasc Interv* 2006; **67**: 366–371.

6 Moussa I, Di Mario C, Moses J *et al.* Coronary stenting after rotational atherectomy in calcified and complex lesions. Angiographic and clinical follow-up results. *Circulation* 1997; **96**: 128–136.

7 Litvack F, Eigler N, Margolis J *et al.* Percutaneous excimer laser coronary angioplasty: results in the first consecutive 3,000 patients. The ELCA Investigators. *J Am Coll Cardiol* 1994; **23**: 323–329.

8 Bilodeau L, Fretz EB, Taeymans Y, Koolen J, Taylor K, Hilton DJ. Novel use of a high-energy excimer laser catheter for calcified and complex coronary artery lesions. *Catheter Cardiovasc Interv* 2004; **62**: 155–161.

9 Tsuchikane E, Katoh O, Shimogami M *et al.* First clinical experience of a novel penetration catheter for patients with severe coronary artery stenosis. *Catheter Cardiovasc Interv* 2005; **65**: 368–373.

10 Nanto S, Ohara T, Shimonagata T, Hori M, Kubori S. A technique for changing a PTCA balloon catheter over a regular-length guidewire. *Cathet Cardiovasc Diagn* 1994; **32**: 274–277.

11 Ali MI, Butman S, Heuser R. Crossing a chronic total occlusion using combination therapy with Tornus and FlowCardia. *J Invasive Cardiol* 2006; **18**: E258–E260.

12 Saito S, Miyake S, Hosokawa G *et al.* Transradial coronary intervention in Japanese patients. *Catheter Cardiovasc Interv* 1999; **46**: 37–41.

13 Saito S, Tanaka S, Hiroe Y *et al.* Comparative study on transradial approach vs. transfemoral approach in primary stent implantation for patients with acute myocardial infarction: results of the test for myocardial infarction by prospective unicenter randomization for access sites (TEMPURA) trial. *Catheter Cardiovasc Interv* 2003; **59**: 26–33.

14 Takahashi S, Saito S, Tanaka S *et al.* New method to increase a backup support of a 6 French guiding coronary catheter. *Catheter Cardiovasc Interv* 2004; **63**: 452–456.

CHAPTER 10

Introduction of a New 0.014-inch CiTop™ Guidewire for CTO: Preclinical Safety and Feasibility Studies

Mickey Scheinowitz, PhD

Neufeld Cardiac Research Institute and Department of Biomedical Engineering Tel-Aviv University, Israel

Chronic arterial occlusions remain the main obstacle of coronary and peripheral interventions. In recent years we have gained more insights on the pathophysiology of chronic total occlusion (CTO), which was accompanied by the introduction of vast technologies and approaches into clinical experimental use. However, these new devices and approaches are still limited and deserve significant improvement before entering into routine use.

We evaluated a new 0.014-inch CiTop™ guidewire designed to cross CTO as a direct channel for over-the-wire catheters and further interventional treatment. We investigated the safety and feasibility of the 0.014-inch CiTop™ guidewire in normal and diseased blood vessels with total occlusions. A 100% success rate was achieved while operating the guidewire in 19 native coronary and peripheral arteries of seven swine. The feasibility to cross total occlusions was tested on human amputations and demonstrated angiographic evidence of arterial occlusion. The overall success rate was 93.3% in recanalizing 15 lesions from 11 human amputations.

Background

Percutaneous coronary intervention (PCI) is one of the most common treatment strategies for patients with coronary artery disease – accounting for more than 1.2 million procedures annually [1]. However, in cases of CTO where the wire fails to cross the occlusion, the success rate of PCI is 50–85% [2,3]. Several novel techniques and devices have been introduced to allow penetration through the occlusions; including anchor balloon technique, contact-wire technique, anterograde and retrograde collateral approaches, Safe-Cross and Flowcardia CROSSER system, and others [4–7]. However, the success rate for the diverse approaches and techniques vary and still do not exceed 80% [5,6]. Most techniques are also limited by operational complexity, flexibility, maneuverability, and operation time [7,8]. Thus, additional techniques or devices are warranted in order to improve the technical and clinical success rate of CTO patients. This chapter describes the safety and feasibility of a new 0.014-inch Ovalum CiTop™ guidewire for the treatment of CTO.

Ovalum CiTop™ guidewire

The Ovalum CiTop™ guidewire (Ovalum Ltd., Rehovot, Israel) is designed to cross chronic arterial occlusions as a direct channel for over-the-wire catheters and further interventional treatment. The 0.014-inch guidewire can be mechanically adjusted into two modes of operation: (1) conventional guidewire with full torquability and steerability control or (2) intra-occlusion/microchannel dilator each time the device is activated. In the CiTop™6 guidewire, the tip dilation reaches 1.0 mm, while in the CiTop™10 guidewire, the tip dilation reaches 1.4 mm.

A control handle at the proximal end is used to control the tip functions. Activating the guidewire shapes the distal tip in a way that dilates the micro-channel to create a 1 mm furrow that allows the CiTop™ guidewire to advance forward (Figure 10.1). A supporting accessory is supplied over the CiTop™ guidewire to provide additional control, and, if needed, steerability, variable flexibility, and torsional strength. The accessory is able to facilitate the CiTop™ guidewire advancement and exchange of wires. The support accessory is a 0.025-inch-OD, 126-cm-long, stainless-steel shaft with helical cut varying pitch to provide gradual flexibility support. It is tapered toward the distal end to provide an atraumatic tip. The supporting accessory can be shaped prior to insertion for up to 30° to facilitate vasculature turns and is visible under fluoroscopy.

We have tested the CiTop™ guidewire in two different sets of experiments: *in vivo* safety experiments and *ex vivo* feasibility experiments. In both cases we used the CiTop™6 guidewire 1.0 mm tip and the CiTop™10 1.4 mm tip.

In vivo safety experiments

In vivo experiments were performed in seven healthy domestic female swine peripheral and coronary arteries after the experimental protocol was approved by the Institutional Animal Care and Use Committee. Cardiac and peripheral catheterizations were performed using a carotid artery approach according to standard procedures. Animals received peri-procedure 5000 U of heparin. The CiTop™ guidewire working element was inserted into the target lumen, then expanded and released by operation of the handle device for approximately 50 times within

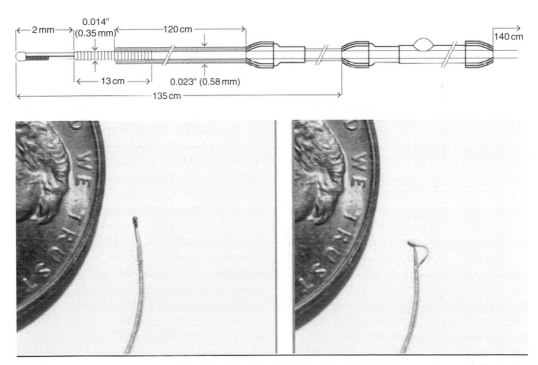

Figure 10.1 Schematic demonstration of the CiTop™ guidewire (top) and the distal tip in its operating mode (bottom).

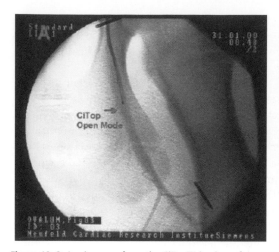
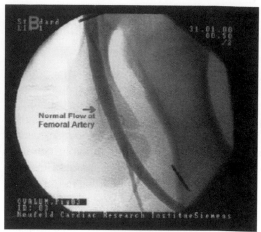

Figure 10. 2 Angiograms from the CiTop™ *in vivo* safety experiment. The CiTop™ inserted within the femoral artery (A) and postprocedure angiography showing normal filling with no angiographic evidence of arterial damage (B).

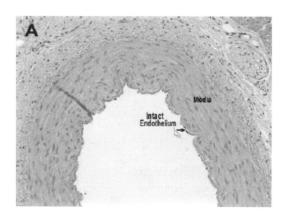
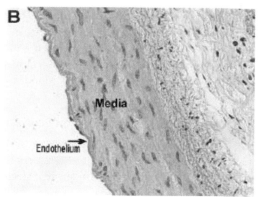

Figure 10.3 Low (×20, panel A) and high (×40, panel B) magnifications of H&E stained slides obtained from the femoral artery of swine treated with the CiTop™. Normal, intact endothelium is evident.

native/normal arteries, while advancing and retracting the device five times along a 15 cm arterial segment in peripheral arteries and 3 cm in coronary arteries under fluoroscopic guidance and monitoring. The CiTop™ guidewire was retrieved out of the animal and postprocedure angiography was recorded to evaluate potential arterial damage. Procedures were repeated over the peripheral and coronary arteries of each swine. Following sacrifice, the hearts and treated arteries were carefully removed, then stained with hematoxylin and eosin (H&E) for histopathological evaluation.

One hundred percent success was achieved as the CiTop™ guidewire operated inside native/ healthy peripheral and coronary arteries without angiographic or histological evidence of damage to arterial wall (Figures 10.2 and 10.3). A total of 19 arteries from seven swine were treated with the following distribution: 6 LAD, 2 marginal, 3 circumflex, 2 diagonal, 6 femoral, and 1 profunda. No angiographic, macroscopic, or microscopic evidence of arterial damage (perforation, hematoma, or hemorrhage) was noted. It was feasible and safe to advance and operate the CiTop™ guidewire in normal peripheral and coronary arteries. Neither arrhythmias nor vasospasm were induced during the device operation within the coronary bed. Visualization of the device was good. Compatibility with standard equipment was good. No operational problems were detected during device insertion or retrieval.

Ex vivo experiments

Ex vivo experiments were performed on amputated human legs (*n* = 11) obtained from patients with documented peripheral vascular disease. Informed consent and approval of the protocol by the Sheba Medical Center Helsinki Committee was obtained. Sheath with introducer canola was inserted into the open-end of the target artery (obtained from either below knee [BK] or above knee [AK] amputations), and a Y-connector was attached, which enabled contrast media injections while the device was in the artery. Contrast media was injected and baseline angiography was recorded to approve or refute the existence of total occlusion, recognize potential segments to be treated, and evaluate degree of the occlusion. After diameter estimation of the target artery, a 0.035-inch standard guidewire was introduced to the target segment. After a failed attempt, the standard guidewire was replaced with the CiTop™ guidewire introduced proximal to the target segment. The CiTop™ guidewire working element was expanded and released by operation of the handle, advancing in steps inside the target segment. Progression of the CiTop™ guidewire inside the target segment was halted when it was progressed smoothly (successfully passed through the occlusion), when it was stuck and could not be progressed any further, or when a procedural problem was noted, such as perforation or slippage from the main course of the artery (to avoid operating in small side branches that are disproportional to the device measures). The CiTop™ guidewire was retrieved from the amputation and postprocedure angiography was recorded to evaluate flow and potential arterial damage. In cases where more than one artery was accessible, the procedure was repeated over the rest of the arteries. Eventually, the treated arterial segments underwent histopathological evaluation.

In 9 out of 15 lesions, the procedures were completed with balloon angioplasty over the CiTop™ guidewire. The remaining procedures were not completed by balloon dilation since it creates additional damage to the vascular wall, and the intention was to isolate the effect of the CiTop™ guidewire during histopathological evaluation.

Out of 11 amputations enrolled in the study, 7 fulfilled the inclusion criteria by having angiographic evidence of total occlusion and severe stenosis. The 4 amputations excluded from the main study included arteries that demonstrated normal filling (*n* = 1), arteries with occlusions that a standard guidewire passed (*n* = 1), and occluded arteries in which the arterial diameter was less than the minimal diameter of 1.5 mm (*n* = 2).

The CiTop™ guidewire was advanced and operated in 5 total occlusions and 4 severe stenoses (mean 94 ± 6%); 4 of which were BK amputations and 11 AK amputations. Occlusion lengths ranged from 9 mm to 104 mm, with an average occlusion length of 30.6 ± 26.7 mm. Arterial diameters were 2.2 to 6.8 mm, with a mean diameter of 3.1 ± 1.2 mm (Table 10.1). The treated arterial segment distribution was: 1 SFA (superficial femoral artery), 5 tibialis anterior, 5 tibialis posterior, 2 peroneal arteries, and 2 popliteal arteries. Average time to cross the occlusion was 3.5 ± 1.6 min. In 14 cases (93.3%), the CiTop™ guidewire successfully passed the occlusions resulting in angiographic evidence of occlusion filling and without significant histological evidence of arterial damage (Table 10.2, Figures 10.4 and 10.5). In one artery (6.7%) there was angiographic evidence of vessel perforation.

Summary and conclusion

There are various animal models mimicking total vessel occlusions, however, these models in most cases contain soft thrombus and are based on acute occlusion, thus do not fulfill the requirements for CTO. Included is the rabbit iliac model for peripheral CTOs generated by drying the endothelium with carbon dioxide gas with or without mechanical injury and/or thrombin administration [9], rabbit and porcine superficial femoral arteries generated by creation of stenosis and injecting autologous blood clot above the stenosis [10], stent implantation with occluded outflow [11], balloon injury to the carotid artery in swine [12], and direct alcohol injection to promote thrombosis [13]. Creating a coronary model is even more

Table 10.1 Vessel description and occlusion characteristics of each treated amputation

Case no.	AK/ BK	Occlusion/ stenosis length (mm)	Angiographic evidence for arterial stenosis (%)	Average arterial diameter (mm)	Crossing time for CiTop™, min	Post-procedure angiographic evidence for perforation	Post-procedure balloon angioplasty	Angiographic success
1	BK	63	100	2.5	18	No	No	Yes
2	BK	21	100	2.7	6	No	No	Yes
3	AK	50	100	3.8	N/A	Yes	No	No
4	AK	26	100	6.8	1	No	No	Yes
5	AK	58	100	4.3	8	No	Yes	Yes
6	AK	13	100	2.3	>1	No	Yes	Yes
7	AK	9	99	2.2	>1	No	Yes	Yes
8	BK	24	95	2.8	1	No	Yes	Yes
9	BK	15	100	2.7	2	No	Yes	Yes
10	AK	23	99	3.3	3	No	Yes	Yes
11	AK	17	100	2.7	2	No	Yes	Yes
12	AK	104	100	2.2	3	No	Yes	Yes
13	AK	10	100	2.5	1	No	Yes	Yes
14	AK	9	85	3.4	2	No	No	Yes
15	AK	18	90	2.8	>1	No	No	Yes

Table 10.2 Angiographic results of the treated arteries from human amputations

No.	CiTop™ passed	Angiographic perforation	Occlusion filling	Distal filling	Collaterals filling
1	+	−	+	+	+
2	+	−	+	−	−
3	+	−	+	+	+
4	+	−	+	+	+
5	+	−	+	−	−
6	+	−	+	−	−
7	+	−	+	−	−
8	+	−	+	−	−
9	−	+	−	−	−
10	+	−	+	−	−
11	+	−	+	−	−
Total	10	1	10	3	3

complicated than a peripheral model and requires aggressive measures such as the use of thermal injury and copper stent implantation [14,15], percutaneous model of CTO using copper-plated stents [16], or placing a microporous poly L-lactic acid polymer into pig and dog coronaries [17]. In our laboratory, we used human amputations previously diagnosed with total peripheral vessel occlusions. The diseased blood vessels showed on histology various plaque morphology with some documentation of hard material containing calcium islets. Nonetheless, this model can not serve as a CTO model (defined as total occlusion >3 months) unless predocumented occlusion is noted with CT/angiography prior to amputation. Thus, the ability of the 0.014-inch CiTop™ guidewire to cross human lesions with documented arterial occlusions has superiority over any existing animal models of chronic arterial occlusion. The protocol in our study included an initial

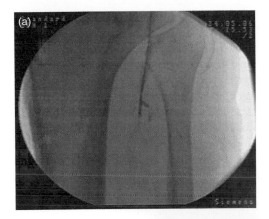
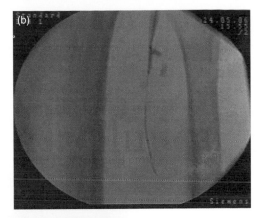
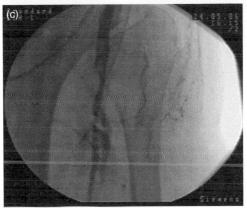

Figure 10.4 Angiograms from the CiTop™ *ex vivo* feasibility evaluation obtained from case #13. Standard guidewire failed to pass the occlusion (a), the CiTop™ passed it (b), and a postprocedure angiogram demonstrating occlusion and distal filling (c).

attempt to cross the occlusion with a conventional 0.035-inch guidewire. Therefore, the CiTop™ guidewire showed a benefit over standard wiring of CTO, as opposed to previous experimental studies that showed no benefit compared with standard wiring of CTO procedure when using Prima laser [18], or low-speed rotational device [19].

The CiTop™ guidewire was designed to be a guidewire and therefore has the advantage of lower perforation risk and higher navigation ability related to mechanical devices of larger diameters. The CiTop™ has proven maneuverable while being navigated in both normal peripheral and coronary arteries, as demonstrated in the *in vivo* swine experiments. The guidewire can be maneuvered just like a standard guidewire by creating a j-shape before inserting it into the artery. An additional advantage of the CiTop™ guidewire is that

once the wire crossed the occlusion, it enabled the introduction of a balloon catheter and completion of the procedure with stent implantation. When using non over-the-wire devices, there is a risk of loosing the newly created path through CTO and angioplasty would not be completed.

Time to cross CTO is an important measure mainly because of the longer procedure time, generally requires more contrast agent with prolongation of radiation exposure. These two factors increase the likelihood of radiation burning [20]. The regular CTO revascularization procedure will normally start with the anterograde approach, during which a relatively soft wire is advanced toward the CTO proximal cap with attempt to cross it. After failure, wires with growing tip stiffness will be attempted. The multiple exchanges of wires prolongs the procedure time and therefore increases

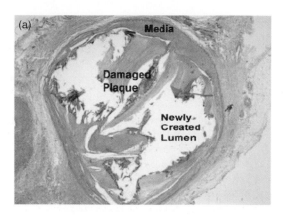

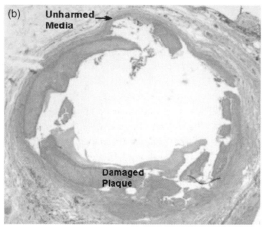

Figure 10.5 Histology of diseased human femoropopliteal artery following the CiTop™ operation stained with H&E. Damage to calcium deposit and newly created lumen is documented in (a) and moderate medial damage is shown in (b).

the radiation exposure to the patient, physician and laboratory staff, and consumes greater resources [21]. In a more recent clinical study, Suzuki and others showed that the average radiation exposure time when treating CTO is 45 ± 24 min compared with a reference level of PCI procedure of 16 min [22]. In cases where the anterograde approach has failed, a retrograde approach could be used [23,24]. A wire is introduced directly into the distal vessel beyond the occlusion usually via a large collateral vessel or a bypass graft that connects with the distal vessel and then steered proximally to approach the end of the convex distal fibrous cap. The retrograde wire can either serve as a marker or create a channel and then be switched with a second wire in an anterograde direction.

Naturally, the procedure time is significantly longer [25]. Using the CiTop™ guidewire, the tip stiffness can be adjusted by advancing the accessory that provides additional support. Adjustment of the tip stiffness of a single CiTop™ guidewire offers a simple alternative to the multiple wires switching in the anterograde approach or to the complex retrograde-kissing approach that results in a shortened procedure time. In our human amputation experiments, the average working time to penetrate and pass the occlusion was 3.5 min, although we had also a case with a working time of 18 min. Nevertheless, it is important to elucidate that our model was an *ex vivo* none flowing/passive system and the accurate time within a real clinical scenario should be tested. Another advantage of the CiTop™ guidewire relates to its ability to "dilate" the occlusion and thereby increase the success to introduce a balloon catheter over the wire, an obstacle that amounts to approximately 10% procedure failure [26].

Safety was demonstrated *in vivo* with 100% success and feasibility was demonstrated *ex vivo* with a 93.3% success rate. Our data show that the device is capable of penetrating total occlusions with minimal risk even when baseline distal flow is not documented. Owing to its minimal size, the CiTop™ guidewire can be suitable for both coronary and peripheral use. It is simple to operate, safe, enables maneuvering through twisted arteries, allows contrast-media injection during the procedure, involves no power source or electrical components, therefore is low cost and disposable, and is over-the-wire, which is important for completing the procedure with a balloon.

See Plates 14 through 18 in the color plate section.

References

1 DeFrances CJ, Hall MJ. 2002 National hospital discharge Survey. *Adv Data* 2004; **21**(342): 1–29.

2 Stone GW, Kandzari DE, Mehran R *et al.* Percutaneous recanalization of chronically occluded coronary arteries: a consensus document: Part I. *Circulation* 2005; **112**: 2364–2372.

3 Prasad A, Rihal CS, Lennon RJ, Wiste HJ, Singh M, Holmes DR Jr. Trends in outcomes after percutaneous coronary intervention for chronic total occlusions: a 25-year experience from the Mayo Clinic. *J Am Coll Cardiol* 2007; **49**: 1611–1618.

4 Hamood H, Makhoul N, Grenadir E, Kusniec F, Rosenschein U. Anchor wire technique improves device deliverability during PCI of CTOs and other complex subsets. *Acute Card Care* 2006; **8**: 139–142.

5 Werner GS, Fritzenwanger M, Prochnau D *et al.* Improvement of the primary success rate of recanalization of chronic total coronary occlusions with the Safe-Cross system after failed conventional wire attempts. *Clin Res Cardiol* 2007; **96**: 489–496.

6 Melzi G, Cosgrave J, Biondi-Zoccai GL *et al.* A novel approach to chronic total occlusions: the crosser system. *Catheter Cardiovasc Interv* 2006; **68**: 29–35.

7 Lukes P, Wihed A, Tidebrant G, Risberg B, Ortenwall P, Seeman T. Combined angioplasty with the Kensey catheter and balloon angioplasty in occlusive arterial disease. A preliminary report. *Acta Radiol* 1992; **33**: 230–233.

8 Muller-Hulsbeck S, Bangard C, Schwarzenberg H, Gluer CC, Heller M. *In vitro* effectiveness study of three hydrodynamic thrombectomy devices. *Radiology* 1999; **211**: 433–439.

9 Strauss BH, Goldman L, Qiang B *et al.* Collagenase plaque digestion for facilitating guide wire crossing in chronic total occlusions. *Circulation* 2003; **108**: 1259–1262.

10 Yoon HC, Goodwin SC, Ko J *et al.* A porcine model of chronic peripheral arterial occlusion. *J Vasc Interv Radiol* 1996; **7**: 65–74.

11 Nikol S, Armeanu S, Engelmann MG *et al.* Evaluation of endovascular techniques for creating a porcine femoral artery occlusion model. *J Endovasc Ther* 2001; **8**: 401–407.

12 Raval AN, Karmarkar PV, Guttman MA *et al.* Real-time magnetic resonance imaging-guided endovascular recanalization of chronic total arterial occlusion in a swine model. *Circulation* 2006; **113**: 1101–1107.

13 Ekelund L, Jonsson N, Treugut H. Transcatheter obliteration of the renal artery by ethanol injection: experimental results. *Cardiovasc Intervent Radiol* 1981; **4**: 1–7.

14 Schwartz RS, Murphy JG, Edwards WD *et al.* Restenosis after balloon angioplasty: a practical proliferative model in porcine coronary arteries. *Circulation* 1990; **82**: 2190–2200.

15 Staab ME, Srivatsa SS, Lerman A *et al.* Arterial remodeling after experimental percutaneous injury is highly dependent on adventitial injury and histopathology. *Int J Cardiol* 1997; **58**: 31–40.

16 Song W, Lee J, Kim H *et al.* A new percutaneous porcine coronary model of chronic total occlusion. *J Invasive Cardiol* 2005; **17**: 452–454.

17 Prosser L, Elliott JJ, Aggrawal M, *et al.* Porcine model of atherothrombotic chronic total occlusion. *J Am Coll Cardiol* 2004; **43**: 56.

18 Serruys PW, Hamburger JN, Koolen JJ *et al.* Total occlusion trial with angioplasty by using laser guidewire, the TOTAL trial. *Eur Heart J* 2000; **21**: 1797–1805.

19 Hartmann A, Kaltenbach M. Reopening of chronic coronary occlusions by low-speed rotational angioplasty. *Cardiol Clin* 1994; **12**: 623–629.

20 Vlietstra RE, Wagner LK, Koenig T *et al.* Radiation burns as a severe complication of fluoroscopically guided cardiological interventions. *J Interv Cardiol* 2004; **17**: 131–142.

21 Stone GW, Colombo A, Teirstein PS, *et al.* Percutaneous recanalization of chronically occluded coronary arteries: procedural techniques, devices, and results. *Catheter Cardiovasc Interv* 2005; **66**: 217–236.

22 Suzuki S, Furui S, Isshiki T *et al.* Patients' skin dose during percutaneous coronary intervention for chronic total occlusion. *Catheter Cardiovasc Interv* 2008; **71**(2): 160–164.

23 Henderson D, Gunalingam B. Retrograde application of the buddy wire technique. *Catheter Cardiovasc Interv* 2007; **70**: 718–720.

24 Ozawa N. A new understanding of chronic total occlusion from a novel PCI technique that involves a retrograde approach to the right coronary artery via a septal branch and passing of the guidewire to a guiding catheter on the other side of the lesion. *Catheter Cardiovasc Interv* 2006; **68**: 907–913.

25 Garcia LA, Carrozza JP. The chronic total coronary occlusion: you can get there from here. *J Invasive Cardio* 2006; **18**: 339–340.

26 Stone GW, Colombo A, Teirstein PS *et al.* Percutaneous recanalization of chronically occluded coronary arteries: procedural techniques, devices, and results. *Catheter Cardiovasc Interv* 2005; **66**: 217–236.

CHAPTER 11

Frontrunner CTO Technology

Chad Kliger, MD, *Steven P. Sedlis,* MD, FACC, FSCAI, *&*
Jeffrey D. Lorin, MD, FACC

New York University School of Medicine, New York, NY, USA
VA New York Harbor Healthcare System, New York Campus, NY, USA

Chronic total occlusions (CTOs) pose a technical challenge for the interventional cardiologist. Percutaneous recanalization is often limited by the inability to fully cross a CTO or to safely gain access to the distal true lumen with conventional guidewires. Increased understanding of CTOs has provided insight and novel means for opening of these lesions. The Frontrunner coronary catheter (Lumend Inc., Johnson and Johnson, New Jersey) recanalizes CTOs by a unique mechanical system focused on intraluminal blunt dissection through the occluded vessel, allowing for further percutaneous intervention.

To understand how the Frontrunner works, it is important to first understand the anatomy and histopathology of a CTO. Chronic coronary occlusions often arise from thrombus formation following repeated plaque rupture in diseased vessels, leading to eventual obliteration of the lumen [1]. The thrombus, along with the lipid-rich cholesterol esters from the fractured plaque, is gradually replaced with collagen and calcium [2]. Calcified, collagen-rich fibrous tissue forms at the proximal and distal ends of a CTO providing a barrier of entry into a softer core of organized thrombus and lipids [3]. With time, the edges of the occluded plaque become progressively more fibrous and calcified [2,4]. It is this hard, fibrous cap that makes crossing with conventional guidewires difficult and successful recanalization a challenge.

Current device strategies to cross CTOs include tapered guidewires that engage luminal microchannels and ablative and mechanical devices designed to dissect through the hard, fibrous cap. The Frontrunner catheter is an example of the latter method, using controlled blunt microdissection to create a channel across the occlusion necessary to facilitate guidewire passage and subsequent adjunctive angioplasty and stent placement. The concept of blunt microdissection inherent to the Frontrunner takes advantage of the differential elastic properties between the intraluminal plaque and the adventitia and allows for preferential disruption of the plaque while maintaining the integrity of the outer adventitial layer of the arterial wall [5].

The Frontrunner catheter is a 3.1 Fr catheter consisting of four parts: an articulating distal tip assembly with actuating jaws (Figures 11.1 and 11.2), a flexible distal shaft which may be manually shaped, a proximal braided shaft for push and torque control, and a proximal handle consisting

Chronic Total Occlusions, 1st edition. Edited by R. Waksman and S. Saito. © 2009 Blackwell Publishing, ISBN: 978-1-4051-5703-2.

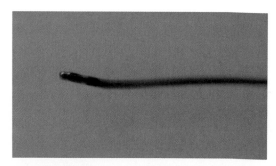

Figure 11.1 The Frontrunner catheter with actuating jaws closed.

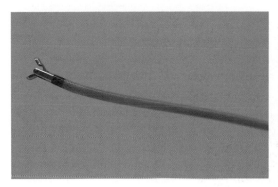

Figure 11.2 The Frontrunner catheter with actuating jaws open.

of a lever, rotator, and a side port for flushing to lubricate the catheter jaws. The handle rotator provides rotational control for the distal shaft and tip assembly and the handle lever provides the adjustment of the actuating jaws allowing for manual opening and closing.

Prior to the introduction of the Frontrunner catheter, visualization of the target lesion and its associated outflow vessels is necessary. In cases where the distal vessels are not well opacified, dual injections of the contralateral coronary arteries providing the collateral flow is usually performed. Once visualization of the CTO is achieved, selective manual shaping of the flexible distal shaft and controlled torque by the handle rotator help to guide the Frontrunner through the coronary vasculature.

The distal assembly of the Frontrunner is advanced with the jaws closed, the handle lever held in the back position, until successful delivery to the proximal portion of the resistant CTO (Figure 11.1). Forward pressure is applied while the distal jaws are then opened (Figures 11.2 and 11.3) via the handle lever pressed into the forward position, creating a 2.3 mm excursion that separates tissue planes and displaces plaque within the occluded segment. If necessary, the distal jaws can be rotated in various orientations to assist in further separation and fracture. Next, the catheter is slightly retracted, as not to snare any dissected tissue, and the distal jaws closed. The distal assembly is finally re-adjusted via the handle rotator towards the direction of the microchannel and the Frontrunner is re-advanced and the technique repeated.

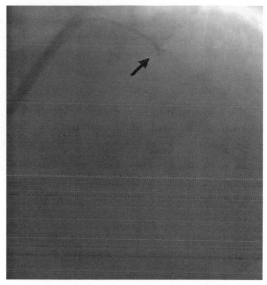

Figure 11.3 The Frontrunner catheter advanced into a chronic total occlusion of an LAD with actuating jaws open.

The separation of tissue planes by the distal jaws, when advanced the entire length of the occlusion, creates a channel either intraluminally through the CTO or around the CTO in the subintimal plane that allows for exchange of a conventional guidewire. In some cases, the Frontrunner is solely necessary for entry through the proximal fibrous cap. Once the guidewire is advanced across the CTO, the Frontrunner catheter is carefully removed and subsequent angioplasty and stenting can be performed.

Creation of a dissection plane through the subintimal space may allow for successful bypass of a CTO as the Frontrunner enters the true lumen of the vessel, usually at a site of a distal bifurcation. Although subintimal angioplasty and stenting have been reported, the introduction of the Frontrunner and guidewire into the subintimal plane may reduce procedure success rates due to the inability to locate the true lumen and may lead to significant vascular complications [6]. Subintimal tracking and re-entry has been recommended for use in prior failed CTO recanalizations, reserved for vessels in which major branches are distally located [7]. This approach can be used for the right coronary artery and potentially the left circumflex artery. Invading the subintimal plane in the left anterior descending artery may dissect the vessel and compromise major downstream branches. If subintimal tracking is used as the last option and the Frontrunner catheter cannot be maneuvered back into the true lumen, giving the vessel time to heal, approximately 4 to 6 weeks, may afford a clearer view of how to access the distal true lumen at a later time [8].

Conventional dual antiplatelet therapy including a loading dose of clopidogrel is given prior to CTO recanalization. The choice of procedural anticoagulation, unfractionated heparin or bivalirudin, remains controversial. The ability to rapidly reverse anticoagulation with protamine favors the use of heparin given the possibility of tamponade in the event of coronary perforation. Glycoprotein IIb/IIIa inhibitors have been used when multivessel stenting is planned, but only after successful, uncomplicated opening of the CTO [9].

Successful Frontrunner catheter recanalization of CTOs considered unsuitable for guidewire attempt or with prior guidewire failure ranges from 50–77% in small series [9–11]. LuMend Inc., in a registry of 107 patients with previously failed CTOs, reported a 56% success rate [12]. This success rate compares with, and in some cases is superior to, many of the other current device strategies [13–15].

An advantage of the Frontrunner catheter is its potential to reduce the risk of coronary dissection and perforation since this catheter provides more control than conventional guidewires over the degree and direction of force applied to the occlusive plaque [9]. Microdissection with the Frontrunner can decrease the number of risky attempts to cross CTOs with stiff or hydrophilic guidewires and the overall controlled blunt approach may further reduce the risk of arterial wall puncture [16]. The current perforation rate is 0.9–6%, with one multicenter trial reporting a 2% incidence of perforation requiring pericardiocentesis [11,12,15]. The dissection rate is approximately 1% [11,12].

The rate of complications is even lower with CTOs resulting from severe in-stent restenosis. Existing stents provide a guide for luminal direction and can act as a protective shell for the vessel wall, minimizing advancement into the subintimal plane and the likelihood of vessel trauma and perforation. Furthermore, the distal tip assembly of the Frontrunner is blunt and in most cases larger than the spaces between the stent struts [17].

Angiographic markers of procedural failure with CTOs include long lesion length, severe calcification, the presence of bridging collaterals, vessel tortuosity greater than 45°, and the morphologic absence of a tapered tip [18,19]. Using the Frontrunner catheter, the presence of some of these characteristics has not been shown to predict procedure failure [10]. It has been suggested, however, that severe vessel calcification, tortuosity, and the presence of other proximal lesions to the CTO may serve as either a mechanical hindrance to passage of the Frontrunner or a site of friction. Increased frictional forces proximal to the CTO can lessen the transmitted forces of the device to the fibrous cap and therefore hinder procedural success.

The Frontrunner has significant limitations. The device is bulky and cannot be delivered to distal vessels or via tortuous or heavily calcified vessels. Small vessels should be avoided. The greatest risk to using the Frontrunner device is perforation, but this risk can be significantly reduced with careful case selection, proper technique, and appropriate anticoagulation that allows for rapid reversal if necessary. The availability of the Frontrunner does not relieve the interventional cardiologist from the responsibility to employ appropriate techniques for CTOs such as dual coronary injections, patient wire manipulation, proper guide selection with strong support, careful inspection of the cine, use of multiple wires, leaving wires in false lumens, and checking of the catheter and wire direction in multiple views.

A reasonable strategy may be trying the Frontrunner when conventional wires appear to deflect away from a hard fibrotic cap. It should be reserved for larger vessels and more proximal total occlusions where there is limited tortuosity and proximal calcification. Longstanding in-stent restenosis may have an extremely hard fibrous cap, where the Frontrunner may provide access through the cap safely. The authors recommend that the procedure is performed using unfractionated heparin, which can be reversed if there is any evidence of perforation. A general principle for CTOs and especially if the Frontrunner can be advanced, but cannot be maneuvered into the true lumen, is to have the patient return in 4–6 weeks for a repeat attempt. Giving the vessel some time to heal may afford a clearer view of how to access the distal true lumen at a later date.

Blunt microdissection through preferential disruption of plaque via the Frontrunner catheter is an alternative device for the treatment of chronic total coronary occlusions, which cannot be opened using conventional guidewires.

References

1 Kandzari DE. The challenges of chronic total coronary occlusions: an old problem in a new perspective. *J Intervent Cardiol* 2004; **17**: 259–267.

2 Srivatsa S, Edwards WD, Boos CM *et al.* Histologic correlates of angiographic chronic total coronary artery occlusions: Influence of occlusion duration on neovascular channel patterns and intimal plaque composition. *J Am Coll Cardiol* 1997; **29**(5): 955–963.

3 Stone GW, Kandzari DE, Mehran R *et al.* Percutaneous recanalization of chronically occluded coronary arteries: A consensus document: Part I. *Circulation* 2005; **112**: 2364–2372.

4 Suzuki T, Hosokawa H, Yokoya K *et al.* Time-dependent morphologic characteristics in angiographic chronic total coronary occlusions. *Am J Cardiol* 2001; **88**(2): 167–169.

5 Yang Y-M, Mehran R, Dangas G *et al.* Successful use of the frontrunner catheter in the treatment of in-stent coronary chronic total occlusions. *Cathet Cardiovasc Intervent* 2004; **63**: 462–468.

6 Bahl VK, Kewal SC, Goswami C, Manchanda SC. Crosswire for recanalization of total occlusive coronary arteries. *Cathet Cardiovasc Diag* 1998; **45**: 323–327.

7 Colombo A, Mikhail GW, Michev I *et al.* Treating chronic total occlusions using subintimal tracking and reentry: The STAR Technique. *Cathet Cardiovasc Intervent* 2005; **64**: 407–411.

8 Lorin JD, Boglioli JR, Sedlis SP. Case report and brief review: successful revascularization of a long chronic total occlusion with blunt microdissection complicated by coronary artery dissection. *J Inv Cardiol* 2004; **16**(11): 673–676.

9 Orlic D, Stankovic G, Sangiorgi G *et al.* Preliminary experience with the frontrunner coronary catheter: Novel device dedicated to mechanical revascularization of chronic total occlusions. *Cathet Cardiovasc Intervent* 2005; **64**: 146–152.

10 Loli A, Liu R, Pershad A. Immediate- and short-term outcome following recanalization of long chronic total occlusions (>50 mm) of native coronary arteries with the frontrunner catheter. *J Inv Cardiol* 2006; **18**(6): 283–285.

11 Whitlow PL, Selmon M, O'Neill W *et al.* Treatment of uncrossable chronic total occlusions with the frontrunner: multicenter experience. *J Am Coll Cardiol* 2002; **39**(Suppl. 1): 29A.

12 Segev A, Strauss BH. Novel approaches for the treatment of chronic total coronary occlusions. *J Intervent Cardiol* 2004; **17**: 411–416.

13 Baim DS, Braden G, Heuser R *et al.* Utility of the safe-cross-guided radiofrequency total occlusion crossing system in chronic coronary total occlusions (results from the guided radio frequency energy ablation of total occlusions registry study). *Am J Cardiol* 2004; **94**(7): 853–858.

14 Serruys PW, Hamburger JN, Fajadet J *et al.* Total occlusion trial with angioplasty by using laser guidewire. The TOTAL trial. *Euro Ht J* 2000; **21**: 1797–1805.

15 Stone GW, Reifart NJ, Moussa I *et al.* Percutaneous recanalization of chronically occluded coronary arteries: A consensus document: Part II. *Circulation* 2005; **112**: 2530–2537.

16 Whitbourn RJ, Cincotta M, Mossop P, Selmon M. Intraluminal blunt microdissection for angioplasty of coronary chronic total occlusions. *Cathet Cardiovasc Intervent* 2003; **58**: 194–198.

17 Ho PC. Case reports: Treatment of in-stent chronic total occlusions with blunt microdissection. *J Inv Cardiol* 2005; **17**(12): E37–E39.

18 Leonzi O, Ettori F, Lettieri C. Coronary angioplasty in chronic total occlusion: angiography results, complications, and predictive factors. *Giornale Ital Cardiol* 1995; **25**: 807–814.

19 Noguchi T, Miyazaki S, Morii I, Daikoku S, Goto Y, Nonogi H. Percutaneous transluminal coronary angioplasty of chronic total occlusions. determinants of primary success and long-term clinical outcome. *Cathet Cardiovasc Intervent* 2000; **49**: 258–264.

IV PART IV
Wires Technique

CHAPTER 12

Use of Two Wires in the Treatment of CTO

Thierry Lefèvre, MD, FESC, FSCAI, *Yves Louvard,* MD, FSCAI, *&*
Marie-Claude Morice, MD, FACC, FESC

Institut Cardiovasculaire Paris Sud, Massy, France

The success rate of chronic total occlusion (CTO) revascularization has greatly improved in recent years thanks to the new angioplasty guidewires (GWs) and dedicated techniques developed by our Japanese colleagues [1–4]. These recent advancements are also attributable to enhanced anatomical and histological knowledge [5] of this lesion type, increasing operator experience and, last but not least, to "mental power" (steadfastness coupled with clear-sightedness), which is required throughout the procedure.

In order to increase the success rate of CTO-PCI (percutaneous coronary intervention), it is important to review carefully the cine film in order to have a complete anatomical understanding of the occluded coronary artery, accurate visualization of the entry and exit point of the occluded site, the severity of potential tortuosities in or proximal to the occluded site, presence and location of calcification that may influence selection of GW, length of the lesion, presence of important side branches that should be protected, and presence of bridging collaterals that may overlap the occluded site [6].

The use of two or more angioplasty GWs is common in this setting and deserves thorough discussion as it is one of the keys to success.

Chronic Total Occlusions, 1st edition. Edited by R. Waksman and S. Saito. © 2009 Blackwell Publishing, ISBN: 978-1-4051-5703-2.

Second wire for guiding catheter stability (anchor wire technique)

When the guiding catheter is unstable or gives poor back support, a first standard PCI GW BMW (balance middle weight type) may be positioned in a proximal small side branch in order to stabilize the guiding catheter and allow the crossing of the occlusion with a dedicated wire. This is a common problem, with proximal occlusion or disease of the right coronary artery (Figure 12.1).

Second wire for side-branch protection

This is a frequent issue in CTO, especially when the occlusion is long or distal to a significant side branch (Figure 12.2). In some cases, it is preferable to position a BMW-type GW in the side branch before dilating the CTO site, because of the risk of side branch occlusion. The discovery of a significant branch in a chronic occlusion is also a frequent occurrence (Figure 12.3) and such branches should be protected as soon as possible by means of a BMW-type GW, before stent placement, and, if possible, prior to aggressive predilatation maneuvres, in order to avoid incomplete recanalization due to the loss of a significant side branch.

Second wire for correction of proximal tortuosities

Since the advent of new dedicated GWs such as the Miracle or Confianza "family," the predictive

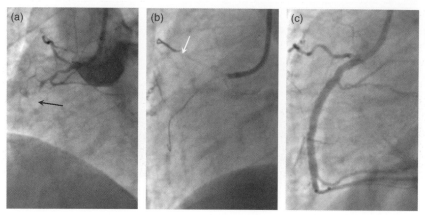

Figure 12.1 Example of anchoring wire technique. (a) Guiding catheter instability with inability to cross the lesion of the right coronary artery (RCA) Black arrow indicates CTO. (b) Successful wiring the occlusion using a whisper wire, after inserting a BMW wire in the proximal side branch (white arrow). (c) Final result.

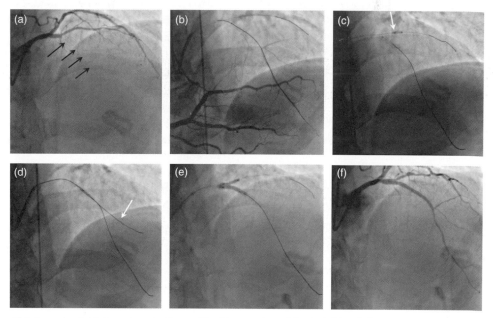

Figure 12.2 Example of side branch protection and buddy wire technique. (a) CTO (black arrows) of the mid-left anterior descending coronary artery (LAD) at the level of previous stent implantation, just distal to the bifurcation with the first diagonal branch. (b) Successful wiring using a Miracle 6. (c) Inability to cross the lesion with a Maverick 2 × 1.5 coaxial balloon despite anchoring balloon technique (white arrow). (d) Use of an Athlete wire (white arrow). (e) Kissing balloon inflation after main branch stenting. (f) final result.

factors of recanalization failure have markedly changed. The significant predictors in 2006 are no longer lesion duration and length, presence of bridging collaterals, and absence of stump distal to a side branch, but rather calcifications and presence of proximal tortuosities, which may cause the operator to lose control of the GW distal segment. The addition of a second stiff GW (BHW type) may help the operator regain control of the GW tip and cross the occlusion.

Need for different types of wire for crossing the lesion

Tissue hardness along the occlusion, from entry to exit point, is extremely variable. It is often

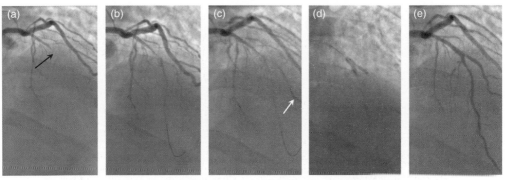

Figure 12.3 Second wire in a bifurcation lesion. (a) CTO (black arrow) of the mid-LAD. (b) Successful wiring and predilatation using a whisper wire and Maverick 2 × 2 mm. (c) BMW wire inserted in the diagonal branch. (d) Kissing balloon inflation after main branch stenting. (e) Final result.

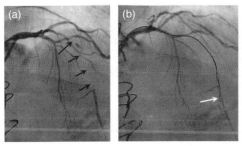
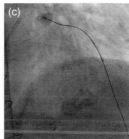
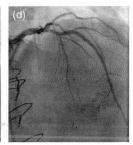
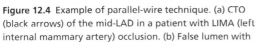

Figure 12.4 Example of parallel-wire technique. (a) CTO (black arrows) of the mid-LAD in a patient with LIMA (left internal mammary artery) occlusion. (b) False lumen with the Miracle 4.5 wire (white arrow), a Miracle 6 wire is used to find the true lumen. (c) Successful crossing with the Miracle 6. (d) Final result.

helpful to use various types of GW to cross the occlusion (for example, starting with a 3 gram Miracle GW to enter the lesion, then continuing with a 6 gram or more GW to cross the distal part of the occlusion or come back to the true lumen before returning to the first wire for entering the distal run-off). As soon as an anterograde flow is visible, especially in the presence of a distal dissection, it may be helpful to shift from a stiff to a flexible GW, whether hydrophilic or not, in order to traverse the distal bed. This multiwire approach is facilitated by the use of a coaxial balloon or a microcatheter.

Two wires or more for parallel-wire technique

It is difficult to differentiate between a false and a true lumen at the occluded site. From a technical point of view, re-entering the distal site through a false lumen is relatively difficult and may result in perforation. When the wire is in a false lumen,

it is preferable to leave it there and use a second wire with a different distal shape and/or a different stiffness in order to find the true lumen. In some instances, it may be helpful to use three wires (Figures 12.4 and 12.5). This technique is one of the major advances in CTO approach and has completely modified the rate of success in our cath lab since it is used systematically when a first GW is in a false lumen even a "large" false lumen.

Side-branch techniques

In the presence of a false lumen, use of a second GW in order to reach a side branch may prove helpful. The result of this maneuver may be assessed through a controlateral injection or a local injection through a microcatheter (or a coaxial balloon), in order to ensure that the wire is in a true lumen. In some instances it may be useful to dilate with a small balloon down to this small branch and then try to advance a second GW through the occlusion, distal to the side branch, step by step

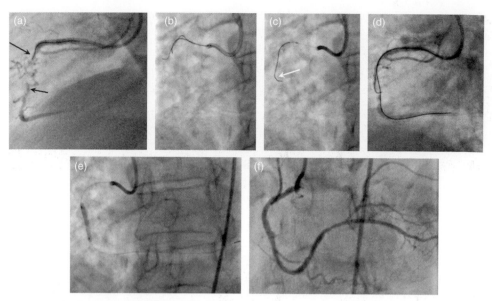

Figure 12.5 Example of multiple wire technique in a patient with bridging collaterals. (a) Whisper wire. CTO indicated by black arrows. (b) Whisper wire and Asahi medium. (c) Whisper wire was able to reach a side branch with coaxial balloon support (white arrow). (d) Use of a Miracle 4 wire to cross the distal part of the lesion. (e) Stenting of the mid right coronary artery . (f) Final result.

towards another distal side branch It may be useful to use more than three wires.

After insertion of a GW into a side branch, distal penetration of the wire is facilitated by orienting the GW towards the carina which is usually the appropriate orientation to find the true lumen.

In the last three indications described above, wire shaping is very important and must be re-adjusted (modified) after crossing failure. Use of a microcatheter or coaxial balloon greatly facilitates the reshaping of the wire. For instance, in order to facilitate the proximal crossing of the artery, we give the wire a secondary longer shape (in addition to the short distal shape) for easier insertion into the side branches or loops. Once the occlusion has been reached, this shape may be modified before advancement of the microcatheter into the lesion, side branch, or dissection.

IVUS guided

When localization of the occlusion entry or re-entry point proves impossible, a second wire may be used for intravascular ultrasound (IVUS) visualization purposes (from the main branch or a side branch), in order to orientate a second wire towards the true lumen.

Buddy wire

This technique has been widely described and consists in inserting a second wire (or more) into the arterial lumen in order to facilitate the passage of a stent in complex lesions. It may prove very helpful in CTO for advancing a balloon downwards especially in stent CTOs (Figure 12.2) or for downwards placement of a stent through another previously deployed proximal stent. The additional(s) wire(s) serves as a rail and facilitates stent passage across calcifications or through a previously implanted stent.

Anchoring-balloon technique

When the balloon catheter cannot be advanced through the lesion due to insufficient backup support, it may be helpful and efficient to insert a second wire into a small branch in order to

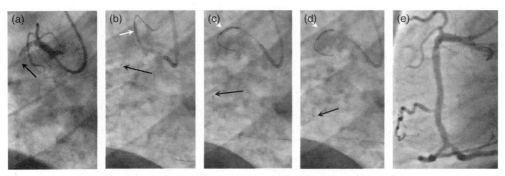

Figure 12.6 Example of anchoring-balloon technique. (a) CTO of the right coronary artery. (b–d) Anchoring balloon in a side branch (white arrow) and progression of the Maverick 1.5 × 15 mm balloon. (e) Final result after stenting. Black arrows in (a)–(d) indicate CTO.

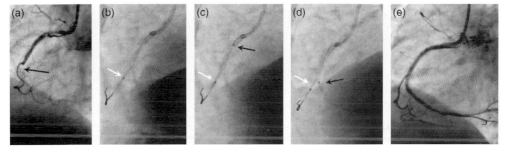

Figure 12.7 Example of anchoring-balloon technique. (a) CTO of the mid right coronary artery. (b–d) Anchoring balloon in a side branch (white arrow) and progression of the Maverick 1.5 × 15 mm balloon. (e) Final result after stenting. Balck arrows in (a), (c) and (d) indicate CTO.

inflate a balloon. This allows the anchoring of the guiding catheter and facilitates balloon passage (and sometimes wire passage) across the occlusion (Figures 12.6 and 12.7). This technique may also be used to advance the stent towards the lesion in complex instances. A 6 Fr guiding catheter can be used when two monorail balloons are used. Otherwise, the operator must select 7 Fr guiding catheters when using over the wire balloons. A variety of this technique consists in placing the anterograde wire upon the wire inserted via the retrograde approach by means of distal balloon inflation, which enables the operator to advance the balloon or stent on the anterograde wire.

Anchoring stent technique

This is a more sophisticated "anchoring technique" used when crossing proves impossible, which consists in "jailing" a wire outside the stent for distal balloon advancement over an other GW.

Conclusion

One of the keys to successful treatment of chronic total occlusion lies in the correct mastering of the multiwire strategy. This approach consists in inserting one or several wires (1) proximal to the occlusion in order to stabilize the guiding catheter when crossing the occlusion and accommodate varying degrees of tissue hardness and tortuosities, "mark" dissections, and protect significant side branches, (2) distal to the occlusion in order to traverse a normal distal bed or find the true lumen in a dissection.

Implementation of this technique requires a thorough acquaintance with the specific features of the numerous wires that may be used in CTO as well as the original techniques that have been developed in this setting.

References

1 Tamai H, Tsuchigane E, Suzuki T *et al.* Interim Results from Mayo, Japan. Investigation for Chronic Total Occlusion (MAJIC). *Circulation* 1998; **68**: I-639.

2 Kinoshita I, Katoh O, Nariyama J *et al.* Coronary angioplasty of chronic total occlusions with bridging collateral vessels: immediate and follow-up outcome from a large single-center experience. *J Am Coll Cardiol* 1995; **26**: 409–415.

3 Noguchi T, Miyazaki MDS, Morii I *et al.* Percutaneous transluminal coronary angioplasty of chronic total occlusions: determinants of primary success and long-term outcome. *Catheter Cardiovasc Intervent* 2000; **49**: 258–264.

4 Giokoglu K, Preusler W, Storger H *et al.* The recanalization of chronic coronary artery occlusions: what factors influence success. *Dtsch Med Wochenschr* 1994; **119**: 1766–1770.

5 Suzuki T, Hosokawa H, Yokoya K *et al.* Time-dependent morphologic characteristics in angiographic chronic total coronary occlusions. *Am J Cardiol* 2001; **88**: 167–169.

6 Tan KH, Sulke N, Taub NA *et al.* Determinants of success of coronary angioplasty in patients with a chronic total occlusion: a multiple logistic regression model to improve selection of patients. *Br Heart J* 1993; **70**: 126–131.

Parallel-Wire Techniques

Jean-François Surmely[1] MD & *Takahiko Suzuki*[2] MD

[1]District General Hospital, Aarau, Switzerland
[2]Toyohashi Heart Center, Toyohashi, Japan

Introduction

In the recent few years, percutaneous treatment of coronary chronic total occlusions (CTOs) has been a field of great interest, leading to increased knowledge about its natural history and prognosis, as well as the development of new techniques and devices [1–3]. With the use of an antegrade approach with a single wire, a successful rate between 50% and 70% can be achieved [4,5]. In the standard antegrade approach with a single wire, a conventional coiled floppy-tipped guidewire or a hydrophilic floppy-tipped guidewire are used for the initial approach in CTO lesions. If it is not successful, wires with stepwise increased stiffness, and eventually tapered wires with hydrophilic coating are then chosen.

The commonest percutaneous coronary interventions (PCI) failure cause for CTOs is the inability to successfully pass a guidewire across the lesion into the true lumen of the distal vessel [6,7]. After penetration of the proximal CTO fibrous cap, the guidewire often enters the subintima, creating a subintimal lumen. Repeated wire manipulations in order to redirect the guidewire into the CTO body can result in extensive subintimal dissection with accompanying extramural hematoma. Such dissections extend circumferentially and longitudinally and can compress the distal true lumen, which makes at times distal true lumen re-entry difficult [4,8]. Another common reason for unsuccessful recanalization is the difficulty to perforate the CTO distal fibrous cap, the guidewire sliding consequently in the subintimal space. The difficulty to redirect a wire into a CTO until it passes to the distal vessel true lumen, as well as the increased complications risks associated to repeated guidewire manipulations in the subintimal space, has led to the development of the parallel-wire technique.

Parallel-wire technique

The parallel-wire technique has two main purposes: redirecting a wire inside the body of the CTO, and puncture of the distal CTO fibrous cap. The parallel-wire technique has been shown to increase the success rate after a failed attempt with the conventional wire technique [7]. An important condition for using the parallel-wire technique is the visualization of the distal true lumen, filled via collaterals, on angiography. Indeed, the visualization of the first guidewire and its relative position to the distal true lumen, as well as its relative position to the second guidewire, using orthogonal angiographic views, is necessary for the success of this technique. A contralateral injection is needed for the visualization of the distal true lumen, apart from cases with autocollaterals. Also of outmost importance is to switch to this technique before a large subintimal dissection occurs, as the chance of successful recanalization by the second guidewire decreases proportionally to the severity of the subintimal dissection induced by the first guidewire.

Technique description

When a wire has entered a false channel, it is left in place in the dissection plane as a marker, and

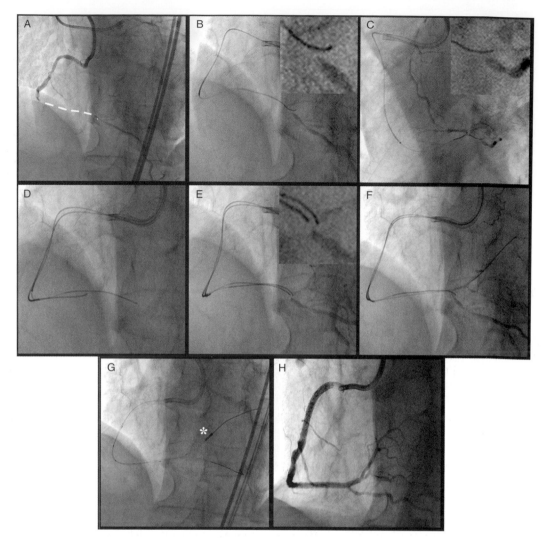

Figure 13.1 Example illustrating the use of the parallel-wire technique. All images are left and cranial views, apart from Panel C, which is a left and caudal view. Bi-lateral contrast injection allows visualizing the distal CTO end, and to imagine the course of the occlusion (dashed white lines) on the baseline angiography (panel A). A first wire could cross the CTO body but was not able to penetrate the CTO distal fibrous cap, sliding at this point into the subintima (panels B and C, with magnification image on the upper right). Parallel-wire technique was thereafter undertaken. A second wire with a different tip curve was brought along the same path (panel D) up to the distal fibrous cap (panel E). The second wire could enter the distal true lumen of the posterior-lateral (panel F). As it was difficult to enter the distal true lumen of the posterior descending artery, an IVUS catheter (*) was brought on the PLA wire to manipulate the first wire into the PDA under direct visualization (panel G). Final result after stent implantations is shown in panel H.

a second guidewire is passed along the same path parallel to the first wire. The main pitfall is the occurrence of the two wires twisting with each others. In order to avoid wires twisting, usage of a support catheter and appropriate wires selection/ handling are necessary.

Use and correct positioning of a support catheter. We can either use an over-the-wire balloon catheter, or a microcatheter. It is important to advance the tip of the support catheter just in front of the proximal CTO cap. We favor the use of the Transit® (Jonhson & Jonhson) or Finecross® (Terumo) microcatheter, as their tips are very flexible, which allows a better wire maneuverability. The use of a support catheter also allows maintaining an acceptable maneuverability of the second wire as well as enables the reshaping of the wire tip easily.

Wires selection and handling: The second wire should be stiffer than the first one, and should have a superior torquability. These characteristics allow a better maneuverability of the second wire, and decrease the risk of wires twisting. The wires that we most commonly use as a second wire are the Miracle 12 g, or a Confianza Pro wire. As the second wire is advanced along the same path parallel to the first wire, we should apply only limited rotation. At best, a 45–90° clockwise rotation followed by a similar degree counterclockwise rotation, and so on, should be performed. The advance of the wire should be check on multiple angiographic views, to confirm the correct location of the second wire (Figure 13.1).

Use of the parallel-wire technique

The parallel-wire technique can be used with different aims, at different stages of the CTO recanalization:

1 *Exchanging wires inside a CTO*: When working with the conventional single wire technique, we often have to exchange the wire for another wire with different characteristics (increased stiffness, hydrophilic coating, tapered tip), or a different tip curve. It is, however, difficult to pass the new wire through the channel made inside the CTO by the previous wire. When we have to exchange a wire, we essentially use the parallel-wire technique as it minimizes the risk of creating new false lumen or perforations.

2 *Finding a new channel inside the CTO body (Figure 13.2)*: When a wire entered a false lumen, it can be difficult to find a new path through the CTO body, as the wire slip repeatedly in the same subintimal path. Leaving the first wire in the subintimal path prevent the second wire to end up in the same subintimal path. It is therefore easier to manipulate the second wire along another path inside the CTO body. This can be achieved via either truly parallel-wire course, or via contact of the second guidewire against the first guidewire which allows adjusting the direction of the second wire.

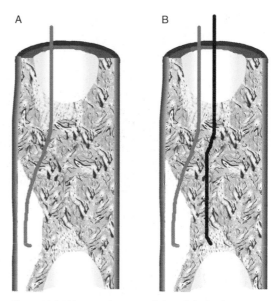

Figure 13.2 When a wire entered the sub-intimal space (panel A), a new channel is not easily created. Leaving the first wire (gray color) in the sub-intimal path, prevent the second wire (black color) to slip in it, and allows redirecting the second wire inside the CTO body.

3 *Puncture of the distal CTO fibrous cap (Figures 13.1 and 13.3)*: The shape of the distal fibrous cap is often dome shaped [9]. When the wire tip reaches this dome shaped distal fibrous cap, it often fails to penetrate and crossing it into the distal true lumen, but instead slides along it into the subintimal space. In this case, we should as well leave the first wire in the subintimal space located around the distal CTO fibrous cap, and bringing a second wire with a different tip curve (acute bend) along the same path up to the distal fibrous cap. This is also recommended in case of tapered distal end of a CTO which is more difficult to penetrate successfully. Visualization of the distal true lumen and its relation to the first wire, as well as a stiffer wire, preferably tapered (Confianza) with a different wire tip curve increase the chance of penetration and successful recanalization.

The parallel-wire technique can be applied to all CTOs, irrespective of individual lesion characteristics. In our center, 181 CTO recanalizations were attempted in 2005. With the use of an antegrade approach with a single wire, successful recanalization was obtained in 54%. The parallel-wire technique was used in 40% of the

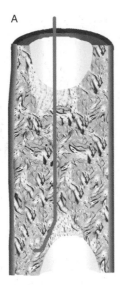
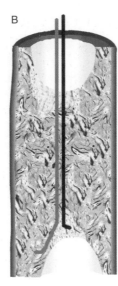

Figure 13.3 Penetrating the distal CTO cap. When a first wire (gray color) traveled through the CTO, but penetration of the distal fibrous cap is unsuccessful (panel A), the bringing of a second wire (black color) with a different tip curve can be very effective (panel B).

cases, and increased the success rate to 78%. Use of advanced techniques such as IVUS- (intravascular ultrasound) guided technique or retrograde approach further slightly improves the overall success rate to 83%. The general benefits of the parallel-wire technique include a decreased fluoroscopy time as you spend less time exchanging wires and trying crossing the lesion, reducing the amount of contrast medium used as you can confirm the position of the wire by looking at the first wire without to have a contrast injection.

Conclusion

When a first wire entered the subintimal space, the parallel-wire technique should be used. The parallel-wire technique increases significantly the success rate in percutaneous CTO recanalization.

See Plates 19 and 20 in the color plate section.

References

1 Stone GW, Colombo A, Teirstein PS *et al.* Percutaneous recanalization of chronically occluded coronary arteries: procedural techniques, devices, and results. *Catheter Cardiovasc Interv* 2005; **66**(2): 217–236.

2 Stone GW, Kandzari DE, Mehran R *et al.* Percutaneous recanalization of chronically occluded coronary arteries: a consensus document: part I. *Circulation* 2005; **112**(15): 2364–2372.

3 Stone GW, Reifart NJ, Moussa I *et al.* Percutaneous recanalization of chronically occluded coronary arteries: a consensus document: Part II. *Circulation* 2005; **112**(16): 2530–2537.

4 Kinoshita I, Katoh O, Nariyama J *et al.* Coronary angioplasty of chronic total occlusions with bridging collateral vessels: immediate and follow-up outcome from a large single-center experience. *J Am Coll Cardiol* 1995; **26**(2): 409–415.

5 Maiello L, Colombo A, Gianrossi R *et al.* Coronary angioplasty of chronic occlusions: factors predictive of procedural success. *Am Heart J* 1992; **124**(3): 581–584.

6 Noguchi T, Miyazaki MS, Morii I, Daikoku S, Goto Y, Nonogi H. Percutaneous transluminal coronary angioplasty of chronic total occlusions. Determinants of primary success and long-term clinical outcome. *Catheter Cardiovasc Interv* 2000; **49**(3): 258–264.

7 Saito S, Tanaka S, Hiroe Y *et al.* Angioplasty for chronic total occlusion by using tapered-tip guidewires. *Catheter Cardiovasc Interv* 2003; **59**(3): 305–311.

8 Kimura BJ, Tsimikas S, Bhargava V, DeMaria AN, Penny WF. Subintimal wire position during angioplasty of a chronic total coronary occlusion: detection and subsequent procedural guidance by intravascular ultrasound. *Catheter Cardiovasc Diagn* 1995; **35**(3): 262–265.

9 Surmely J-F, Katoh O, Tsuchikane E, Nasu K, Suzuki T. Coronary septal collaterals as an access for the retrograde approach in the percutaneous treatment of coronary chronic total occlusions. *Catheter Cardiovasc Interv* 2007; **69**(6): 826–832.

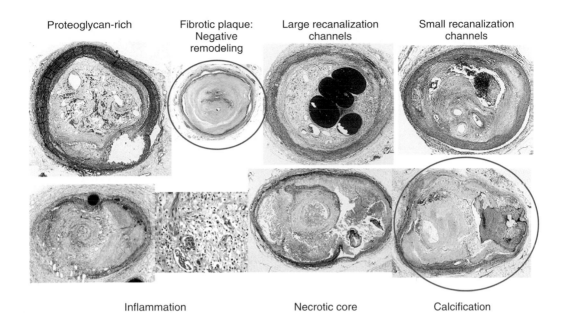

| Proteoglycan-rich | Fibrotic plaque: Negative remodeling | Large recanalization channels | Small recanalization channels |

| Inflammation | Necrotic core | Calcification |

Plate 1a The spectrum of lumen morphology in CTO: clinical challenges of a fibrotic plaque.

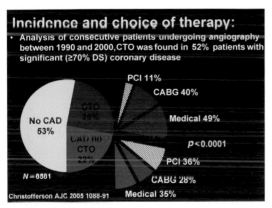

Plate 2a Incidence and choice of therapy.

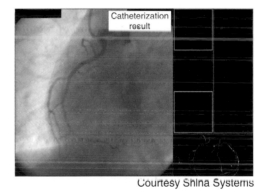

Courtesy Shina Systems

Plate 4 Catheterization result.

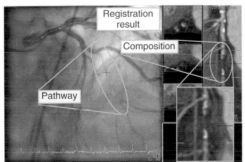

Courtesy Shina Systems

Plate 4a Integrating angiography & CT data.

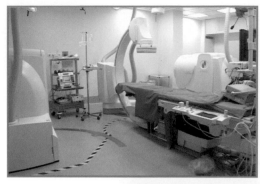
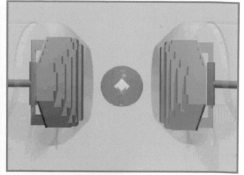

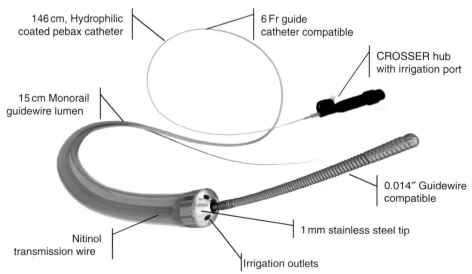

Plate 5a Magnet platform.

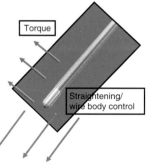

- 0.014″ Guidewire containing a single magnet
- Torque is applied by directing the magnetic field at varying angles to the wire
- Straightening – apply field in direction of wire and it will resist angulation
- "Dynamic control" provides no greater force than manual intervention

Torque

Straightening/ wire body control

Plate 5b Stereotaxis: guidewire control.

CROSSER CATHETER

- 1.0 mm tip
- Monorail
- Hydrophilic coating
- 0.014″ guidewire compatible
- 6 Fr guide compatible

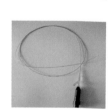

Plate 6a The CROSSER™ system.

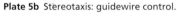
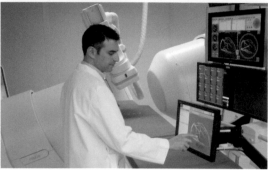

146 cm, Hydrophilic coated pebax catheter

6 Fr guide catheter compatible

CROSSER hub with irrigation port

15 cm Monorail guidewire lumen

0.014″ Guidewire compatible

1 mm stainless steel tip

Nitinol transmission wire

Irrigation outlets

Plate 6b CROSSER™ 14 catheter for coronary CTOs.

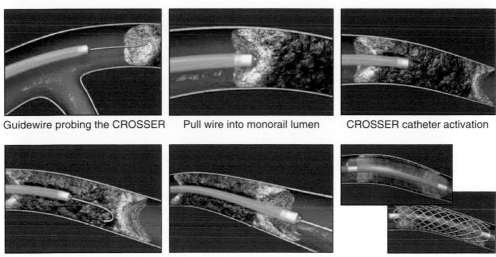

Guidewire probing the CROSSER   Pull wire into monorail lumen   CROSSER catheter activation

Optional: wire probe mid-lesion   CROSSER through, wire advanced   Therapy over existing wire

Plate 6c Procedural steps.

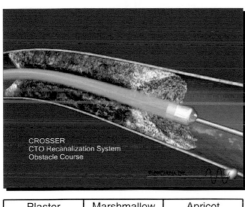

CROSSER
CTO Recanalization System
Obstacle Course

| Plaster | Marshmallow | Apricot |
| = Calcific CTO | = Thrombus | = Fibrotic CTO |

Plate 6d Bench-top efficacy model – simulated CTO morphology.

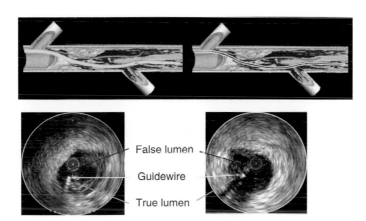

False lumen

Guidewire

True lumen

Plate 6e IVUS-guided crossing of guidewire.

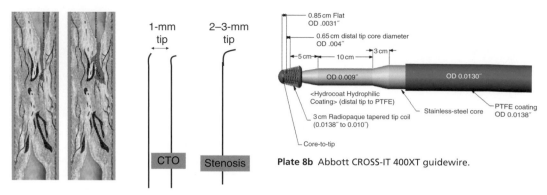

Plate 7a Wire tip for CTO.

Plate 8b Abbott CROSS-IT 400XT guidewire.

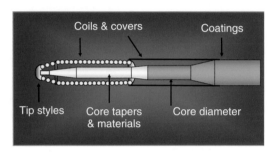

Plate 8a Anatomy of guidewires.

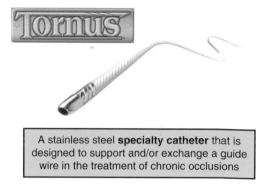

A stainless steel **specialty catheter** that is designed to support and/or exchange a guide wire in the treatment of chronic occlusions

Plate 9a Tornus catheter.

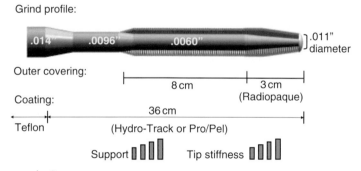

Plate 9b Medtronic persuader 9.

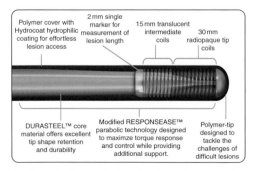

Plate 10a Abbott PILOT guidewires (50, 150, and 200).

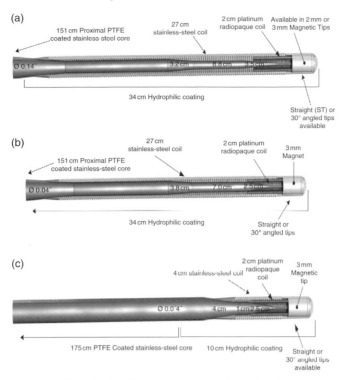

(a)

151 cm Proximal PTFE coated stainless-steel core

27 cm stainless-steel coil

2 cm platinum radiopaque coil

Available in 2 mm or 3 mm Magnetic Tips

Ø 0.14"

3.2 cm   8.8 cm   3.5 cm

34 cm Hydrophilic coating

Straight (ST) or 30° angled tips available

(b)

151 cm Proximal PTFE coated stainless-steel core

27 cm stainless-steel coil

2 cm platinum radiopaque coil

3 mm Magnet

Ø 0.04"

3.8 cm   7.0 cm   2.5 cm

34 cm Hydrophilic coating

Straight or 30° angled tips

(c)

4 cm stainless-steel coil

2 cm platinum radiopaque coil

3 mm Magnetic tip

Ø 0.0'4"

4 cm   1 cm 2.5 cm

175 cm PTFE Coated stainless-steel core

10 cm Hydrophilic coating

Straight or 30° angled tips available

Plate 11a The Titan™ magnetic guidewire family. (a) *Titan Soft Support*: General workhorse navigation device 2-mm angled tip for small angulated vessels. (b) *Titan Assert*: Stiffer tipped crossing situations. (c) *Titan Super Support*: Added shaft support.

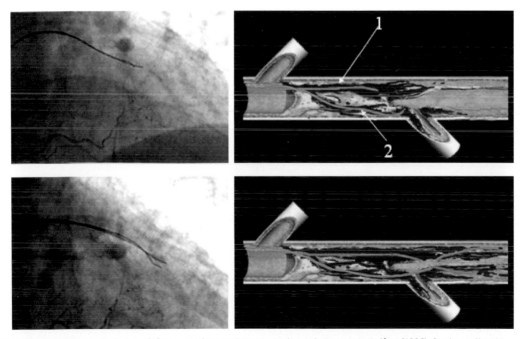

Plate 13a Parallel wire technique (after several passes into wrong lumen). *Source*: N. Reifart (1996), further refined by O. Katoh

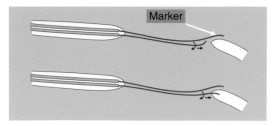

Plate 13b Seesaw wiring parallel wire method with double support catheters.

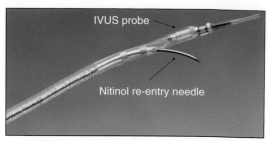

❖ Designed to facilitate true lumen re-entry

Plate 15a Pioneer TransAccess catheter.

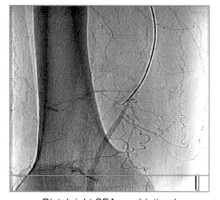

Distal right SFA – subintimal

Plate 15b Re-entry from subintimal space.

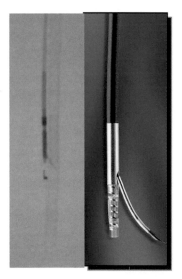
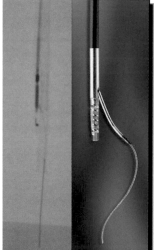

Plate 16a Subintimal return technique (Outback LTD Catheter).

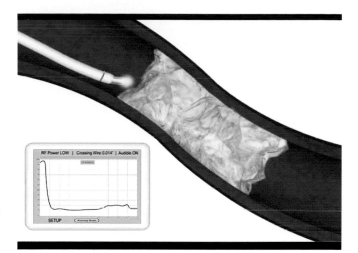

Plate 19a SafeCross – OCR plus RF.

Hemodynamic support	Seal perforation
• Volume, Inotropes	• Reverse heparin
• Echocardiogram	• Balloon occlusion
	• Platelets (abciximab)
• Delayed echo may be necessary	• Embolization (coil, gel foam, thrombin)
• Pericardiocentesis	• Covered stent
• IABP	• Surgery

Javaid. *Am J Cardiol* 2006; 98:911–914.

Plate 25a Management of coronary perforation.

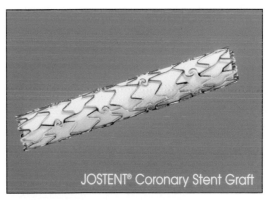

JOSTENT® Coronary Stent Graft

Plate 25b JOSTENT® coronary stent graft.

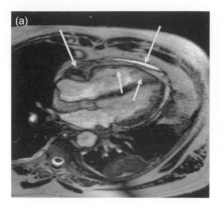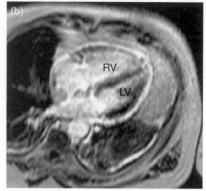

Plate 25c Cardiac MRI. (a) Hematoma in AV groove. (b) Pericardial effusion.

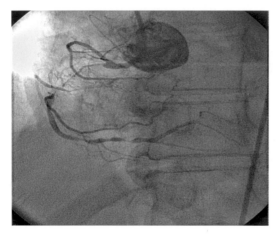

Plate 25d PCI of RCA CTO.

CHAPTER 14

Wire Control Handling Technique

Shigeru Saito, MD, FACC, FSCAI, FJCC

Shonan Kamakura General Hospital, Kamakura, Japan

Introduction

Even after the introduction of new revolutionary devices, the conventional guidewire techniques, which have been developed mainly by Japanese physicians, are essential and most important in percutaneous coronary interventions (PCI) for chronic total occlusion (CTO) lesions. The main handling techniques of the conventional guidewires are classified into "drilling" and "penetrating" techniques. For the adjunctive techniques, we have double or triple guidewire, side-branch, or open-sesame techniques. While using these different techniques, the most important point is how clearly we can identify the distal anatomy. Bilateral simultaneous angiography is essential. If you want to treat "real" CTO lesions, never trust the touch and feeling at the tip of the guidewire. You can trust in only what you can see. This is an important principle.

Selection of guidewires

Pathological examination of CTO lesions revealed that there were small vascular channels of 160 to 230 μm in diameter, which were connection to the proximal free space of the occlusions. These small vascular channels cannot be identified by fluoroscopic or cine-angiographic observations, because their diameter is too small, and contrast dye cannot fill in the lumen [1]. If we try to positively utilize these small vascular channels, it is better to use tapered-tip guidewires. In fact, our previous data show that the use of the tapered-tip guidewires was the most significant predictor in successful angioplasty for CTO lesions [2]. However, the ASAHI INTECC Company has devoted itself to the improvement of CTO guidewires. Nowadays, we can use good nontapered CTO guidewires, which are safer than tapered-tip ones in terms of the possibility of guidewire perforation.

We examined which guidewire finally passed through the 72 successful CTO lesions of >3 months of age in our hospital during July 2004 and January 2005. Among these lesions, Miracle 3 guidewire was successful in 45 lesions (62.5%). However, those stiff guidewires like Miracle 12, Conquest-Pro, or Conquest-Pro 12 were necessary to cross in 19 lesions (26.4%). From this important observation, we can reasonably declare that we first start from Miracle 3 or equivalent stiffness guidewires. If they are not successful to cross the lesion, it is better to change the guidewire to stiff guidewires like Miracle 12, Conquest-Pro, or Conquest-Pro 12.

Spring-coil nontapered guidewires
Miracle 3 or equivalent guidewires are the first-choice guidewire for CTO lesion. By use of these wires, even if we cannot cross the lesions, we can know the touch of the proximal cap and its rigidity.

Spring-coil tapered-tip guidewires
The penetration power of a guidewire is determined by three factors: tip stiffness (tip load), tip cross-sectional area, and tip lubricity. Thus, the use of tapered-tip guidewires increases the risk of

Chronic Total Occlusions, 1st edition. Edited by R. Waksman and S. Saito. © 2009 Blackwell Publishing, ISBN: 978-1-4051-5703-2.

guidewire perforation. These guidewires cannot be the front-line wires for CTO lesions.

Hydrophilic guidewires

The use of hydrophilic guidewires is generally not recommended, since they can easily advance into the subintimal space and expand it. However, after crossing the main part of the CTO lesion, if there is a tortuous anatomy, you may take these wires in order to negotiate the severe tortuosity.

These guidewires are mainly used for retrograde approach in modern techniques.

Unique physical properties of CTO guidewires

CTO guidewires have different overall characteristics from normal floppy guidewires. Everybody has to be familiar with these differences.

Torque transmission

Torque transmission is normally better in stiffer guidewires compared to floppy guidewires. However, if it is positioned in the proximal tortuous anatomy, stiffer guidewires lose their torque transmission ability more than normal guidewires. Figure 14.1a and b shows *in vitro* experiments. It is very important in order to keep the torque transmission smooth for CTO guidewires that we straighten the peripheral arteries by inserting stiff long introducers in case of the peripheral tortuous arteries. Otherwise, the torque transmission will be lost and the PCI will result in failure.

Tip stiffness

The tip load against the lesion is normally changing according to the length extended from the tip of a microcatheter. This change is different between CTO and normal guidewires. In CTO guidewires, the tip load dramatically increases if the length extended becomes shorter as in Figure 14.1c and d. Thus, we have to be very careful for not applying too much heavy load against the lesion by shortening the length extended from the microcatheter.

How to shape the tip of the guidewire

If you imagine the CTO lesions as an artery with no lumen size, you can easily understand that

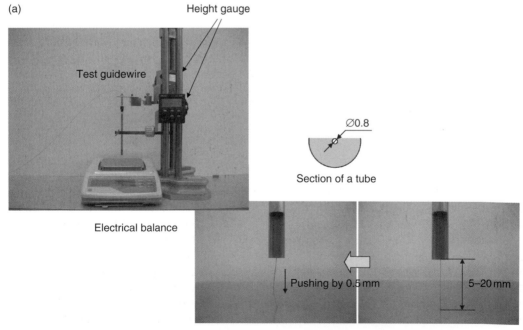

Figure 14.1 (a) Measurement of tip stiffness according to the length extending from a microcatheter. (b) Effect of microcatheter on guidewire stiffness. (c) Measurements of torque transmission. (d) Torque transmission is lost in a tortuous artery.

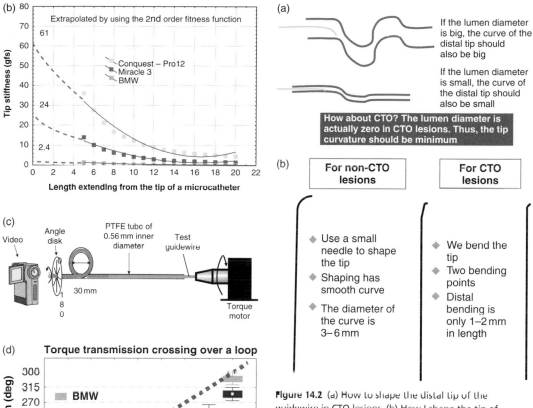

(b)

Tip stiffness (gfs) vs Length extending from the tip of a microcatheter

Extrapolated by using the 2nd order fitness function

Conquest – Pro12
Miracle 3
BMW

(c)

Video — Angle disk — PTFE tube of 0.56 mm inner diameter — Test guidewire — Torque motor

30 mm

(d) Torque transmission crossing over a loop

Distal rotation (deg) vs Proximal rotation (deg)

BMW
Miracle 3

Figure 14.1 (Continued)

(a)

If the lumen diameter is big, the curve of the distal tip should also be big

If the lumen diameter is small, the curve of the distal tip should also be small

How about CTO? The lumen diameter is actually zero in CTO lesions. Thus, the tip curvature should be minimum

(b)

For non-CTO lesions	For CTO lesions
◆ Use a small needle to shape the tip ◆ Shaping has smooth curve ◆ The diameter of the curve is 3–6 mm	◆ We bend the tip ◆ Two bending points ◆ Distal bending is only 1–2 mm in length

Figure 14.2 (a) How to shape the distal tip of the guidewire in CTO lesions. (b) How I shape the tip of guidewires?

It is specifically designed for retrograde approach negotiating the cork-screw tortuosity of collateral small vessels. The length of soldering is less than 1 mm. Thus, we can bend the tip of this guidewire very short.

Use of an over-the-wire system

As described above, the tip load of CTO guidewires can be changed according to the length extended from the tip of an over-the-wire (OTW) system. We can utilize these characteristics in order to adjust the tip stiffness. If we want to increase the stiffness, we put the tip of the OTW system more closely to the tip of the guidewire. When you want to change the shape of the guidewire or even want to exchange it to the different stiffness ones, you can leave the OTW system and easily do them. Thus, you leave the OTW system in front of the CTO lesion, pull out the guidewire, and then you can change the shape or exchange

the tip bend should be short. This short tip bend can find the softest part within the CTO lesion. Normally, we make the second mild bend 3 to 6 mm proximal to the tip (Figure 14.2a and b). This second bend can work as a navigator, which transfers the tip of the guidewire near the CTO lesion. How short you can make the tip bend is dependent on the length of the soldering of the spring coil at the tip of the guidewire. Normally, the length is more than 1 mm. Thus, the shortest tip bend you can make is 1 mm. However, the situation is different for Fielder X-treme guidewire.

to another guidewire. The use of an OTW system is essential in PCI for CTO lesions. Between small-size OTW balloon catheter and micro-catheters, the latter ones are favored, since their tip is softer than the former. This means it is easier for microcatheters to achieve the better coaxial alignment with the lesion.

When you want to change the shape of the guidewire or even want to exchange it to the different stiffness ones, you can leave the OTW system and easily do them.

How to handle the guidewires

In the "drilling" technique, the guidewire is rotated clockwise and counterclockwise while the tip is pushed modestly against the CTO lesion.

The guidewire is introduced into the lesion while traversing the softest part. In the "penetrating" technique, the operator aims at the target with the tip of the guidewire without clockwise and counterclockwise rotation.

The drilling technique should be applied first, because the risk of guidewire perforation and creating the intimal dissection is lower compared to the penetrating technique, and it works well even through the tortuous artery. Miracle series guidewires are better for the drilling technique than Conquest series. However, if the proximal cap of the CTO lesion is very hard, we need to penetrate it. In this purpose, the tapered-tip guidewires are adequate, since the penetration ability is dependent on the tip stiffness, tip cross-sectional area, and the slippery coating. The majority of CTO lesions can be passed through by using Miracle 3 guidewire. However, some lesions need very stiff guidewires like Conquest-Pro 12, in which a penetration technique is necessary.

Drilling technique

The basic concept of this technique is essentially not drilling but rather sneaking or slipping into the CTO lesion. By applying clockwise and counterclockwise rotation, the short tip bent of a stiff guidewire can find the loosest part of the lesion and advance into the true lumen while avoiding the hardest plaque or vessel wall. The important

tip in this technique is that you do not push the guidewire very hard. If the tip of the guidewire does not advance any more with gentle pushing, it is better to exchange the wire to stiffer one rather than to push it. If you push the wire hard, it will easily go into the subintimal space.

Penetrating technique

Since the penetration power of Conquest or Conquest-Pro series guidewires is so high, these guidewires behave like needles. In order to use the penetrating technique, the target has to be clearly identified by using the multiangle projections with bilateral simultaneous dye injection. You cannot trust in the tip feel but you can trust only in what you can see.

Adjunctive techniques

Double- or triple-guidewire technique (Figures 14.3 and 14.4)

Even if you handle the guidewire carefully, it often goes into the subintimal space. In this case, you must not pull out the guidewire from the subintimal space. While leaving the first wire in the position, you can take the second guidewire. You can navigate the second wire more easily into the true lumen. Rationale for this approach includes (1) the first wire can occlude the entry for the false lumen, (2) the first wire can change the geometry of the tortuous artery, and (3) the first wire plays as a landmark for the second wire.

If double-wire technique does not work, you can take the third wire while leaving two wires in the artery. This triple-wire technique works sometimes. However, too many guidewires interfere with each other and reduce the free guidewire manipulation ability.

The tips for double- or triple-guidewire technique are: (1) you have to take the next guidewire of equal or stiffer strength compared to the first guidewire, because the stiffer guidewire has better torque control ability; (2) do not manipulate the first wire too much, since it will expand the false lumen, and (3) use one or tow OTW systems together in order to avoid the guidewire twisting.

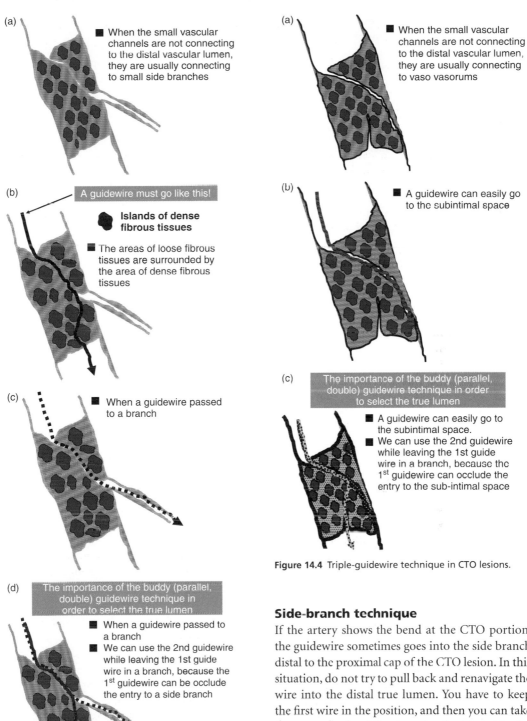

(a) When the small vascular channels are not connecting to the distal vascular lumen, they are usually connecting to small side branches

(b) A guidewire must go like this!

● **Islands of dense fibrous tissues**

■ The areas of loose fibrous tissues are surrounded by the area of dense fibrous tissues

(c) ■ When a guidewire passed to a branch

(d) The importance of the buddy (parallel, double) guidewire technique in order to select the true lumen

■ When a guidewire passed to a branch
■ We can use the 2nd guidewire while leaving the 1st guide wire in a branch, because the 1st guidewire can be occlude the entry to a side branch

Figure 14.3 Double-guidewire technique in CTO lesions.

(a) ■ When the small vascular channels are not connecting to the distal vascular lumen, they are usually connecting to vaso vasorums

(b) ■ A guidewire can easily go to the subintimal space

(c) The importance of the buddy (parallel, double) guidewire technique in order to select the true lumen

■ A guidewire can easily go to the subintimal space.
■ We can use the 2nd guidewire while leaving the 1st guide wire in a branch, because the 1st guidewire can occlude the entry to the sub-intimal space

Figure 14.4 Triple-guidewire technique in CTO lesions.

Side-branch technique

If the artery shows the bend at the CTO portion, the guidewire sometimes goes into the side branch distal to the proximal cap of the CTO lesion. In this situation, do not try to pull back and renavigate the wire into the distal true lumen. You have to keep the first wire in the position, and then you can take the second wire following the double-guidewire technique.

Also, you can take a 1.5 mm balloon, put it along the guidewire in the side branch, and inflate it. Then, this balloon dilatation will break the proximal hard plaque, which enables for the second wire to advance into the distal true lumen.

Open-sesame technique

If a very hard plaque is obstructing the proximal entry point, even the most stiff guidewire like Conquest-Pro 8:20 cannot penetrate it. Even a small hard plaque can block the guidewire passage. If there is a side branch, which is diverting from the main branch just in front of the proximal cap, you can put a stiff guidewire and/or a balloon catheter into the side branch. This maneuver results in the distortion of the geometry between the hard plaque and the true lumen, which enables a guidewire advancing into the distal true lumen. This is the concept of "open-sesame technique."

Conclusion

Still in the era of retrograde approach for CTO lesions, the antegrade approach is essential. It needs a lot of expertise. All of the operators have to be familiar with these guidewire handling techniques.

References

1 Katsuragawa M, Fujiwara H, Miyamae M, Sasayama S. Histologic studies in percutaneous transluminal coronary angioplasty for chronic total occlusion: comparison of tapering and abrupt types of occlusion and short and long occluded segments. *J Am Coll Cardiol* 1993; **21**: 604–611.

2 Saito S, Tanaka S, Hiroe Y *et al*. Angioplasty for chronic total occlusion by using tapered-tip guidewires. *Catheter Cardiovasc Interv* 2003 ; **59**: 305–311.

CHAPTER 15

Subintimal Angioplasty

Masashi Kimura, MD, PhD, *Antonio Colombo,* MD,
Eugenia Nikolsky, MD, PhD, *Etsuo Tsuchikane,* MD, PhD,
& George Dangas, MD, PhD

Cardiovascular Research Foundation, New York, NY, and Columbia University Medical Center, New York, NY, USA

Successful recanalization of chronic total occlusions (CTO) in native coronary arteries is no doubt one of the most technically challenging lesion subsets. New technologies, such as drug-eluting stents (DES), dramatically reduced restenosis rates in a variety of complex or simple lesions. Similar to non-CTO angioplasty, complications of CTO angioplasty arise from different sources, including perforation, tamponade, guide-catheter dissection, vessel or aortic root, shearing off collateral circulation, distal embolism (due to debris or air), side-branch occlusion, arrhythmia, intramural hematoma, extensive dissection, and subacute vessel reocclusion during or following CTO procedures. In this chapter, we focus on issues related to major technical complications and solutions.

Major complications

Death and myocardial infarction may occur during percutaneous coronary interventions (PCI) of totally occluded arteries by shearing off the collateral circulation, damaging the proximal epicardial coronary artery or proximal side branches, thrombus formation, arrhythmia, air embolism, or perforation [1–4]. Emergency bypass graft surgery may be required for trauma of nondiseased vessels (such as the left

main), side-branch occlusion, guidewire fracture with entrapment, and perforation [5].

Even with extensive operator experience, periprocedural myocardial infarction may occur in >2% of cases, emergency bypass surgery may be required in 1%, and death may occur in 1% of patients [6]. One of the most common, serious complications during CTO procedures is coronary perforation that may be significantly associated with different type of major adverse cardiac events (MACE) and cardiac tamponade. Coronary artery perforation is of particular significance and necessitates physician awareness, early recognition, and management. Coronary perforation accounts for approximately 10% of the total referrals for emergent cardiac surgery, but it is most commonly managed in the catheter laboratory with different types of intervention. According to published data from several large PCI series, the incidence of coronary perforation occurs in less than 1% of the procedures, ranging from 0.29% to 0.93% [7].

Perforation or rupture
Causes of perforation

Coronary artery perforation represents a disruption of the vessel wall through the intima, media, and adventitia. Risk factors for coronary perforation during standard PCI can be classified as patient-related, procedure-related, and device-related (Table 15.1). In general, patients with CTO lesions classified as more atherosclerotic and AHA/ACC (American Heart Association/American

Chronic Total Occlusions, 1st edition. Edited by R. Waksman and S. Saito. © 2009 Blackwell Publishing, ISBN: 978-1-4051-5703-2.

Table 15.1 Risk factors for coronary perforation

Risk factors		
Patient related	Procedure related	Device related
Female gender	High balloon-stent ratio	Stiff wire
Older age	High inflation pressure	Hydrophilic-coated wire
	Extremely distal location of the guidewire	Cutting balloon
		Atheroablative devices IVUS

College of Cardiology) Type C lesions are more difficult to treat because they require a higher level of technique and more specialized device compared to regular lesions.

In terms of patient-related risks, several studies found that older age and female gender are associated with an increased incidence of coronary perforation [7–11]. In a multicenter study by Ellis and colleagues [7], patients who developed perforation were almost 10 years older than those who had no perforation; in the same study, women represented 46% of the patients with perforation compared with 16% of women among patients without this complication [7].

In terms of procedure-related risks, the use of oversized compliant balloons coupled with relatively high inflation pressure to achieve full stent expansion to minimize residual stenosis after stent implantation may cause vessel wall perforation. Several mechanisms may be involved, including overstretching of the most compliant coronary artery segment, a high-pressure jet due to balloon rupture, and outward pushing of a stent strut through the vessel wall. Procedural success and complication rates as a function of balloon-to-vessel ratio and high inflation pressure has been shown in several studies. In a study by Tobis [12], the use of a high balloon-to-vessel ratio (1.2:1) with a mean pressure of 12 atm for the treatment of coronary stenosis in 60 patients was associated with a mean final percentage stenosis of 8% with 1 case of coronary rupture. In the same study, usage of similar balloon-to-vessel ratio which a higher inflation pressure (a mean of 15 atm) applied in

the next 300 patients, yielded a slight improvement in the final percentage stenosis (mean 10%), but at the expense of an increase the incidence of vessel rupture and major dissections (3.4%). Finally, in the different subgroup, usage of a smaller balloon-to-vessel ratio of only 1.0 but with a higher mean pressure (16 atm) applied in 162 patients, yielded a percentage of residual stenosis of 1% with a rate of coronary rupture reduced to 0.7%. Likewise, in a series by Ellis *et al.* [7], the mean balloon inflation pressure in patients treated with plain balloon angioplasty was significantly higher in those that developed coronary perforation compared with those who did not (1.19 ± 0.17 versus 0.92 ± 0.16, $p = 0.03$); the same observation was made by Stankovic *et al.* [10] where a high balloon-to-artery ratio was associated with a 7.6-fold increase in the odds of coronary perforation ($p = 0.001$).

Coronary perforation as a result of forceful injection of contrast media has also been reported [13].

Regarding device-related risks, there are reports describing coronary perforations caused by guidewire, balloon rupture, intravascular ultrasound (IVUS) catheter, embolic protection device, and guiding catheter [10,14–16]. Recently, stiffer wires for CTO procedures have been developed to dramatically enhance the ability to cross the lesions. Vessel perforation has become particularly important with the introduction of stiff wires for penetrating the proximal and distal caps of the total occlusion. Dilating a subintimal channel may not only result in vessel occlusion or perforation but may also prohibit future surgical grafting of the coronary artery. Special care must also be taken when hydrophilic wires are used due to their propensity for subintimal passage and perforation of end capillaries. These wires may easily enter thin-walled vasa vasorum, which are prone to perforation either directly from the wire or from subsequent dilatations. The possibility of wire dissection can be avoided by meticulous angiography (including dual injections) and observing the path of the wire in orthogonal projections. It is important to recognize that in certain circumstances wire dissection and subintimal tracking can provide a unique opportunity for exiting the occluded vessel proximally and entering it distally via the STAR technique [17].

Aggressive guidewire manipulation may result in guidewire entrapment [5], a complication that can be avoided by never rotating the wire >180° in one direction, and may sometimes be relieved by super-selective injections of nitroglycerin or verapamil via the over-the-wire balloon or support catheter.

Incidence of perforation

The true incidence of guidewire-related coronary perforation is most likely higher than reported because some instances remain unrecognized and are self-limited. According to the published literature, the rates of coronary perforation due to guidewire were 0.21% in the series by Dippel and colleagues [8] and 0.36% in the series by Fukutomi and colleagues [18] In the latter series, perforation occurred at the treatment site in 12 cases, in a distal vessel in 10 cases, and could not be localized in 5 cases [18]. In the series by Witzke and colleagues [19], coronary perforation due to guidewire use was observed in 20/39 cases of perforation (51%). Of these cases, perforations occurred while trying to cross the lesion with the guidewire in 11 patients (55%), with the distal wire in 7 patients (35%) and as a result of wire fracture in 2 patients (10%). Based on these data, the authors emphasize that the distal migration of the guidewire is an important factor contributing to coronary perforation, and that meticulous care of the guidewire should be taken, especially in patients treated with platelet GP IIb/IIIa receptor inhibitors [19] Several wires are known to increase the risk of perforation. In a study by Dippel and colleagues [8], 10 of 13 cases of guidewire-induced coronary perforations occurred with the same coronary guidewire (Super Soft Stabilizer, Cordis, Miami Lakes, FL); the wire was subsequently redesigned to enhance flexibility of the distal segment. Stiff guidewires (Athlete and/or Confianza-Conquest, Asahi Intec, Nagoya, Japan) provide the ability to steer, shape, and push, thus allowing accurate advancement through hard fibrous tissue. Because of the high risk of vessel perforation using stiff wires, visualization of the distal vessel is of paramount importance. Hydrophilic guidewires (Choice PT, Boston Scientific Scimed, Natick, MA; Crosswire, Terumo Medical Corporation, Somerset, NJ; Shinobi, Cordis, Miami Lakes, FL) represent floppy wires with a hydrophilic coating; they possess excellent gliding characteristics and reduced friction. However, these wires are known for their limited ability to steer and push. This increases the risk of creating a dissection and/or perforation [19]. These wires, therefore, should always be used carefully and never pushed against resistance.

It is worth noticing that the rate of coronary perforation was 2 to 10 times higher in all published series using atheroablative techniques (directional atherectomy, excimer laser, rotablator, and transluminal extraction catheter) than plain balloon angioplasty with/without stenting [20,21]. The excimer laser probably carries the highest risk of coronary perforation (up to 3%) [7,22,23]. However, the device-related learning curve may also explain the higher rates of complications. For example, in one series, coronary perforation in conjunction with excimer laser use occurred in 1.2% of 3000 consecutive patients, but decreased to 0.3% in the last 1000 patients [23].

Classification of the coronary perforation

A classification of coronary perforations related to the angiographic appearance of blood extravasation (Table 15.2) was created based on the analysis of prospectively recorded data of a total of 12,900 PCI procedures from 11 US sites during a 2-year period [7]. Coronary perforation occurred in 62 patients (0.5%). Type II perforation was the most frequent perforation type in this series (31/62; 50%), followed by type III (16/62; 25.8%) and type I (13/62; 21%); the minority of cases were characterized by cavity spilling (2/62; 3.2%) (Figure 15.1) [7].

In addition, other studies evaluated the proposed classification system as a tool to predict

Table 15.2 Classification of coronary perforation

Type I	Extraluminal crater without extravasation
Type II	Pericardial or myocardial blush without contrast jet extravasation
Type III	Extravasation through frank (≥1 mm) perforation
Cavity spilling	Perforation into anatomic cavity chamber, coronary sinus, etc.

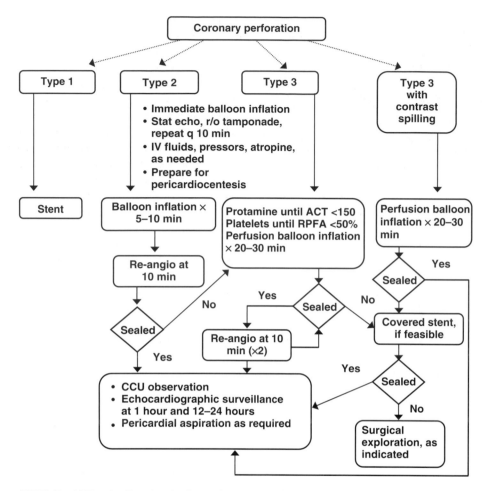

RPFA, Rapid Platelet Function Analyzer, Accumetrics, San Diego, CA; **CCU,** Coronary Care Unit; **ACT,** activated clotting time; **IV,** intravenous.

Adapted from: Dippel EJ *et al. Catheter Cardiovasc Interv* 2001; **52**(3): 279–286.

Figure 15.1 Treatment algorithm for the management of coronary perforation.

outcome and as the basis of management [7,24–26]. Analyses showed that:

1 Type I perforations rarely result in tamponade or in myocardial ischemia.

2 Type II perforations have high treatment success rates when managed with prolonged balloon inflation, and commonly have a low occurrence of persistent contrast extravasation, consequently resulting in a low incidence of adverse sequelae [24].

3 Type III perforations are associated with rapid development of hemodynamic compromise and life-threatening complications, including abrupt tamponade, the need for emergent bypass surgery, and very high mortality. Notably, type III perforation with contrast spilling into either the left or right ventricle or coronary sinus does not have catastrophic consequences and is commonly benign [25,26].

Management and treatment for perforation

Coronary perforation carries a significant mortality risk. Therefore, management and treatment are quite important and used to be initiated very rapidly. The strategy for treating coronary perforation is best determined by specific angiographic type and clinical circumstances. Based on the angiographical classification, a treatment

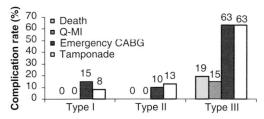

Figure 15.2 Rates of death, Q-wave myocardial infarction (Q-MI), emergent coronary artery bypass grafting, and tamponade in patients with different types of coronary perforation

algorithm for coronary perforations was proposed by Dippel and colleagues (Figure 15.2) [7,8].

If extravasation is limited (Type I perforation) and due to guidewire perforation, then the guidewire should be retrieved to a more proximal location in the vessel. In many of these conditions, prolonged proximal balloon inflations (if tolerated) may help to solve the problem. When limited pericardial effusion occurs as in Type I or II perforation, serial echocardiography may suggest clues to ongoing leakage as evidenced by changes in the effusion size. Early diastolic right ventricular collapse and late diastolic right atrial collapse are early signs of cardiac tamponade and precede the onset of hypotension.

In Type I perforations, the management is commonly limited to careful observation for 15 to 30 min with repeated injections of contrast media. If the degree of extravasation does not enlarge or if it diminishes, no further action is required. If the extravasation enlarges, heparin-neutralizing protamine sulfate (1 mg per 100 units heparin) should be given intravenously, with subsequent dose titration guided by anticoagulation status (target activated clotting time <150 s) [18]. Direct antithrombin agents (such as bivalirudin) may be more problematic as there is no antidote for this class of agents. Platelet glycoprotein IIb/IIIa inhibitor infusions are not usually used during CTO procedure. Regarding protamine usage, while its effectiveness and safety has been demonstrated following bare metal stenting, little is known about the risk of protamine administration following DES implantation.

In Type II perforations, the first step in management is placement of a perfusion balloon catheter to seal the perforation [8,27]. Echocardiographic assessment should be performed without delay.

Reversal of anticoagulation with protamine sulfate and platelet transfusion in patients who have received abciximab along with urgent pericardiocentesis should be performed in patients with signs of tamponade [8,18]. Emergent cardiac surgery is reserved for those patients who do not achieve hemostasis with these conservative measures.

In Type III perforations, an immediate aggressive treatment strategy is required, including adequate volume resuscitation, administration of catecholamines, and, frequently, urgent pericardiocentesis. Immediate reversal of anticoagulation with intravenous protamine and platelet transfusion in abciximab-treated patients is critical. According to the algorithm proposed by Dippel and associates, the treatment of Type III perforation should start from the standard balloon catheter inflation at the site of perforation for at least 5–10 min to provide time for preparation of a perfusion balloon catheter and to perform pericardiocentesis [8]. Subsequent prolonged perfusion balloon inflation (for 20–30 min) may successfully seal a Type III perforation or can provide time to prepare an autologous vein, radial artery, or a polytetrafluoroethylene (PTFE)-covered stents. The site of coronary perforation must be completely sealed by these therapeutic modalities and confirmed by angiogram performed at least 10 min following treatment. Intermittent or continuous pericardial catheter aspiration should be employed overnight [8]. Furthermore, the authors recommend in-hospital observation for an additional 24 hours with repeat echocardiography prior to discharge or on the day following pericardial catheter removal [8].

Reversal of anticoagulation with protamine should also be considered unless the operators employed bivalirudin as anticoagulation regimen during PCI. In this last instance waiting at least one hour or administering cryoprecipitates are the only possible solutions.

Specific devices and materials for perforation

Several devices and materials for sealing the perforation site, such as plugs, coils, glues, beads and deployment of covered stents. These are summarized in Table 15.3.

Plugs, coils, glues, and beads are usually used for small perforation (Type I or II) or distal

Table 15.3 Devices and materials for treatment of the coronary perforation

	PTFE covered stent	Microsphere	Coils	Coils
Company	Abbott	Bioshere Medical™	Abbott	Boston Scientific
Device name	JOSTENT®	Embospheres		GDC® 360° Detachable Coils
Diameter	3.0–5.0 mm		3–20 mm	3–6 mm
Length	12–26 mm		2–15 cm (extended embolus length)	

perforation due to guidewire which we can not seal with covered stent. For pinhole more) is useful. After defining the perforation on angiogram, we recommend to re-inflated balloon used in the procedure with low pressure at the perforation site. Dilation with perfusion balloon should be with minimum pressure capable of ensuring hemostasis. In general, long balloon inflation (10–30 min or more) with 2–3 atm is required to plug the extravascular flow. When the perforation persists, coil embolization is one of the options for the treatment. For the distal perforation caused by guidewire, the injection of the gel foam strips through an infusion catheter is the another option.

If ischemic effect of the patients develops (hypotension), the balloon can be change to a perfusion balloon. If cardiac tamponade and low blood pressure ensure, pericardiocentesis and drainage with pigtail catheter are required. One important point to consider is the need to use two guiding catheters in order to be able to control the perforation with the inflated balloon while being ready to advance a covered stent if needed. When extravascular flow is observed on angiogram despite of prolonged perfusion balloon inflation, a covered stent should be used to stop the leakage. However, preparing these covered stents is technically difficult and the delay of preparation could affect patients' hemodynamics. The small-size covered stents are compatible with a 6 Fr catheter, but advance more easily and have less chance to dislodge when a larger catheter is used sue to bigger inner lumen and greater passive support.

If a life-threatening perforation occurs while working with a smaller guide requiring the covered stent for sealing, a balloon angioplasty catheter (or stent delivery balloon) should immediately be inflated across the tear in the coronary vessel to provide temporary hemostasis. Another guide catheter should then be introduced from the contra-lateral femoral artery access and used to cannulate the coronary ostium after gently disengaging the another guide. The covered stent should be introduced into the new guide over a second guidewire and passed just proximal to the occluding balloon, which is then deflated and retracted, allowing passage of the new guidewire and the covered stent for definitive closure of the perforation [28].

Covered-stent device description

The covered-stent device was first approved by the Food and Drug Administration in 2001. According to recent reports, the use of a PTFE-covered stent can reduce the mortality related to coronary perforation to <10% [10]. The currently available Coronary Stent Graft is a balloon expandable, slotted-tube stent; it consists of two co-axially-aligned tubular stainless-steel stents, with an ultrathin microporous layer (75 µm) of expandable PTFE placed between the two stents and welded at its ends, creating a sandwich-like configuration [28]. Available lengths of the stent are 9, 12, 19, and 26 mm, with diameters of 3.0–5.0 mm. The main limitations of the stent are enhanced propensity for stent thrombosis which may be diminished by high-pressure prolonged balloon inflation (for optimal expansion, the recommended inflation pressure is 14–16 atm during for at least 30 seconds to allow for complete expansion of the stent), intravascular ultrasound evaluation for proper implantation, and prolonged (6 months) antiplatelet therapy that includes aspirin and thienopyiridines.

According to data from a multicenter international registry that studied the use of

PTFE-covered stents in either native coronary arteries (77.8%) or saphenous vein grafts (22.2%) in a total of 35 patients with coronary perforation (32/35 patients), arteriovenous fistula (2/35), or large aneurysm (1/35), the deployment of covered stent was successful in 100% of patients; 2 patients in this series required more than one covered stent to seal the perforation [29]. There were no cases of procedural or in-hospital death, Q-MI, or emergent CABG (coronary artery bypass graft), despite 13.9% of the patients having tamponade before the use of covered stent. Based on the comparison of outcomes of coronary perforations in two Milan centers before and after 1998, Stankovic et al. [10] showed that the use of the covered stent was associated with a significant reduction of in-hospital MACE (death, any myocardial infarction, and target vessel revascularization) in class III perforations (from 91% to 33%), but had no impact on the clinical course of class II perforations. A two-center study in Europe reported 49 cases of coronary perforation complicating a total of 10,945 PCI procedures (0.45%) [30]. Adequate sealing of the perforation was not achieved by conventional methods (perfusion balloon, reverse of anticoagulation, platelet transfusion with/without pericardiocentesis) in 29 of 49 patients. The first 17 of 29 patients in this series were treated with a Palmaz-Schatz stent (attempted in 5 patients and successful in only 2 patients) and/or with emergent cardiac surgery (15 patients). In the subsequent 12/29 patients, perforation was treated with a PTFE-covered stent: in 11 patients, the stent was uneventfully deployed at the perforation site within a mean time of 10 ± 3 min (range: 4–15 min) using a mean pressure of $15 + 4$ atm (range: 12–18 atm), and ruptures were successfully sealed. TIMI-3 (thrombolysis in myocardial infarction) flow was achieved in all but 1 case; in 1 patient the use of the stent was not feasible following distal location of the ruptured site. Thus, in this series, PTFE-covered stents successfully sealed 91% of coronary perforations after other conservative approaches failed. In the same series, pericardial effusion without hemodynamic impairment was identified less frequently in patients receiving PTFE-covered stents compared with those receiving another stent and/or undergoing urgent cardiac surgery ($p < 0.0001$). At mean follow-up of 14 ± 4 months,

10 of 12 patients treated with a PTFE-covered stent were MACE-free. Angiographic restenosis at 6 ± 2 months was found in 2 of 7 patients (29%). Although PTFE-covered stents are considered to be the device of choice in the treatment of coronary perforations, in some situations the use of this stent is technically impossible due to its limitations (limited flexibility and trackability, especially in diffusely diseased vessels) and the distal site of the perforation with a relatively small luminal diameter. In this specific situation, the amount of myocardium supplied by small vessels is rather small, and an attempt may be made to cause distal vessel thrombosis to prevent further blood extravasation and/or tamponade. Successful treatment of two cases of perforation with intracoronary injection of thrombin has been described by Fischell et al. [31].

Prognosis

For the patients with major perforation in hospital, careful observation with frequent monitoring of the hemodynamics is required after the procedure and follow-up angiographic examination should be done the next day. After making sure of no adverse findings, patients can be discharged.

Sequelae of coronary perforations range from none to devastating, and are fraught with early (often instant) and/or late complications. Based on the series by Ellis and associates [7], a clear correlation exists between the angiographic type of coronary perforation and early complications (Figure 15.3). In this series, mortality and Q-MI were entirely limited to type III perforations. The majority of cases of emergent CABG and tamponade were also associated with Type III perforation (63% for both complications), while emergent CABG and tamponade were remarkably lower in type I (15% and 8%, respectively) and type II coronary perforation (10% and 13%). Other series confirmed the validity of Ellis' classification in relation to early sequelae and treatment modality. In the series by Dippel and colleagues [8] clinical outcomes were quite favorable in patients with type II perforation: there were no cases of death or emergency CABG, with only 1 patient (5.3%) requiring pericardiocentesis. Importantly, these

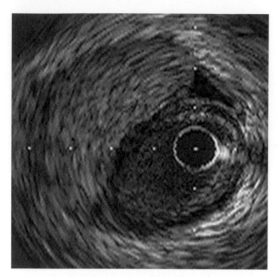

Figure 15.3 Devices and materials for the treatment of coronary perforation.

outcomes were achieved despite fairly infrequent reversal of procedural anticoagulation (21.1%), platelet transfusion (15.8%), or the use of prolonged perfusion balloon catheter infusions (26.3%), although the majority of patients (73.7%) received abciximab during PCI. In contrast, patients with type III perforation had high rates of mortality (21.4%), pericardial tamponade (42.9%), and emergent CABG (50.0%), despite more aggressive therapies including the use of protamine (64.3%), platelet transfusion (50.0%), and prolonged perfusion balloon catheter inflation (85.7%). Similarly, in a series by Stankovic and colleagues, all cases of in-hospital death and/or emergency CABG (13 of 28 patients; 46.4%) were associated exclusively with Type III coronary perforation.

A number of reports have emphasized that pericardial tamponade may develop several hours after coronary perforation. In a series by Ellis and colleagues [7], there was a 5–10% incidence of delayed (24 hours or more post-PCI) tamponade, arguing for careful patient monitoring especially during that time period. Delayed pericardial tamponade typically results from a guidewire-related perforation and occurs not infrequently in patients undergoing recanalization of a chronic total occlusion. In a series by Fukutomi and

colleagues [18], 5 cardiac tamponade occurred in a total of 25 patients; in 12 patients, the signs of tamponade emerged immediately after coronary perforation, while tamponade had a delayed presentation (after a mean time of 4.9 ± 3.4 hours) in 13 patients who were all treated for chronic total occlusion. In the same series, a guidewire caused coronary perforation in 8 of 13 patients (61.5%) with delayed development of pericardial tamponade. Furthermore, the series by von Sohsten and colleagues [32], which analyzed 15 cases of cardiac tamponade complicating a total of 14,927 diagnostic and 6,756 interventional procedures within a 2-year period, showed that 6 patients (40%) developed signs of tamponade during the procedure, while 9 patients (60%) had delayed tamponade presentation (≥2 hours post-procedure; maximum, 36 hours) [32]. Finally, in a series by Fejka 20 and associates analyzing 31 cases of cardiac tamponade occurring in a total of 25,697 procedures (0.12%) during a 7-year period, tamponade was diagnosed during the procedure in 17 patients (55%) at a mean time of 18 min from the start of PCI; in 14 patients (45%) tamponade presented later (mean time 4.4 hours post- PCI, range: 2–15 hours). The same series demonstrated clearly that cardiac tamponade related to coronary perforation was associated with high rates of mortality; 13 of 31 patients (42%) in this series died. Mortality was especially high for those patients who developed cardiac tamponade during PCI compared with those who developed delayed tamponade (59% versus 21% in patients).

Other complications

In the past few years, some newer devices (Tornus®, Frontrunner®, etc.) have been approved and rotational atherectomy and the excimer laser have been used for PCI of CTO lesions. Although all interventions share some general management principles, newer devices and new techniques involve some new complications.

Entrapment of a device inside a lesion

CTO lesions are one of the toughest lesions with severe calcifications. As technology advances, operators have tried crossing and clearing more difficult CTO lesions. In several cases, our group could not advance any dilating devices, although a stiff wire crossed the CTO lesions. In such cases, if pushing the device may have resulted in the device becoming stuck. In particular, the Rotablater® bar and Tornus® became stuck more often. This complication prolongs the procedure time and increases the amount of contrast media and affects patient prognosis. The solution to this complication is:

1 Advancing another stiff wire forward in the subintimal space beside the trapped device.

2 Advancing goose neck Snare® just proximal to the lesion and snaring the trapped device.

3 Retrieving the entire devices including guiding catheter and guidewire together.

During the retrograde approach, it may be possible that the catheter becomes entrapped in collaterals due to severe spasm.

Perforation in collateral artery

In some cases, the CTO can not be successfully crossed from an antegrade approach. In this case, we sometimes use a retrograde approach including a controlled antegrade and retrograde subintimal tracking technique (CART) [33]. With these new techniques requiring dilatation of a collateral artery, it is possible to cause a perforation in the small collaterals. Coronary artery perforation could cause a fistula into the ventricle if occurring in septal collaterals or tamponade if occurring in epicardial collaterals.

Coronary thrombosis

Recently, the introduction of more specialized technique (retrograde approach and CART) has increased the complexity of the procedure with the added risk of coronary thrombosis due to prolongation of the procedure and creation of dissection planes. Careful observation in angiogram (small defect etc.) can help us to rule out early phase of coronary thrombus. In such situations, we strongly recommended to check ACT at least each 0.5 to 1 hour and keep ACT (activated clotting time) more than 250 seconds during procedure. If visible thrombus is observed, we should remove the thrombus with aspiration devices and avoid embolize with thrombus in another non culprit vessel. If impossible to remove, we should stop the procedure.

Intramural hematoma

When manipulating the stiff guidewire for CTO lesions, guidewires often enter into the subintimal space. Rough manipulation with wire could induce the intramural hematoma (Figure 15.3). Intramural hematoma leads lumen narrowing at the proximal portion to CTO site that we sometime need to treat in rare conditions intramural hematoma can cause compression of other vessel. The managements of intramural hematoma are different on its severity. After detecting the intramural hematoma by IVUS, if you do not see any lumen narrowing, we do not need to treat. If lumen narrowing occurred extends axially, stent implantation is required. In general, lumen narrowing and axial extension proximal to the lesion do not progress to critical condition.

Summary

Chronic total occlusion is the last frontier in the field of interventional cardiology. Despite the development of new devices and techniques, certain complications still persist. One of the most common, serious complications during CTO procedures is coronary perforation. The angiographic spectrum of coronary perforation ranges from small-size extravasations with no hemodynamic consequences to life-threatening events including cardiac tamponade, myocardial infarction, emergent cardiac surgery, and death. Treatment of coronary perforation depends largely on the angiographic type of perforation. Types I and II perforations may be effectively treated with the reversal of anticoagulation and prolonged balloon inflations. Type III perforations should be treated with PTFE-covered stent grafts, demonstrated to be an alternative to surgery. Given the delayed development of cardiac tamponade, a high index of suspicion for tamponade should be maintained for patients with unexplained hypotension after PCI. Once complications occur, careful management and adequate treatment are indispensable. A complete understanding of appropriate decision-making and skills for managing this life-threatening complication should be mandatory for all interventional cardiologists.

See Plates 21 and 22 in the color plate section.

References

1 Suttorp MJ, Laarman GJ, Rahel BM *et al.* Primary Stenting of Totally Occluded Native Coronary Arteries II (PRISON II): a randomized comparison of bare metal stent implantation with sirolimus-eluting stent implantation for the treatment of total coronary occlusions. *Circulation* 2006; **114**(9): 921–928.

2 Stewart JT, Denne L, Bowker TJ *et al.* Percutaneous transluminal coronary angioplasty in chronic coronary artery occlusion. *J Am Coll Cardiol* 1993; **21**(6): 1371–1376.

3 Leonzi O, Ettori F, Lettieri C, Metra M, Maggi A, Niccoli L. Coronary angioplasty in chronic total occlusion: angiography results, complications, and predictive factors. *G Ital Cardiol* 1995; **25**(7): 807–814.

4 Orford JL, Fasseas P, Denktas AE, Garratt KN. Anterior ischemia secondary to embolization of the posterior descending artery in a patient with a chronic total occlusion of the left anterior descending artery. *J Invasive Cardiol* 2002; **14**(9): 527–530.

5 Safian RD, McCabe CH, Sipperly ME, McKay RG, Baim DS. Initial success and long-term follow-up of percutaneous transluminal coronary angioplasty in chronic total occlusions versus conventional stenoses. *Am J Cardiol* 9 1988; **61**(14): 23G–28G.

6 Suero JA, Marso SP, Jones PG *et al.* Procedural outcomes and long-term survival among patients undergoing percutaneous coronary intervention of a chronic total occlusion in native coronary arteries: a 20-year experience. *J Am Coll Cardiol* 2001; **38**(2): 409–414.

7 Ellis SG, Ajluni S, Arnold AZ *et al.* Increased coronary perforation in the new device era. Incidence, classification, management, and outcome. *Circulation* 1994; **90**(6): 2725–2730.

8 Dippel EJ, Kereiakes DJ, Tramuta DA *et al.* Coronary perforation during percutaneous coronary intervention in the era of abciximab platelet glycoprotein IIb/IIIa blockade: an algorithm for percutaneous management. *Catheter Cardiovasc Inter* 2001; **52**(3): 279–286.

9 Gruberg L, Pinnow E, Flood R *et al.* Incidence, management, and outcome of coronary artery perforation during percutaneous coronary intervention. *Am J Cardiol* 2000; **86**(6): 680–682, A688.

10 Stankovic G, Orlic D, Corvaja N *et al.* Incidence, predictors, in-hospital, and late outcomes of coronary artery perforations. *Am J Cardiol* 2004; **93**(2): 213–216.

11 Fasseas P, Orford JL, Panetta CJ *et al.* Incidence, correlates, management, and clinical outcome of coronary perforation: analysis of 16,298 procedures. *Am Heart J* 2004; **147**(1): 140–145.

12 Tobis J. *Techniques in Coronary Artery Stenting.* London: Martin Dunitz Ltd; 2000.

13 Timurkaynak T, Ciftci H, Cemri M. Coronary artery perforation: a rare complication of coronary angiography. *Acta Cardiol* 2001; **56**(5): 323–325.

14 Michael A, Solzbach U, Saurbier B *et al.* Bypass perforation by stent implantation: complication management. A case report. *Z Kardiol* 1998; **87**(3): 233–239.

15 Pasquetto G, Reimers B, Favero L *et al.* Distal filter protection during percutaneous coronary intervention in native coronary arteries and saphenous vein grafts in patients with acute coronary syndromes. *Ital Heart J* 2003; **4**(9): 614–619.

16 Mauser M, Ennker J, Fleischmann D. Dissection of the sinus valsalvae aortae as a complication of coronary angioplasty. *Z Kardiol* 1999; **88**(12): 1023–1027.

17 Colombo A, Mikhail GW, Michev I *et al.* Treating chronic total occlusions using subintimal tracking and reentry: the STAR technique. *Catheter Cardiovasc Interv* 2005; **64**(4): 407–411; discussion 412.

18 Fukutomi T, Suzuki T, Popma JJ *et al.* Early and late clinical outcomes following coronary perforation in patients undergoing percutaneous coronary intervention. *Circ J* 2002; **66**(4): 349–356.

19 Witzke CF, Martin-Herrero F, Clarke SC, Pomerantzev E, Palacios IF. The changing pattern of coronary perforation during percutaneous coronary intervention in the new device era. *J Invasive Cardiol* 2004; **16**(6): 257–301.

20 Fejka M, Dixon SR, Safian RD *et al.* Diagnosis, management, and clinical outcome of cardiac tamponade complicating percutaneous coronary intervention. *Am J Cardiol* 1 2002; **90**(11): 1183–1186.

21 Cohen BM, Weber VJ, Relsman M, Casale A, Dorros G. Coronary perforation complicating rotational ablation: the U.S. multicenter experience. *Cathet Cardiovasc Diagn.* 1996; Suppl 3: 55–59. http://www.ncbi.nlm.nih.gov/pubmed/8874929?ordinalpos=3&itool=EntrezSystem2.PEntrez.Pubmed.Pubmed_RVDocSum.

22 Bittl JA, Ryan TJ, Jr, Keaney JF, Jr *et al.* Coronary artery perforation during excimer laser coronary angioplasty. The percutaneous Excimer Laser Coronary Angioplasty Registry. *J Am Coll Cardiol* 1993; **21**(5): 1158–1165.

23 Litvack F, Eigler N, Margolis J *et al.* Percutaneous excimer laser coronary angioplasty: results in the first consecutive 3,000 patients. The ELCA Investigators. *J Am Coll Cardiol* 1994; **23**(2): 323–329.

24 Del Campo C, Zelman R. Successful non-operative management of right coronary artery perforation during percutaneous coronary intervention in a patient receiving abciximab and aspirin. *J Invasive Cardiol* 2000; **12**(1): 41–43.

25 Korpas D, Acevedo C, Lindsey RL, Gradman AH. Left anterior descending coronary artery to right

ventricular fistula complicating coronary stenting. *J Invasive Cardiol* 2002; **14**(1): 41–43.

26 Hering D, Horstkotte D, Schwimmbeck P, Piper C, Bilger J, Schultheiss HP. Acute myocardial infarct caused by a muscle bridge of the anterior interventricular ramus: complicated course with vascular perforation after stent implantation. *Z Kardiol* 1997; **86**(8): 630–638.

27 Maruo T, Yasuda S, Miyazaki S. Delayed appearance of coronary artery perforation following cutting balloon angioplasty. *Catheter Cardiovasc Interv* 2002; **57**(4): 529–531.

28 Lansky AJ, Yang YM, Khan Y *et al.* Treatment of coronary artery perforations complicating percutaneous coronary intervention with a polytetrafluoroethylene–covered stent graft. *Am J Cardiol* 1 2006; **98**(3): 370–374.

29 Lansky AJ SG, Grube E, Proctor B *et al.* A multi-center registry of the JoStent PTFE stent graft for the treatment of arterial perforations complicating percutaneous coronary interventions. *J Am Coll Cardiol* 2000; **35**(26): A825.

30 Briguori C, Nishida T, Anzuini A, Di Mario C, Grube E, Colombo A. Emergency polytetrafluoroethylene-covered stent implantation to treat coronary ruptures. *Circulation* 19 2000; **102**(25): 3028–3031.

31 Fischell TA, Korban EH, Lauer MA. Successful treatment of distal coronary guidewire-induced perforation with balloon catheter delivery of intracoronary thrombin. *Catheter Cardiovasc Interv* 2003; **58**(3): 370–374.

32 Iga K, Fujikawa T, Ueda Y, Miki S, Konishi T. Massive hemopericardium as a first manifestation of coronary aneurysm: successful surgical management. *Am Heart J* 1996; **131**(3): 618–620.

33 Surmely JF, Tsuchikane E, Katoh O *et al.* New concept for CTO recanalization using controlled antegrade and retrograde subintimal tracking: the CART technique. *J Invasive Cardiol* 2006; **18**(7): 334–338.

CHAPTER 16

Re-entry Technique – Pioneer Catheter

Nicolaus Reifart, MD, PhD, FESC, FACC, RANS

Johann Wolfgang Goethe University Frankfurt and Main Taunus Kliniken, Bad Soden, Germany

Although one or more totally occluded coronary vessels is identified in as many as one-third of diagnostic cardiac catheterizations, recanalization of a chronic total occlusion (CTO) is attempted in only 8–15% of the patients undergoing percutaneous coronary interventions (PCI) [1–4]. In the Emory Angioplasty versus Surgery Trial (EAST), the presence of a CTO was the most common reason for referral to bypass surgery [5]. Similarly, in the Bypass Angioplasty and (BARI, bypass angioplasty revascularization investigation) trial, of the 12,530 patients that were clinically eligible for randomization to angioplasty versus bypass graft surgery, 8000 patients were deemed angiographically ineligible, with the most common reason being the presence of one or more CTOs (68% of patients) [5].

The technical and procedural success rates of PCI in chronic total coronary occlusions have steadily increased over the last 15 years due to greater operator experience, improvements in equipment and procedural techniques [6]. Despite this fact, CTOs remain the lesion subtype in which angioplasty is most likely to fail. In a series of 1074 consecutive patients [7] undergoing PCI, the primary success rate was 90% in non-occluded lesions, 78% in functional total occlusions (TIMI flow grade 1), and 63% in true CTOs [8]. In recent contemporary series, procedural success rates have ranged from 70% to 80%, with the variability reflecting differences in operator technique and experience, availability of advanced guidewires, CTO definition, and case selection [9].

The most common PCI failure mode for CTOs is inability to successfully pass a guide wire across the lesion into the true lumen of the distal vessel [8,10]. In a recent large series by Kinoshita and others, reasons for procedural failure included inability to cross the lesion with a guidewire (63% of cases), long intimal dissection with creation of a false lumen (24%), dye extravasation (11%), failure to cross the lesion with the balloon or dilate adequately (2%), and thrombus (1.2%) [8]. We evaluated the most common reasons why the first attempt to recanalize a CTO was unsuccessful in 200 consecutive patients referred for a second procedure in 1998–2002 at our institution in Bad Soden, Germany [11]. Failure to successfully cross the occlusion with the guidewire was the most common cause (89%), followed by inability to cross the lesion with the balloon (9%), and inability to dilate the lesion (2%). In an estimated 10% of cases, the operator aborted the procedure because of uncertainty about the vessel course.

Several techniques had been described how to improve the success rate of penetrating CTOs and how to complete the procedure successfully. Among those are the use of stiffer and tapered wires over low-profile exchange catheters or balloons, parallel-wire technique and the recrossing technique, and

Chronic Total Occlusions, 1st edition. Edited by R. Waksman and S. Saito. © 2009 Blackwell Publishing, ISBN: 978-1-4051-5703-2.

the dissection re-entry technique (STAR [subintimal tracking and re-entry] and CART [controlled antegrade and retrograde subintimal tracking]) [12,13], the CART technique being the most successful and predictable.

The recrossing technique may be applied with and without the visual assessment of the true lumen with intravascular ultrasound (IVUS) [14]. It is noteworthy that it appears far more efficient in identifying the direction where to guide the puncturing wire compared to angiographic orientation only which aim the wire tip in a more arbitrary fashion.

The Pioneer re-entry catheter (formerly TransAccess™) is a unique device designed to introduce a guidewire from one layer or vessel to another with precision and control. The Pioneer catheters are guided through vascular segments using fluoroscopy and targeting the needle is performed using an integrated intravascular ultrasound guidance system.

The catheter was first used in animals and humans by S. Oesterle and N. Reifart [15]. With the Percutaneous *in situ* venous arterialization (PICVA™) they used a series of unique catheter-based devices to arterialize isolated segments of coronary vein, forcing retroperfusion of severely ischemic myocardium. In a series of animals this procedure had been shown to reduce ischemia and myocardial damage in an infarction model. In the PICVA European Safety trial, 11 percutaneous applications of catheter-based coronary bypass in humans revealed feasibility of the technique in highly symptomatic non-option patients [16]. Because of a broad spectrum of anatomical variations and problems in reliably steering the needle and guidewire through calcifications, the procedure was abandoned.

First attempts to use the catheter in coronary arteries for controlled re-entry into true lumen, once the wire had advanced into a false lumen, appeared not very promising, mainly because of the bulky size that needs further miniaturization for coronary application.

The catheter, however, was used quite successfully for re-entering from false into true lumen in peripheral arterial occlusions and aortic dissections (Figures 16.1 and 16.2).

The peripheral application in chronic occlusions and aortic dissections was first described by

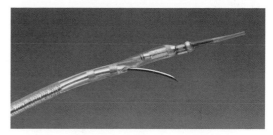

Figure 16.1 The Pioneer™ catheter is a 6.2-F dual lumen catheter combining a 20 MHz IVUS transducer with a preshaped extendable, hollow 24-G nitinol needle. This coaxial needle allows real-time IVUS-G puncture of the target lumen and after successful re-entry a 0.014 guidewire may be advanced through the needle into the target lumen.

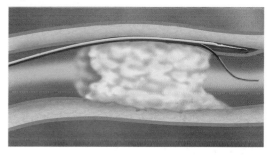

Figure 16.2 Upon entry of the false lumen the Pioneer catheter is advanced into the wrong lumen, under IVUS control, the site of the nitinol needle will be directed toward the true lumen and after puncturing the true lumen, a guidewire will be advanced.

Saket [17]: 10 patients with lower extremity ischemia from CTOs ($n = 7$) or true lumen collapse from aortic dissections ($n = 3$) were treated. Subintimal access and controlled re-entry of the CTOs were performed with the Pioneer catheter. In the CTOs, antegrade flow was restored in all, and the patients were free of ischemic symptoms at up to 8-month follow-up. In the aortic dissection cases, the fenestrations equalized pressures between the lumens and restored flow into the compromised vessels. There were no complications related to the use of this device in any of the 10 patients.

In the same year Saketkhoo published successful re-entry using the same catheter in 6 patients with lower extremity ischemia from CTOs [18].

More recently R. Kickuth described 7 patients who were treated for aortic dissection and 5 patients (with failed previous attempts at subintimal recanalization) for chronic arterial occlusion.

The technical success rate using the Pioneer catheter was 100% [19].

Also in 2006, Jacobs described 87 chronic occlusions (58 iliac and 29 superficial femoral arteries) in whom the true lumen could not be re-entered by using standard catheter and wire techniques. Intravascular ultrasound-guided true lumen re-entry using the Pioneer catheter was applied in 21 of these CTOs with 100% success [20].

Conclusion

The Pioneer re-entry catheter, initially designed to retrogradely perfuse myocardium via arteriovenous connections, was recently successfully applied to re-enter the true lumen of occluded iliac and femoral arteries as well as to percutaneously treat aortic dissections.

The application for coronary occlusions appears not promising unless the current 6 F device is further miniaturized.

See Plate 23 in the color plate section

References

1 Cohen HA *et al.* Impact of age on procedural and 1-year outcome in percutaneous transluminal coronary angioplasty: a report from the NHLBI Dynamic Registry. *Am Heart J* 2003; **146**(3): 513–519.

2 Anderson HV *et al.* A contemporary overview of percutaneous coronary interventions. The American College of Cardiology-National Cardiovascular Data Registry (ACC-NCDR). *J Am Coll Cardiol* 2002; **39**(7): 1096–1103.

3 Williams DO *et al.* Percutaneous coronary intervention in the current era compared with 1985–1986: The National Heart, Lung, and Blood Institute Registries. *Circulation* 2000; **102**(24): 2945–2951.

4 Srinivas VS *et al.* Contemporary percutaneous coronary intervention versus balloon angioplasty for multivessel coronary artery disease: a comparison of the National Heart, Lung and Blood Institute Dynamic Registry and the Bypass Angioplasty Revascularization Investigation (BARI) study. *Circulation* 2002; **106**(13): 1627–1633.

5 King SB, 3rd, *et al.* A randomized trial comparing coronary angioplasty with coronary bypass surgery. Emory Angioplasty versus Surgery Trial (EAST). *N Engl J Med* 1994; **331**(16): 1044–1050.

6 Suero JA, MS, Jones PG *et al.* Procedural outcomes and long-term survival among patients undergoing percutaneous coronary intervention of a chronic total occlusion in native coronary arteries: a 20-year experience. *J Am Coll Cardiol* 2001; **38**(2): 409–414.

7 de Feyter PJ *et al.* Percutaneous transluminal angioplasty of a totally occluded venous bypass graft: a challenge that should be resisted. *Am J Cardiol* 1989; **64**(1): 88–90.

8 Kinoshita I *et al.* Coronary angioplasty of chronic total occlusions with bridging collateral vessels: immediate and follow-up outcome from a large single-center experience. *J Am Coll Cardiol* 1995; **26**(2): 409–415.

9 Carlo Di Mario GSW, Sianos G, Alfredo R *et al.* European perspective in recanalisation of chronic total occlusions: consensus document from the EuroCTO-club. *Eurointervention* 2007; **3**(9): 30–43.

10 Safian RD *et al.* Initial success and long-term follow-up of percutaneous transluminal coronary angioplasty in chronic total occlusions versus conventional stenoses. *Am J Cardiol* 1988; **61**(14): 23G–28G.

11 Stone GW *et al.* Percutaneous recanalization of chronically occluded coronary arteries: a consensus document: Part I. *Circulation* 2005. **112**(15): 2364–2372.

12 Colombo A *et al.* Treating chronic total occlusions using subintimal tracking and reentry: the STAR technique. *Catheter Cardiovasc Interv* 2005; **64**(4): 407–411.

13 Surmely JF *et al.* New concept for CTO recanalization using controlled antegrade and retrograde subintimal tracking: the CART technique. *J Invasive Cardiol* 2006; **18**(7): 334–338.

14 Ito S *et al.* Novel technique using intravascular ultrasound-guided guidewire cross in coronary intervention for uncrossable chronic total occlusions. *Circ J* 2004; **68**(11): 1088–1092.

15 Oesterle SN *et al.* Percutaneous *in situ* coronary venous arterialization: Report of the first human catheter-based coronary artery bypass. *Circulation* 2001; **103**(21): 2539–2543.

16 Oesterle SN *et al.* Catheter-based coronary bypass: A development update. *Catheter Cardiovasc Interv* 2003; **58**(2): 212–218.

17 Saket RR, Razavi MK, Padidar A, Kee ST, Sze DY, Dake MD. Novel intravascular ultrasound-guided method to create transintimal arterial communications: Initial experience in peripheral occlusive disease and aortic dissection. *J Endovasc Ther* 2004; **11**(3): 274–280.

18 Saketkhoo RR *et al.* Percutaneous bypass: subintimal recanalization of peripheral occlusive disease with IVUS guided luminal re-entry. *Tech Vasc Interv Radiol* 2004; **7**(1): 23–27.

19 Kickuth R *et al.* Guidance of interventions in subintimal recanalization and fenestration of dissection membranes using a novel dual-lumen intravascular ultrasound catheter. *Rofo* 2006; **178**(9): 898–905.

20 Jacobs DL *et al.* True lumen re-entry devices facilitate subintimal angioplasty and stenting of total chronic occlusions: initial report. *J Vasc Surg* 2006; **43**(6): 1291–1296.

CHAPTER 17

Bilateral Approach

Jean-François Surmely, MD *& Osamu Katoh,* MD

Toyohashi Heart Center, Toyohashi, Japan

Techniques using a retrograde approach for the percutaneous revascularization of coronary chronic total occlusions (CTOs) have increased the rate of successful CTO recanalization. As a general rule, retrograde approach should be used jointly with an antegrade approach. Only in a few cases is the retrograde approach used alone. Techniques via an antegrade approach are explained in details in other chapters of this book. We will therefore focus in this chapter on the description of techniques performed via bilateral approach (combined antegrade and retrograde approach).

A retrograde approach means that the coronary lesion is approached from its distal end through the best collateral channel from any other patent coronary artery. The retrograde approach was first introduced in the late 1980s for the percutaneous treatment of non-occlusive coronary artery disease [1]. Its application for the percutaneous treatment of CTOs was performed in the early 1990s. Since then, increased knowledge and practical experience as well as improved percutaneous coronary interventions (PCI) materials and devices have led to refined strategies in its application. The most common failure reason for percutaneous CTO treatment by an antegrade approach is the inability to successfully pass a guidewire across the lesion into the true lumen of the distal vessel [2].

In order to understand the benefit of techniques using a bilateral approach, it is important to remember that the histopathologic features are different at the proximal and distal fibrous cap. The concentration of collagen-rich fibrous tissue is particularly dense at the proximal CTO part and loose at its distal end, making its penetration easier [3–5]. Besides, the distal fibrous cap is usually tapered. When looked from the proximal side, the distal fibrous cap has therefore a convex shape, which explains the penetration difficulty. On the other hand, when looked from the distal side as during the retrograde approach, it has a concave shape, which prevents the wire sliding in the subintimal space and facilitates successful penetration inside the CTO body. In the following paragraphs, we will focus on the two main aspects of techniques using a retrograde approach, namely the access route and crossing the CTO.

Access route: Reaching the distal end of the CTO with a retrograde wire

The retrograde approach requires a channel between the occluded coronary artery and another patent coronary artery, which enables to reach the distal CTO site retrogradely. The intercoronary channel can be either an epicardial collateral, a septal collateral, or a bypass graft. One study evaluating collaterals by angiography showed that the anatomical course of the principal collateral is

Chronic Total Occlusions, 1st edition. Edited by R. Waksman and S. Saito. © 2009 Blackwell Publishing, ISBN: 978-1-4051-5703-2.

through septal connections in 44%, atrial epicardial connections in 32%, distal interarterial connections in 18%, and bridging connections in 6%. In order to be used as a retrograde channel for a percutaneous CTO intervention, the collateral need to be visualized throughout its course, which is a common finding in CTOs (86%) [6]. We think that septal collaterals are the safer and most appropriate access route. Septal collaterals have either an intra-muscular course or run under the endocardium. Perforation of a septal collateral which is surrounded by myocardium will in most cases stop bleeding after a long balloon inflation or even spontaneously. When the septal collateral is running subendocardially, perforation can creates a communication with the left or the right ventricle. Such a communication will result in a physiologically non significant shunt, and will probably disappear due to the differences of pressure between the ventricles and the septal collateral. Due to the small size of septal collaterals, a pre-dilatation with a small 1.25-mm-size balloon is necessary to allow its delivery up to the distal CTO site. We reported the feasibility and safety of the percutaneous dilatation of coronary septal collaterals to be used as an access for retrograde approach to PCI of CTOs in 21 patients [7]. In this study, successful wire crossing and balloon dilatation of septal collaterals

was achieved in 90% and 81% respectively, and no major complications occurred.

The procedure requires the placement of two guiding catheter: a first guiding catheter is placed in the vessel with the occlusion, and a second guiding catheter in the coronary artery from which the collateral channel arises. Procedure steps are shown in Figure 17.1 and described in the figure legend. We would like to emphasize three points: (1) A super-selective contrast injection via a microcatheter or OTW balloon catheter is mandatory to confirm the channel course as well as its continuous character, (2) the chosen intercoronary channel should be located at least a few millimeters more distally than the distal CTO end; this allows having a co-axial position of the wire tip and the CTO, and (3) specific materials are required because of the increased intra-arterial length the wire and balloon catheter need to do. We recommend either a short 85 cm guiding catheter, or balloons with long shaft (150–155 cm).

Crossing the CTO lesion

Once the retrograde wire reached the distal CTO end, techniques via a bilateral approach (CART technique: controlled antegrade and retrograde subintimal tracking technique; kissing wire

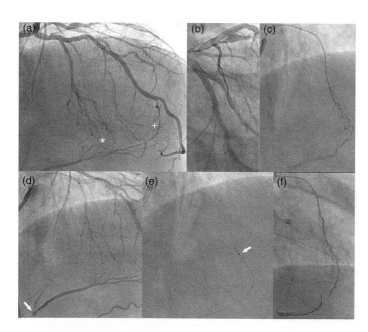

Figure 17.1 Please see opposite page for caption.

technique; knuckle-wire technique) will be used in most cases. In a limited number of cases will techniques via only a retrograde approach (retrograde single-wire technique) be used.

Techniques via a bilateral approach

The safest and most successful technique available is the *CART technique*. This technique combines the simultaneous use of antegrade and retrograde approach. The basic concept of the CART technique is to create a subintimal dissection with limited extension, only at the site of the CTO. We recently published the initial experience of this technique in 10 patients [8]. Successful CTO recanalization was obtained in all cases. No complications such as perforation or occlusion occurred in the collateral channel. In all cases, the subintimal dissection was limited in the CTO region.

As mentioned above, the basic concept of the CART technique is to create a subintimal dissection with limited extension, only at the site of the CTO (Figure 17.2). First a wire is advanced antegradely from the proximal true lumen into the CTO, then into the subintimal space at the CTO site. Next the retrograde wire is advanced from the distal true lumen into the CTO, then into the subintimal space at the CTO site. In order to enable the two wires to meet, a balloon is brought on the retrograde wire and inflated from the subintimal space to the distal end of the CTO. The two subintimal dissections tend to spontaneously expand toward each others and to connect (Figure 17.3). To keep the dissection open, it is important to leave the deflated balloon inside the subintimal space. Then we manipulate the antegrade wire targeting the deflated balloon. Procedure steps are shown and explained in Figures 17.2 and 17.4.

The *bilateral kissing wire technique* combines the simultaneous use of antegrade and retrograde approach. It is a kind of parallel-wire technique. The two wires are in parallel planes and therefore will not necessarily meet. Currently this technique is only used if the CART technique can not be performed due to failure of bringing an OTW balloon catheter through the intercoronary channel.

In the *bilateral knuckle-wire technique*, a loop at the tip of the retrograde wire allows to push it into the CTO or subintimal plane. This results in extensive and uncontrolled dissection inside the CTO or subintimal space, and can sometimes facilitates the antegrade wire passage. However, this technique is linked with an increased risk of complication due to the uncontrolled nature of the dissection, and is therefore no more recommended.

Techniques via a retrograde approach

The *retrograde single-wire technique* uses a retrograde approach with a single wire, without

---

Figure 17.1 Case illustration of the procedure steps for septal collateral dilatation.

Step 1: (a) Meticulous review of the angiography, frame by frame, for the identification of a suitable collateral channel. The septal collateral course is difficult to identify on a non-selective injection of the contralateral patent coronary artery, due to superposition with other collaterals. Two continuous collaterals can be seen. The targeted collateral originates from a septal perforator in the proximal left anterior descending artery (*), a second collateral (+) originates from the distal left anterior descending artery.

Step 2: (b) A hydrophilic floppy wire is advanced in the proximal portion of the septal branch from which originates the most suitable collateral.

Step 3: (c) The microcatheter is advanced until the tip of the wire, and the wire is pulled out. A super-selective contrast injection of the septal collateral is then performed.

Step 4: The hydrophilic floppy wire is then advanced through the septal collateral with the micro-catheter, in order to protect the channel from injury as well as to get a better wire maneuverability.

Step 5: (d) A contra-lateral nonselective injection proves the intra-luminal location of the wire which reached the distal end of the CTO (white arrow).

Step 6: (e) The microcatheter is pulled out, and a small 1.25 mm balloon (white arrow) is then advanced in the septal collateral, where sequential low pressure dilatation (2–3 atm) are performed.

Step 7: (f) A super-selective contrast injection is recorded at the end of the procedure.

(*Source*: Surmely JF, Katoh O, Tsuchikane E, Nasu K, Suzuki T. Coronary septal collaterals as an access for the retrograde approach in the percutaneous treatment of coronary chronic total occlusions. CCI, in press.)

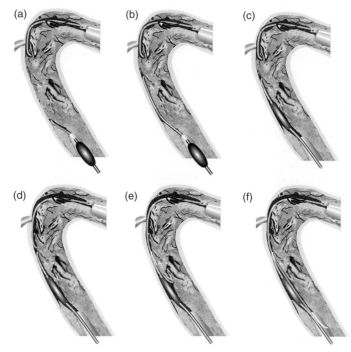

Figure 17.2 Schema of the different steps for the CART technique.

Step 1: (a) Firstly, a wire is advanced antegradely from the proximal true lumen into the CTO, then into the subintimal space at the CTO site.

Step 2: (a) Then a retrograde wire with an over the wire balloon is advanced retrogradely from the distal true lumen into the CTO.

Step 3: (b) The retrograde wire is further advanced into the subintimal space at the CTO site.

Step 4: (c) Balloon dilatation of the subintimal space and also on the course from this subintimal space to the distal end of the CTO.

Step 5: The deflated balloon is left in place.

Step 6: (d and e) The antegrade wire is further advanced in the subintimal space, targeting the deflated balloon.

Step 7: (f) The antegrade wire is advanced through the channel done by the retrograde wire into the distal true lumen.

(*Source:* S Surmely JF, Tsuchikane E, Katoh O *et al.* New concept for CTO recanalization using controlled antegrade and retrograde subintimal tracking: the CART technique. *J Invasive Cardiol* 2006; **18**(7): 334–338. Reprinted with permission from the *Journal of Invasive Cardiology*. Copyright HMP Communications.)

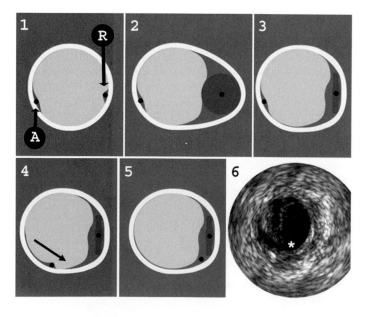

Figure 17.3 Cross-sectional schema illustrating the spontaneous expansion of the subintimal dissections, which tend to get together. With the CART technique, the antegrade wire (A) and retrograde wire (R) lie in the subintimal space, but are not necessarily connecting (panel 1). The subintimal space is expanded via balloon inflation over the retrograde wire. The two subintimal dissections tend to spontaneously expand toward each others and to connect (panel 2). To keep the dissection open, it is important to leave the deflated balloon inside the subintimal space (panel 3). Then we manipulate the antegrade wire targeting the deflated balloon (panel 4, black arrow) until both wires meet (panel 5). A corresponding greyscale IVUS image is shown in panel 6. The connection between both subintimal dissections is shown with an asterisk.

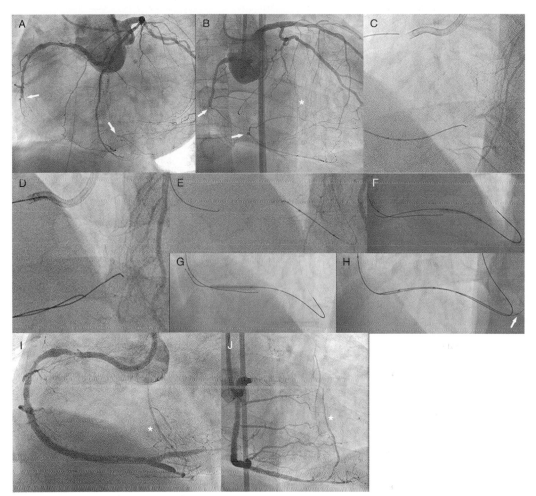

Figure 17.4 Example of a CTO treated by the CART technique where a septal collateral is used as intercoronary channel. Baseline finding obtained by bilateral injection show a long RCA CTO. White arrows show the proximal and distal occlusion end (panel A: LAO view: panel B: RAO view; * indicates the septal collateral used later for the retrograde approach). An antegrade approach was first attempted with a single wire (c) and then with the parallel wire technique (d), but failed puncturing the distal CTO cap. A retrograde wire was advanced through a septal collateral channel up to the distal CTO end (e). Penetration of the CTO end was achieved, and balloon dilatations at the bifurcation of the distal RCA with the PDA, as well as in the distal RCA segment were performed over the retrograde wire (f and g). Thereafter the antegrade wire (white arrow) was advanced targeting the deflated balloon, and could be placed easily in the PDA of the RCA (H). The rest of the procedure was then performed in an antegrade manner with balloon dilatation of the CTO site followed by stent implantation. Final result is shown on panels (I and J). The dilated septal collateral used for the retrograde approach is clearly seen (*) on those final views.

simultaneous antegrade approach. The CTO is crossed only in a retrograde manner. Due to the long access route of the retrograde wire via an intercoronary channel, its maneuverability is poor, and it is difficult to lead it through the CTO lesion, resulting in a low success rate of about 30%. Besides, dissection occurring in the proximal vessel part can compromise important side branch. This technique is nowadays largely abandoned, apart in the case of ostial CTOs, where it still has a role to play.

Conclusion

The shape and characteristics of the distal fibrous cap increases significantly the chances of successful CTO recanalization with techniques using a bilateral approach. Increased knowledge and practical experience as well as improved PCI materials and devices have led to refined strategies in the application of the retrograde approach for the percutaneous treatment of CTOs since its introduction in the early 1990s. Key points for a safe and successful application of a bilateral technique using both antegrade and retrograde approach, have been the use of septal collaterals as an access route to the distal CTO end, and the concept of the CART technique for the CTO recanalization. Techniques using a retrograde approach are advanced techniques and should be attempted in case of the presence of a favorable anatomy, only after unsuccessful recanalization attempt via an antegrade approach.

Reference

1 Kahn JK, Hartzler GO. Retrograde coronary angioplasty of isolated arterial segments through saphenous vein bypass grafts. *Catheter Cardiovasc Diagn* 1990; **20**(2): 88–93.

2 Kinoshita I, Katoh O, Nariyama J *et al.* Coronary angioplasty of chronic total occlusions with bridging collateral vessels: immediate and follow-up outcome from a large single-center experience. *J Am Coll Cardiol* 1995; **26**(2): 409–415.

3 Katsuragawa M, Fujiwara H, Miyamae M, Sasayama S. Histologic studies in percutaneous transluminal coronary angioplasty for chronic total occlusion: comparison of tapering and abrupt types of occlusion and short and long occluded segments. *J Am Coll Cardiol* 1993; **21**(3): 604–611.

4 Srivatsa S, Holmes D, Jr. The Histopathology of Angiographic Chronic Total Coronary Artery Occlusions N Changes in Neovascular Pattern and Intimal Plaque Composition Associated with Progressive Occlusion Duration. *J Invasive Cardiol* 1997; **9**(4): 294–301.

5 Srivatsa SS, Edwards WD, Boos CM *et al.* Histologic correlates of angiographic chronic total coronary artery occlusions: influence of occlusion duration on neovascular channel patterns and intimal plaque composition. *J Am Coll Cardiol* 1997; **29**(5): 955–963.

6 Werner GS, Ferrari M, Heinke S *et al.* Angiographic assessment of collateral connections in comparison with invasively determined collateral function in chronic coronary occlusions. *Circulation* 2003; **107**(15): 1972–1977.

7 Surmely JF, Katoh O, Tsuchikane E, Nasu K, Suzuki T. Coronary septal collaterals as an access for the retrograde approach in the percutaneous treatment of coronary chronic total occlusions. *Catheter Cardiovasc Interv* 2007.

8 Surmely JF, Tsuchikane E, Katoh O *et al.* New concept for CTO recanalization using controlled antegrade and retrograde subintimal tracking: the CART technique. *J Invasive Cardiol* 2006; **18**(7): 334–338.

diligent 勤苦的

fine-tune 使调整好 .

subspecialty

unrevascularized

stenosis = stenoses
restenosis .

aversion 讨厌 反感 .

vibrating penetrating
catheter guidewire system.

CTOs
CTO ~~technology~~ technology

EndNote®
...Bibliographies Made Easy™

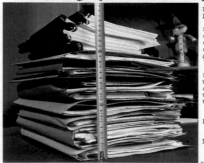

Recent Developments in Personal Bibliographic Software: a Critical Review
By J.W. Bloggs

Since the 1980s, there have been a variety of software products on the market which can be classified under the general heading of Personal Bibliographic Software (see also Budd, 1988). All of these products perform the same two basic functions: they allow the user to maintain a database of bibliographic references and they permit the generation of a bibliography containing some or all of those references (Hall, 1999 p. 11).

Substantial developments have taken place in the functionality of personal bibliographic software. Today it is not difficult to find a product that can automatically import references from a CD-ROM or web database and format both in-text citations and a list of references in a wide variety of styles (Izett, 1987). This has been demonstrated by Barnes (1988).

References

Barnes, C. R. (1988). The proposed Cambrian-Ordovician global boundary stratotype and point (GSSP) in Western Newfoundland, Canada. *Geological Magazine, 125*(4), 381.
Budd, D. A. (1988). Aragonite-to-calcite transformation during fresh-water diagenesis of carbonates - Insights from pore-water chemistry. *Geological Society Of America Bulletin, 100*(8), 1260.

Go from this   *to this!*

Thursday, June 16
3:00 PM – 4:30 PM
Library & LRC (C520K)

- Creating an EndNote library
- Import citations from PubMed
- Using EndNote with Microsoft Word

Register online:
www.texasheart.org/education/library
Look for the ▮REGISTER NOW▮ link.
or contact Sara Ranger
x 54128, sranger@heart.thi.tmc.edu

Presented by: THI Library & LRC

CHAPTER 18

Tips and Tricks of the CART Technique

Osamu Katoh, MD

Toyohashi Heart Center, Toyohashi, Japan

There are a lot of tips and tricks in the retrograde and bilateral approaches to CTOs because those approaches have the long history. In this chapter the tips and tricks only for the CART (controlled antegrade and retrograde subintimal tracking) technique [1,2], which is a novel technique in bilateral approach and the most essential technique among CTO wire techniques to ensure wire crossing in CTOs, are decribed.

Considerations in CART technique

There are some key points to keep in mind for the CART technique. First, it requires very strong guiding catheter backup. Second, there is a need to improve the maneuverability of the retrograde wire. Furthermore, it is required to navigate in a retrograde way through the CTO while avoiding perforation. In addition, it is also required to make a retrograde subintimal dissection. This would appear easy; however, it should be recognized that there are some cases in which this is considerably difficult. The most important point is how to make a connection from the antegrade subintima to the retrograde subintimal dissection. And lastly, after crossing with the antegrade wire, you can use the antegrade balloon in the anchor technique for facilitating antegrade balloon crossing.

Chronic Total Occlusions, 1st edition. Edited by R. Waksman and S. Saito. © 2009 Blackwell Publishing, ISBN: 978-1-4051-5703-2.

Tips and tricks

Backup force from guiding catheter

In the cases performed in the early days of the CART technique a 6 F guiding catheter was often used. However the retrograde balloon could still not pass through septal channel due to insufficient backup even if the 6 F Amplatz was used. We have not used any of 6 F guiding catheters for a retrograde access since these unsuccessful cases.

How to improve the maneuverability of the retrograde wire

After advancing the balloon into the recipient artery, the balloon is inflated inside that recipient artery. In other words, this is fixing the balloon in the vessel (anchor technique). The reasons for poor maneuverability of the retrograde wire are the long retrograde access route, multiple curves plus the beating of the heart. In order to reduce these difficulties, the balloon catheter is anchored to the vessel wall and this works very well in improving wire maneuverability. An over-the-wire (OTW) balloon is usually advanced and inflated to about 8 atm for better wire maneuverability. There is always a junction point along the septal channel of the access route with an acute bend on the side of the RCA (right coronary artery). Furthermore, when accessing the RCA retrogradely through the LAD (left anterior descending artery), it is necessary to cross the RCA bifurcation which has a bend of 90°. Even before the bifurcation, there are many cases with bends of 90° or sharper at the point where the septal branch joins the PD (posterior

descending) branch. So, since there are two 90°
bends here, it is very important in an emergency
that the balloon shaft covers these junction points
in order to stretch out this access route as much
as possible.

Next is wire manipulation within a CTO. Here
it is often helpful to ensure good wire manipulation by first advancing the retrograde balloon
into the CTO as far as possible. There are a cases
where it is very difficult to deliver a retrograde
balloon into the CTO body. This is almost always
due to the friction between the balloon and the
vessel wall. One way to overcome this difficulty
in balloon delivery is to exchange the balloon for
a new balloon, in this case, a monorail balloon.
Then, since a polymer wire was used to cross the
septal channel, there is insufficient support and it
is exchanged for a support wire. It is possible to
exchange wires using Tornus. Also, backup can
be improved by inserting the wire as far as possible. In the case of RCA access, by advancing the
wire towards PL (postero-lateral) branch and not
proximally, you can advance the wire deeply which
will improve backup.

Anchor technique

Figure 18.1 shows an example where utilizing the
anchor technique with a retrograde balloon was
effective in improving wire maneuverability. There
is a bifurcation at the distal end of the occlusion.
As you can see on the right, the retrograde wire
was severely bent by the beating of the heart

during its manipulation. As in this case, the beating
of the heart strongly affects wire manipulation. In
order to overcome this situation, we advanced the
balloon as close to the CTO as possible and dilated
the balloon at that position. By doing so, good
backup was obtained from the balloon catheter and
we successfully broke into the CTO body. A Miracle
12 g was eventually used in this case as a retrograde
wire, but it would not have been successful without
this kind of backup from the catheter.

Wire maneuverability within a CTO

Figure 18.2 indicates the effectiveness of advancing a retrograde balloon into the CTO body as
deeply as possible. In this case, a retrograde balloon
was advanced and reached the point as seen in the
left figure. However, since the maneuverability of
the retrograde wire still deteriorated with this balloon position, the balloon was advanced into the
CTO body little by little, and got to the position as
seen in the right most figure. The maneuverability
of the retrograde wire was finally improved with
this balloon position. In short, it is very important
to get strong backup from the balloon catheter.

As a strategy for improving wire maneuverability, not only do you need to forcefully advance
the balloon into the CTO, but also inflate the balloon inside the CTO. In Figure 18.3, the maneuverability of the retrograde wire deteriorates
from bends as indicated by this arrow in the right
figure, but retrograde wire maneuverability can be
improved by balloon inflation.

Retrograde wire navigation through CTOs

The first thing to be emphasized is not to use a stiff
wire as a first choice of a retrogarde wire because
Miracle 3 g wire can work for retrogradely entering
into CTOs and for the navigation through CTOs
in most of the cases. Poor maneuverability of the
wire indicates that it is difficult to get the feeling
from the wire tip and to confirm if any perforation has been created or not. Since it is also true
that there are some cases in which a floppy wire
successfully gets into the CTO body. Instead of a
stiffer wire or a tapered wire, it is recommended
to deliver an over-the-wire balloon system close to
the distal end of CTO in order to get a backup for a
guidewire.

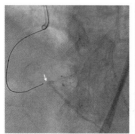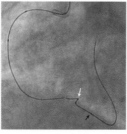

Figure 18.1 If CTO distal end is located at bifurcation and
has no stump like this case (arrow on the left), it is usually
difficult to get into CTO with retrograde wire. For those
cases strong backup from balloon catheter is imperative
to control the retrograde wire. The white arrow on
the right indicates the bend made by heart beating on
the retrograde wire and the black arrow indicates the
retrograde balloon.

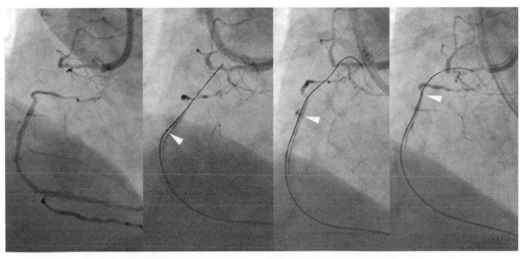

Figure 18.2 In case of the curved CTO located in proximal RCA, the maneuverability of retrograde wire is always deteriorated. In this case, the maneuverability was improved by insertion of retrograde balloon into CTO body. The white arrow indicates the retrograde balloon maker.

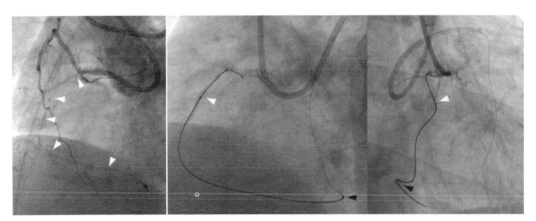

Figure 18.3 The maneuverability of retrograde wire was poor because of acute bend and diffuse disease in distal true lumen (white arrow on the left). In this case deep insertion of retrograde balloon (white arrow) into CTO and the balloon inflation improved wire maneuverability in spite of the acute angle (black arrow).

Making a retrograde dissection
Considerations

There are some points to keep in mind when you make a retrograde subintimal dissection in the CTO body. First, in regards with how to check if a retrograde wire gets into the subintima, it is important to use a relatively soft wire like the Miracle 3 g. You are able to confirm if the retrograde wire gets into the subintima from the motion of the wire or resistance from the wire tip in most of the cases. In addition, a 2 mm balloon or larger, usually a 2.5 mm balloon should be used in order to make an adequate subintimal space. In some occasions, a bigger balloon such as 3.5 mm is necessary. However, the vessel wall sometimes becomes thin after the retrograde balloon inflation in the subintimal space, therefore it should be taken into consideration that a perforation can be easily made by a tapered or stiff antegrade wire in that situation.

Using a bigger retrograde balloon

The upper left in Figure 18.4 is after inflation with a 1.5 mm retrograde balloon, but the antegrade

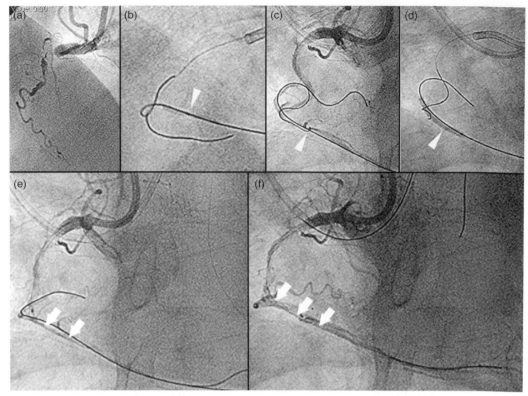

Figure 18.4 (a) Pre-stenting. (b) The dilation of 1.5 mm retrograde balloon (white arrow). (c) The antegrade wire (white arrow) is not in the retrograde dissected lumen. (d) The dilation of 2.5 mm retrograde balloon (white arrow). (e) The 2.5 mm balloon expanded the dissected lumen (white arrow). (f) The antegrade wire got into the retrograde dissected lumen (white arrow).

wire could not penetrate into the space created by the retrograde balloon. So then, we used a bigger, 2.5 mm retrograde balloon as seen on the right in order to expand the subintimal space more, and the antegrade wire was able to penetrate into the subintimal space as seen on the lower left. In the figure, on the lower right after crossing with the antegrade wire, the dissection lumen created by the retrograde balloon can be seen and the antegrade wire is running to the outside of the dissection lumen. However, since antegrade and retrograde subintimal spaces were connected, the antegrade wire successfully crossed.

For RCAs with diameters as large as this shown in Figure 18.5, a 2.5 mm retrograde balloon is too small, so a 3.5 mm balloon was used as shown on Figure 18.5b and we were eventually able to create a subintimal space connection. In this case, after inflation of a 3.5 mm balloon, the wire was advanced towards the balloon markers and successfully crossed.

Making a connection between the antegrade and the retrograde dissection

As one may expect, the Miracle 3 g wire should be the first choice for the antegrade wire. Although, there are cases in which it is necessary to perforate into the retrograde subintimal space using an antegrade wire. The Confianza Pro is useful for this. In this case, we can advance the wire towards the deployed retrograde balloon. In principle, one should use as soft a wire as possible. Regarding how to confirm whether the antegrade wire has made it to the retrograde subintimal space, one method is to inflate the retrograde balloon. By doing so, you can confirm the space between

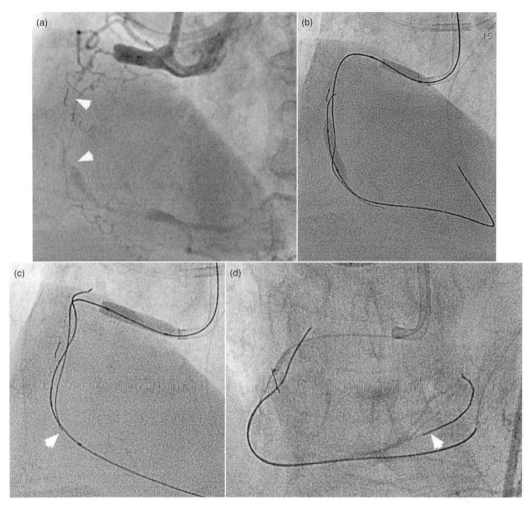

Figure 18.5 (a) Pre-stenting (white arrow). (b) The 3.5 mm retrograde balloon. (c and d) The antegrade wire gets the dissected lumen made by the 3.5 mm balloon (white arrow).

the retrograde balloon and the antegrade wire. Angiographically, if you see a shadow between them, the wire is not in the subintimal space. Rotational angiography is useful in such a situation. The next method is to pull the deflated retrograde balloon little by little while pushing the antegrade wire. Also, there are some cases where the antegrade wire does not cross unless a tapered wire such as Confianza Pro is made to penetrate. In such a case, even after successfully entering the retrograde subintimal space, the tapered wire may easily slip into another false lumen distally. In that case, it is usually effective to insert a Tornus to the retrograde subintimal space and exchange the tapered wire for a polymer wire. This facilitates

wire crossing into the distal true lumen. For a difficult case to make a connection of subintimal spaces, it is another way to change the position of the retrograde balloon. An optimal balloon position is at the bend point. It is advantageous to advance an antegrade wire like puncturing a deflated balloon in an acute angle and this often leads to the result that the wire tip hits the balloon wing and slides into the retrograde subintimal space automatically. Furthermore, using a bigger retrograde balloon to make a bigger subintimal space may enhance the chances of making a successful connection. As the final method, it is useful to inflate the retrograde balloon to less than 1 atm and aiming for the balloon with a tapered wire like the Confianza Pro to puncture the balloon. This is a technique to make the penetration target larger. And as a special technique, one can also make a connection between the subintimal spaces by simultaneously inflating the antegrade and retrograde balloons for a kissing inflation at the same location.

Antegrade wire

With regards to the question of which wire is the best antegrade wire, the answer is that the Miracle 3 g is the best wire when looking for a retrogarde subintimal space. However, it is sometimes

necessary to break open a fibrous or calcified layer in order to make a connection. In that case, do not hesitate to use a stiff wire because the balloon markers are easily visible on fluoroscopy. It is necessary to be careful because the subintima may be easily perforated after expanding it with the retrograde balloon, but this method is still highly recommended to experienced physicians.

How to check if antegrade wire gets into retrograde subintima/distal true lumen

Figure 18.6 shows a representative example in which the antegrade wire successfully crossed by

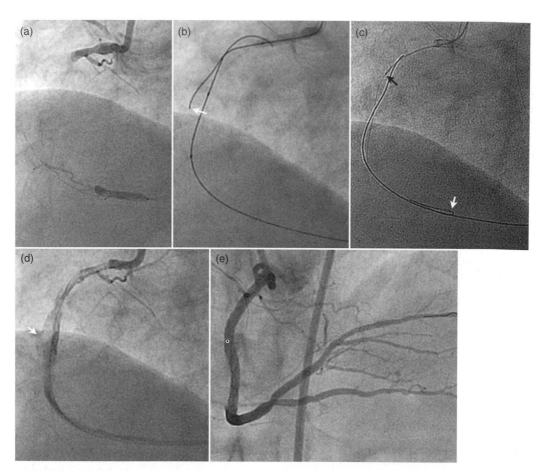

Figure 18.6 (a) Even if the antegrade wire seems to be separated from the deflated retrograde balloon (b – white arrow indicates the tip of antegrade wire (Miracle 12G)), the antegrade subintimal dissection can be connected to the retrograde subintimal dissection like this case. However, you should exchange the stiff wire for floppy wire (polymer wire is often used, c – white arrow indicates the knuckle antegrade wire). For the exchange Tornus is most useful under this kind of situation. The black arrow indicates the tip of Tornus. (d) The connection site with deep dissection, probably subintimal dissection, is seen (white arrow). (e) Post-stenting.

making a connection between the subintimal dissections. It is necessary to check if the antegrade wire tip enters into the retrograde subintimal dissection while advancing the antegrade wire. Otherwise, it may create an antegrade spiral dissection up to the distal site. In this case, by using a Miracle 12 g, it was advanced to the point as shown in Figure 18.6b. This portion has already been expanded by the retrograde balloon, but the wire tip seems to be greatly separated from the balloon. As explained in the chapter regarding the principles of the CART technique, an antegrade wire would cross easily if the both subintimal dissections are connected. This case is a representative example of that. The antegrade wire seemed to be separated

largely from the balloon, nevertheless the Tornus was advanced up to the wire tip and the Miracle 12 g was exchanged for a polymer wire, and though the polymer wire tip was knuckled, the antegrade wire tip crossed easily to the distal true lumen as shown on Figure 18.6c. This phenomenon would not have be seen if a Miracle 12 g had been continuously used, but it can occur only when it is exchanged for a floppy wire. In Figure 18.6d, the deep dissection is seen along with the connection site after recanalization by balloon. If a connection is successfully made like in this case, you can advance the floppy wire to the distal true lumen and it should be avoided to use a stiff wire. Of course, the dissection must be treated

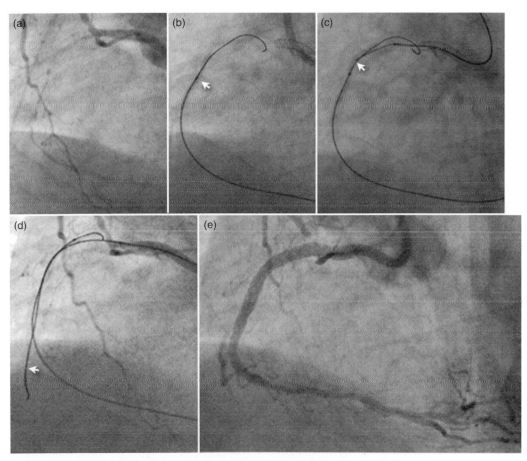

Figure 18.7 (a) A curved CTO is seen in the proximal RCA. In the curved CTO the retrograde balloon inflation does not facilitate antegrade wire crossing. (b) By changing deflated balloon position to the bent site, the antegrade wire easily passed along the deflated balloon (white arrow). (c) The white arrow indicates the tip of antegrade wire. (d) Antegrade wire crossing (white arrow). (e) Post-stenting.

and a Cypher stent may be deployed for these occasions. Some physicians may be concerned about aneurysm formation in these situations, but it is still unknown.

Changing the position of the deflated retrograde balloon

In Figure 18.7 case a diffuse lesion up to the distal part and a curve in the CTO body with calcification are seen (Figure 18.7a). With the first retrograde balloon position in Figure 18.7b, the antegrade wire was not able to get into the retrograde dissected lumen. Therefore by changing the balloon position to the more proximal side to cover the bent site, the balloon was inflated and then deflated and left in position (Figure 18.7c). The balloon wing covered the bent site. By advancing the antegrade wire tip as if to touch the balloon wing, the antegrade wire easily slips into the retrograde dissected lumen (Figure 18.7d). This method becomes very effective with this type of case. It is effective to change the balloon position when the wire does not enter into the retrograde subintima in a straight segment.

Anchor technique for an antegrade balloon crossing

The anchor technique as a by-product of the CART technique is useful when backup of a guiding catheter is not sufficient at the time of advancing the antegrade balloon. By inflating the retrograde balloon at the position to catch the antegrade wire, you can get the sufficient back up for balloon crossing. It is so called an anchor technique. After the antegrade wire crossing, you can use this technique if you leave the retrograde balloon.

References

1 Surmely JF, Tsuchikane E, Katoh O *et al*. New concept for CTO recanalization using controlled antegrade and retrograde subintimal tracking: the CART technique. *J Invasive Cardiol* 2006; **18**: 334–338.

2 Surmely JF, Katoh O, Tsuchikane E, Nasu K, Suzuki T. Coronary septal collaterals as an access for the retrograde approach in the percutaneous treatment of coronary chronic total occlusions. *Catheter Cardiovasc Interv* 2007.

V PART V
Devices Technology

CHAPTER 19

Radio Frequency

Richard Heuser, MD, FACC, FACP, FESC

St. Luke's Medical Center, University of Arizona College of Medicine, Phoenix, Arizona, USA

Introduction

Chronic total occlusion (CTO) of peripheral arteries can cause claudication or even critical limb ischemia [1]. Occlusions are at least three times more common in the femoropopliteal arteries. For the patient with critical limb ischemia, multilevel disease with occlusion of some or all of the infrapopliteal arteries is typical. Patients with long infrainguinal occlusions generally tend to have coronary disease and bypass grafting in this population is often associated with a considerable procedure-related morbidity and mortality. Surgical intervention is usually reserved for patients with critical limb ischemia and consequently, many patients with long, chronic superficial femoral artery (SFA) occlusions remain untreated with a significant limitation in their lifestyle.

While treatment of short CTO lesions of the iliac and femoropopliteal vessels with endovascular techniques has become the standard approach, longer complex lesions intervention can be extremely challenging. Iliac and femoropopliteal CTOs traditionally had high failure rate ranging 5–35% [2,3] and 15–25% [4] respectively. Fortunately, technical skills and devices needed to successfully cross and treat the occlusion continue to improve significantly. Nowadays, an initial

endovascular approach can achieve limb salvage rates equivalent to surgical bypass [4,5].

Pathology of total occlusion

CTOs consist of various degrees of fibroatheromatous plaque and thrombus depending on the mechanism of occlusion and its duration. A tough fibrous cap is often present at the proximal and distal margins of the CTO, with softer material in between. When the fibrous occlusion is long, densely organized and homogenous, guidewire passage is very difficult and subintimal approach in this type of lesion is likely to be more successful.

Patient selection

Revascularization procedures are indicated for patients with disabling claudication, who have failed medical therapy, ischemic rest pain, or impending limb loss. At the present time, for infrainguinal occlusions, the patency rates for long, complex disease are lower than the patency rates for open bypass [6]. The rapid advances in interventional devices have inspired interest in tackling these long occlusions with an endovascular approach with the option of open surgery still remaining if the intervention fails. Recently published guidelines state that the effectiveness of the use of stents, atherectomy, cutting balloons, thermal devices, and lasers for the treatment of infrainguinal lesions (other than to salvage a suboptimal result from balloon dilation) is not well established, and primary stent

Chronic Total Occlusions, 1st edition. Edited by R. Waksman and S. Saito. © 2009 Blackwell Publishing, ISBN: 978-1-4051-5703-2.

placement is not recommended in these arteries. In these guidelines, stent implantation is categorized under one broad definition and includes self-expandable, balloon-expandable, spiral-shaped, and covered stents [7].

Lesion assessment

Initial imaging of patients with iliac and femoral occlusions can be done with computed tomography angiography (CTA) or magnetic resonance angiography (MRA). This allows for excellent definition of the aortic, iliac, and femoral occlusions and the status of the femoral artery for access in case of iliac occlusions and helps in deciding on an antegrade vs. retrograde contralateral femoral access for infrainguinal lesions. A limitation to percutaneous treatment is occlusive disease of the common femoral artery at the site of access. In this situation, open femoral access can be used when treating iliac or femoral-popliteal disease with endovascular techniques.

Angiographically, lesions should first be assessed with appropriate angiographic views, for example, 35° ipsilateral lateral angiogram. Most long SFA occlusions begin with a proximal stump followed by distal vessel reconstitution by collaterals from the profunda femorus artery. Special attention must be paid to the length of the proximal stump and the location of the distal reconstitution as it clearly influences device selection. A flush occlusion at the SFA origin or an extension of an occlusion to the popliteal trifurcation is not suitable for endovascular treatment, especially with antegrade approach [8]. Diffuse, irregular, eccentric, calcified occlusions are much more difficult to recanalize and have less long-term success [9]. Lesion length is an important factor when determining long-term success though it probably plays lesser role in deciding between endovascular and surgical approach.

Crossing total occlusions

Femoral-popliteal CTOs are effectively treated with contralateral techniques, whereas iliac lesions are often best approached via ipsilateral retrograde femoral access. In order to provide the support needed to cross long infrainguinal lesions, a long 6 or 7 F sheath like Ansel or Raabe (Cook Inc.,

Bloomington, IN) is placed over the iliac bifurcation with the tip into the superficial femoral artery. Once the access is obtained, the patient is anticoagulated with either heparin or bivalirudin. Conversely, some operators do not anticoagulate until the CTO is traversed. We often use a combination of a hydrophilic guidewire such as a 0.035-inch Glidewire (Terumo, Somerset, NJ), and a support catheter such as the 4–5 F angled Glidecath as initial approach for crossing a CTO. The procedure from this point on requires roadmap imaging to visualize the distal vessel as angiographic imaging through the support catheter is largely unhelpful. It is important that the hydrophilic guidewire enters the occlusion with the tip straight without any spiraling as this allows for the proper tip engagement into the lesion. At this point one can either attempt crossing intraluminally or looping the wire purposely to enter subintimal space. Despite the counterintuitive nature of starting a subintimal plane intentionally, the technique is relatively simple and usually more successful (70–90% of cases) than intentional true lumen passage for long-segment CTOs [10].

Some interventionalists prefer retrograde approach over antegrade puncture for infrainguinal angioplasty. In a randomized study of 100 consecutive patients, retrograde puncture was found to be technically easier with a tendency to fewer complications like hematoma, but resulted in a higher radiation dose [11].

Subintimal angioplasty

Once the wire enters the occlusion, it often loops back on itself for several centimeters with the 180° turn. One should try to maintain the width of the distal wire loop to remain smaller than or equal to the width of the native vessel as widening of the loop tip signifies more subintimal vessel dissection. This can limit successful re-entry of wire into the distal vessel true lumen. To avoid widening of the wire loop, one can push the support catheter to catch up over the proximal unlooped part of the Glidewire and then pull the wire back into the catheter to straighten the tip. After straightening the wire, it is re-advanced with a small width loop as described previously [12]. If the support catheter is gets trapped in the subintimal space and does not follow the glide wire, a smaller diameter 0.035-inch compatible catheter, such as the Quickcross catheter (Spectranetics Corporation, Colorado Springs, CO) may be used. Finally, the wire is re-entered into the distal true lumen under direct visualization. The support catheter is then advanced into the distal segment, beyond the occlusion, and confirmation of true lumen is done with contrast injection through this catheter. If there is difficulty in reentering the true lumen, re-entry devices like the Outback catheter or Pioneer catheter are used as described below. Alternatively, lower-profile 0.014-inch torqueable stiff wires (e.g., Confianza Wire, Abbott Vascular, Redwood City, CA), with or without over-the-wire angioplasty balloon or coronary support catheters can sometimes be used successfully to achieve true lumen entry. It is preferable to try re-entry devices over vigorous attempts to re-enter the lumen with wire alone as this may lead to worsening of subintimal dissection and progression of dissection plane below the knee compromising distal collaterals.

Primary patency rates of subintimal angioplasty range from 60% to 80% at 6 months and 60% to 70% at 12 months [13]. In critical limb ischemia, limb salvage is achieved in approximately 80% to 90% of patients. Secondary interventions are usually quick and simple and approach does not interrupt subsequent bypass options.

Re-entry devices

The key factor to subintimal success is having a relatively healthy, noncalcified target for re-entry in the distal vessel. Lesions with dense calcification, diffuse disease of the distal target, and small-caliber lumens often prove difficult to gain successful reentry. In addition, in some cases re-entry is not achieved until subintimal passage to a site significantly remote from the level of patent vessel lumen. This causes subintimal angioplasty or stenting of unintended target beyond the diseased segment and may jeopardize important collaterals. In these cases, re-entry tools such as the Pioneer catheter (Medtronic Vascular) or the Outback (Cordis Corporation, a Johnson & Johnson Company, Miami, FL) can be used [14]. It is important to remember that a large enough sheath (7–8 Fr) is necessary for these devices.

Pioneer catheter

The Pioneer catheter is a 7 F phased-array 20 MHz intravascular ultrasound (IVUS) catheter and is connected to a Volcano (Volcano Corporation, Rancho Cordova, CA) IVUS console. The catheter has two monorail 0.014-inch compatible wire ports, one with a curved retractable nitinol 24G needle distally. The catheter is gently maneuvered under ultrasound guidance until the tip of the nitinol needle is oriented toward the true lumen and is lined up at the 12 o'clock position on the ultrasound image. The needle tip is then carefully advanced and deployed. A floppy tip extra-support 0.014-inch guidewire is then passed through the needle into the distal vessel and is confirmed with angiography. The needle is then retracted, and the Pioneer catheter is removed, leaving the wire behind with distal end in the true lumen. At this point secondary interventions are performed with standard techniques (Figure 19.1).

Outback catheter

The Outback catheter (Lumend Inc.) is a 5 F multipurpose-type catheter with 22-gauge nitinol cannula that can be advanced or retracted from the end of the catheter to penetrate from the dissection plane to the true lumen. With the help of two orthogonal fluoroscopic views, the angle of the catheter is adjusted to point the end toward the true lumen. The proprietary locate, tune, and deploy technique is used to deploy needle through the intima to the true lumen. A 0.014-inch wire is then advanced into the true lumen and Outback catheter is then removed. Secondary interventions are then performed either on this wire or after exchanging it with a 0.35-inch wire system (Figure 19.2).

Angioplasty and stenting

Common iliac artery occlusions are routinely stented with balloon-expandable stents because of their high radial force and precise placement. When both sides are occluded, the kissing technique is essential with balloon expandable stents. In the external iliac, one can use either the balloon-expandable or self-expanding stents depending upon the lesion characteristics and location. Femoral or popliteal occlusions are treated with primary angioplasty with long balloons at nominal

(a)

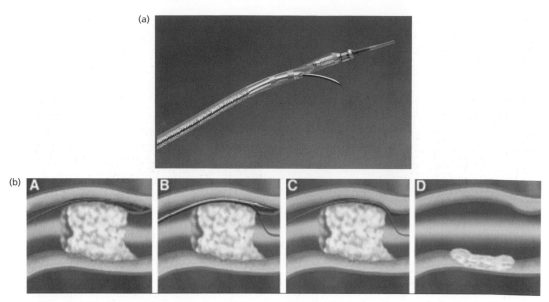

(b)

Figure 19.1 (a) Pioneer catheter with integrated 20 MHz phase array transducer and 24 G nitinol curved needle. (b) The Pioneer facilitating the true lumen re-entry. (A) Wire trapped in a sub-intimal location. (B) Pioneer catheter is advanced to the target segment, where the needle is deployed under ultrasound guidance. (C) The guidewire is then passed through the needle into true distal lumen and the Pioneer is removed. (D) The lesion is treated successfully with an angioplasty device advanced over the wire.

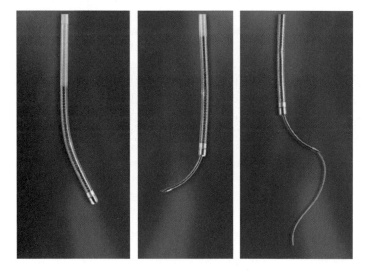

Figure 19.2 Outback catheter from Lumend Inc.

or greater pressures and longer inflations up to 2–3 min. If there is presence of a flow-limiting dissection, then self-expanding bare nitinol stents should be deployed. Some interventionalists have also used laser, thermal or atherectomy devices in this setting to treat residual lesions after angioplasty (Figure 19.3).

Complications

The major complication related to the treatment of chronic total occlusion is vessel rupture secondary to catheter manipulation or angioplasty. Long or calcified lesions are often more prone to such complication. The true lumen re-entry devices itself may not result in perforation related to the

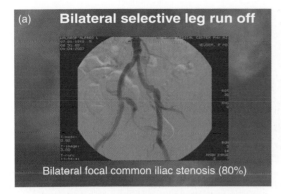

(a) **Bilateral selective leg run off**

Bilateral focal common iliac stenosis (80%)

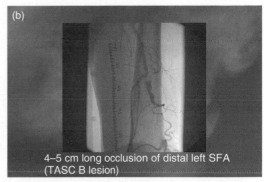

(b)

4–5 cm long occlusion of distal left SFA
(TASC B lesion)

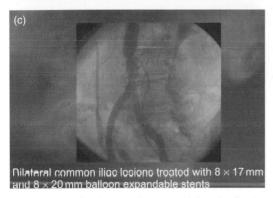

(c)

Bilateral common iliac lesions treated with 8 × 17 mm
and 8 × 20 mm balloon expandable stents

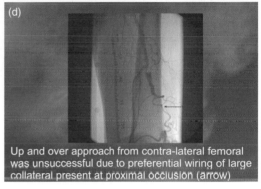

(d)

Up and over approach from contra-lateral femoral
was unsuccessful due to preferential wiring of large
collateral present at proximal occlusion (arrow)

Figure 19.3 Popliteal approach. 66 M with h/o claudication walking 2–3 blocks. Can't play tennis any more. Risk factors: HTN, dyslipidemia, obesity, 40-pack years smoking. Meds: Lotrel, Lipitor, ASA. Exam: BP 120/85, HR 96, RR 16, wt 197 lb. CVS: s1, s2 normal, no murmur. Ext Pulses 1+, no edema. Right ABI 0.88, Left ABI 0.82. (a) Angio reveals bilateral common iliac artery stenosis. (b) The left SFA was an occlusion. (c) Angio after iliac stenting. (d) Contralateral approach to recanalize the SFA was unsuccessful.

needle deployments, but these devices are often used in complex difficult to cross lesions that have increased risk of rupture with angioplasty. It is imperative that covered stents be available in the cath lab at the time of CTO intervention. The other important complication of intervening total occlusions is thromboembolism that can occur in of 1–4% of cases. Adequate anticoagulation is therefore necessary during the procedure.

CTO devices

Because of often complex and long occlusions, more than 80% of patients usually need a more specialized crossing technique over standard technique. Recently, several devices have entered the market that may enable treatment of these difficult lesions. These devices cross the calcified plaque using different physical principles, such as blunt microdissection, optical coherence reflectometry, or laser. Some of the devices like magnum wires, rotational atherectomy, Kensey catheter, and Rotacs are already of historical significance only and will not be described any further in this chapter.

Excimer laser

The photoablative effect of excimer laser can be used to recanalize total occlusions by debulking atherosclerotic and thrombotic material. In addition, it can facilitate subsequent balloon dilation at lower pressure to prevent dissection and reduce the risk of thromboembolic events. An excimer laser produces photons of ultraviolet light at a unique wavelength of 308 nm that is readily absorbed in human tissues, including atherosclerotic material and clot (Figure 19.4).

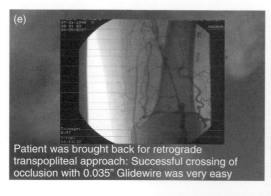

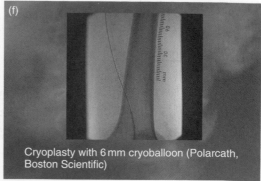

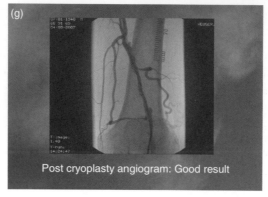

Figure 19.3 (e) The popliteal approach was successful. (f) Cryoplasty treatment was delivered. (g) The post cryoplasty angiogram revealed a good result. Patient had no recurrence of claudication for 2 years and his ABI's are now over 1.0.

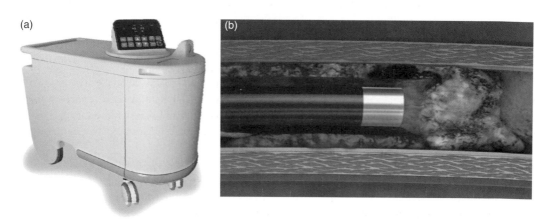

Figure 19.4 (a) The Spectranetics CVX-300® Excimer Laser System and (b) TURBO elite laser ablation catheter (FDA approved October 2006).

The activated laser catheter must be advanced very slowly, not exceeding 1 mm/s. Fluoroscopic road mapping is used throughout to verify alignment of guidewires and catheters to the vessel lumen. Improvements in saline-infusion techniques with lasers have resulted in lower incidence of dissection. Thorough flushing the vessel with saline effectively facilitates transmission of the laser light to the atherosclerotic tissue. In addition, effective removal of contrast medium prevents

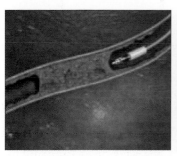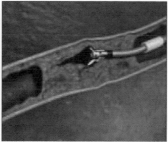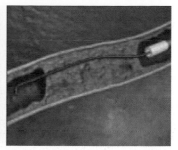

Figure 19.5 Schematic of blunt microdissection with Frontrunner device.

formation of shock waves that can result in dissections of the vessel wall. There also appears to be direct platelet aggregation inhibition with the use of excimer lasers, making it an attractive tool for treating chronic thrombotic lesions [15].

The mid-term outcomes of patients with long chronic iliac artery occlusions after excimer-laser-assisted interventional recanalization were recently reported in 43 patients after 4-year follow-up. The primary technical success rate was 95.3%, with a major complication rate of 6.9% and clinical improvement in 97.6% of cases. The overall primary and secondary patency rate as determined by ankle brachial index and duplex ultrasound was 86.1% and 95.4% respectively [16]. This is similar to the patency rates of short stenoses. In a study of laser-assisted recanalization of chronic SFA (superficial femoral artery) occlusions in 318 consecutive patients over 1 year, the primary and secondary patency rate was 83.2% and 90.5% respectively [17]. There are data supporting use of laser in tibioperoneal region as well. In the LACI (laser angioplasty in chronic ischemia) prospective, multicenter, clinical registry patients with poor surgical risk with critical limb ischemia were treated with excimer laser in the SFA, popliteal, and/or infrapopliteal arteries with adjunctive PTA (percutaneous transluminal angioplasty), and optional stenting. Patency with distal flow to the foot was achieved in 89% of patients and the rate of limb salvage was 93% at 6 months [18].

Blunt microdissection

New catheter technology has recently been developed to recanalize CTOs through a process of blunt microdissection. The Frontrunner X39 CTO Catheter (LuMend, Inc., Redwood City, CA) is a single-use catheter consists of an articulating, distal tip assembly. This tip features a crossing profile of 0.039 inch with actuating jaws that open to 2.3 mm and is remotely actuated by a manual rocker handle to facilitate blunt microdissection of the plaque (Figure 19.5). The Frontrunner catheter is commonly used in combination with the 4.5 F Frontrunner Micro Guide Catheter that provides additional support and acts as a conduit for a more rapid wire exchange once the frontrunner crosses the CTO. The microdissection can be performed in various planes to separate tissue in the target vessel segment.

Though originally designed for coronary intervention, the Frontrunner CTO Catheter has now been used extensively to facilitate guidewire placement across peripheral CTOs. In a prospective study of 36 patients with 44 symptomatic CTOs (2 terminal aortic, 24 iliac, 16 femoral, and 2 popliteal), blunt microdissection was carried out with this type of catheter. Procedural success, evaluated angiographically, was achieved in 91% with no complications related to blunt microdissection itself [19].

Vibration angioplasty

Vibrational angioplasty is based on the concept of using high-frequency, mechanical vibrational energy to help recanalize chronic total occlusions. The CROSSER system consists of a generator, a transducer and the single use CROSSER Catheter [6]. The generator converts AC power into high-frequency current. This high-frequency current is then converted into vibrational energy by piezoelectric crystals contained within the transducer. The Crosser catheter is a nitinol core standard 0.014 inch and 0.018-inch guidewires monorail catheter system with a stainless steel tip. Mechanical vibrations are transmitted to this stainless steel tip at approximately 20 kHz or 20,000 cycles per second. This vibrational energy provides mechanical impact at a stroke depth of approximately 20 μm and pulverizes the solid CTO tissue. In addition, high-frequency vibration creates vapor filled microbubbles in the blood. These microbubbles expand and implode producing liquid jets that can break the molecular bonds and cause erosion of the CTO tissue helping recanalization of an occluded artery.

This system has already been used safely and effectively in coronary artery total occlusions [20–22]. Recently, the PATRIOT (Peripheral Approach To Recanalization In Occluded Totals) data on 40 patients was presented in TCT 2006 meeting.

The average CTO length was 10.6 cm with half of the attempted occlusions in the SFA and the remainder in the popliteal artery or below. CROSSER activation time averaged 2.5 min. Procedure time (PT) and fluoroscopy time were 2 hours and 39 min respectively. There were no procedural complications and no clinical perforations. Technical success (successful passage of a guidewire into the true distal lumen) was achieved in 78% of the occlusions attempted. Improvement in ABI (arterial brachial index) (>0.10) was achieved in 85% of patients with successful recanalization.

Optic coherence reflectometry with radio frequency ablation

All the new technologies described above are unable to see the true lumen of the vessel. Optical Coherent Reflectometry with radio frequency ablative energy (Safe-Cross wire, Intraluminal Therapeutics, CA) is a forward-looking system that has been utilized to treat CTO [23]. Using near-infrared light, this guidewire system can distinguish calcified from noncalcified plaque and atherosclerotic lesions from arterial wall and display the signals on a monitor in real time. Green bar indicates lumen and radio frequency ablative energy is enabled. Red bar means wire is against the vessel wall and RF energy is disabled (Figure 19.6 also see the Color Plate section).

There are some technical limitations with the current system. The wire tip cannot be manually shaped or bent without risking the fracture of optical fibers inside the wire. The wire itself is not easily steerable though this problem has been significantly improved in the latest generation of Safe-Cross wire.

The GRIP registry study is one of the first peripheral-device studies to focus on total occlusion recanalization with Safe-Cross system [24]. The device success rate, defined, as the achievement of distal lumen position, was 76%, For the 56 lesions that were recanalized, the mean preprocedural ABI was 0.59; the mean postprocedural ABI was 0.86. In another study, Dippel and others demonstrated a 72.7% success rate in recanalizing CTO in the peripheral vasculature following failure of conventional techniques.

Thrombolytic therapy

While thrombolytic therapy is still the treatment of choice in acute and subacute arterial occlusions and graft thrombosis, there are a few reports regarding thrombolytic therapy in chronic arterial occlusions [25–27] (Figure 19.7). In a series reported by Motarjeme, 276 arterial occlusions (lesion length 3–66 cm) were treated in 268 patients with thrombolytic therapy. Though the duration of the occlusion based on angiography was undetermined in majority of patients, seventeen patients had arterial occlusions older than 2 years and half the patients had intermittent claudication from 8 months to 10 years. Surprisingly, 80% of CTOs including iliac and infrainguinal occlusions responded favorably to thrombolysis.

Most arterial occlusions (more than a few centimeters in length) are associated with some degree of arterial thrombosis, and thus may be amenable to thrombolysis. Advances in the availability of smaller catheters (3 F and 4 F) and development of an open-end injectable guidewire have increased the rate of success due to both a better delivery system and fewer complications. In the absence of bleeding complications, lytic therapy can be continued as low-dose prolonged infusion until complete clot lysis is achieved.

Medical management

Though the detailed medical management is beyond the scope of this chapter, role of medical therapy in patients with advanced PVD (peripheral

(a)

(b)

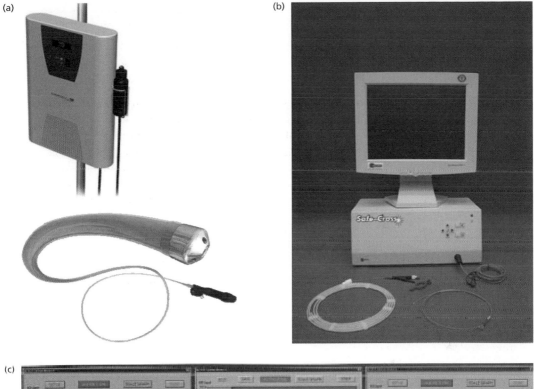

(c)

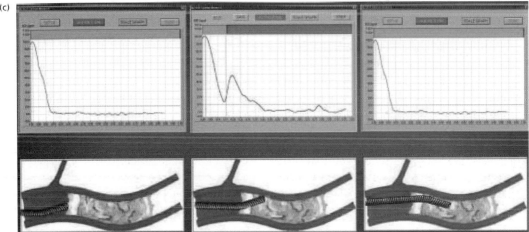

Figure 19.6 (a) The Crosser system generator – high-frequency current is converted into vibrational energy (top). Crosser Catheter – mechanical vibration at 20,000 cycles/s (bottom). (b) Safe-cross system.

(c) Optical coherence reflectometry-guided radiofrequency ablation-waveform display. See Plate 24 in Color Plate section.

vascular disease) should not be underestimated. Even in patients requiring invasive intervention, medical management has been proven to improve outcome, prolong the success of the intervention, improve functional capacity, and prolong life. One must address all modifiable risk factors including smoking, hypertension, dyslipidemia, obesity, physical inactivity, and diabetes. In addition, the appropriate use of beta-blockers, antiplatelet therapy, angiotensin-converting enzyme (ACE) inhibitors and statins are recommended for patients with peripheral vascular disease.

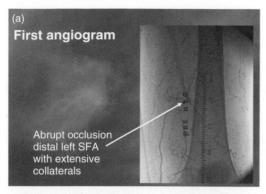

(a) First angiogram

Abrupt occlusion distal left SFA with extensive collaterals

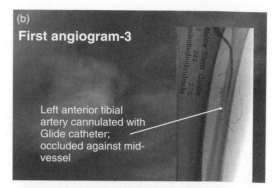

(b) First angiogram-3

Left anterior tibial artery cannulated with Glide catheter; occluded against mid-vessel

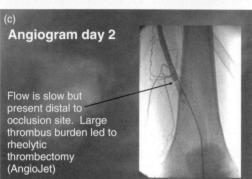

(c) Angiogram day 2

Flow is slow but present distal to occlusion site. Large thrombus burden led to rheolytic thrombectomy (AngioJet)

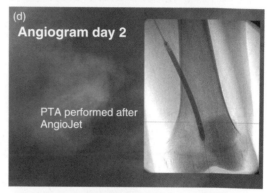

(d) Angiogram day 2

PTA performed after AngioJet

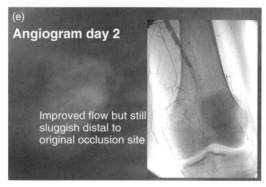

(e) Angiogram day 2

Improved flow but still sluggish distal to original occlusion site

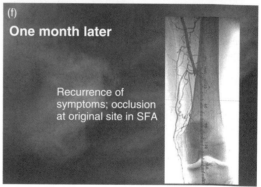

(f) One month later

Recurrence of symptoms; occlusion at original site in SFA

Figure 19.7 Thrombolytic therapy. (a, b) 54 Y/O African–American male presented with a month long history of claudication of the left leg. Over the last few weeks the patient noted resting leg pain. The patient noted a non-healing ulcer ½ cm in diameter on his small toe. (c) Glide catheter left in the left anterior tibial artery overnight. Reteplase was infused via the sheath in the left common femoral artery and the glide catheter. Returned for repeat angiography the next day. (d) PTA and stenting in the distal SFA performed using self-expanding stents. Lytics again given intra-arterially. Symptoms improved. (e) Patient had relief of claudication. Foot was now warm. Good dorsalis pedal pulse on left. ABI on Right 0.75. ABI on Left 0.69. (f) The patient returned one month later with increased claudication.

Future technologies

There are many new innovative technologies on the horizon to treat chronic vessel occlusions. Omniwave technology using acoustic energy, Cronus stereotaxis wire for magnetic navigation [28] and collagenase infusion [29,30] are few of such novelties under investigation. Recent advances

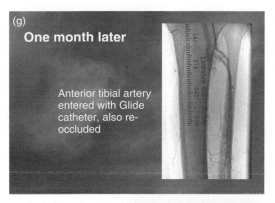

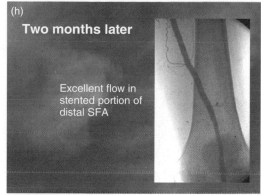

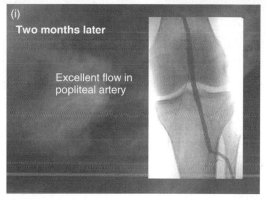

Figure 19.7 (g) The vessel was reinserted with a glide catheter and re-infusion of thrombolytics was successful in restoring flow. (h) The patient returned a month later for stenting of the popliteal artery. (i) The popliteal flow is now preserved with one vessel run off.

in rapid imaging, along with development of special catheter devices visible under MRI, have made real-time MRI (rtMRI) guided therapeutic interventions feasible [31]. Recently Raval and others demonstrated successful real-time MRI-guided recanalization of a long peripheral artery CTO in a swine model [32]. This technology may offer advantage in future human peripheral artery visualization during CTO traversal, while avoiding x-ray radiation and nephrotoxic contrast agents.

Conclusions

At present, endovascular intervention is generally well accepted as an effective treatment modality in majority of occlusive iliac artery lesions, but its role in the femoropopliteal region is still debatable.

A successful intervention of chronic total occlusions depends a lot on operator's patience, technique, and experience. New technologies, including Frontrunner catheter, Safe-Cross system and re-entry catheters, have significantly improved our success of crossing long total occlusions. These innovations along with ever increasing operator experience have considerably enhanced long-term patency in even the most complex chronic occlusions. In the future, more patients will have the opportunity for a less invasive treatment for their arterial disease.

See Plate 24 in the color plate section.

References

1 Heuser RR, Henry M. *Textbook of Peripheral Vascular Interventions*, 2 Edn., 2008 Informa UK Ltd. (15): 92.

2 Uher P, Nyman U, Lindh M, Lindblad B, Ivancev K. Long-term results of stenting for chronic iliac artery occlusion. *J Endovasc Ther* 2002; **9**(1): 67–75.

3 Carnevale FC, De Blas M, Merino S, Egana JM, Caldas JG. Percutaneous endovascular treatment of chronic iliac artery occlusion. *Cardiovasc Intervent Radiol* 2004; **27**(5): 447–452.

4 Lofberg AM, Karacagil S, Ljungman C *et al.* Percutaneous transluminal angioplasty of the femoropopliteal arteries in limbs with chronic critical lower limb ischemia. *J Vasc Surg* 2001; **34**(1): 114–121.

5 Leville CD, Kashyap VS, Clair DG *et al.* Endovascular management of iliac artery occlusions: extending treatment to TransAtlantic Inter-Society Consensus class C and D patients. *J Vasc Surg* 2006; **43**(1): 32–39.

6 Yilmaz S, Sindel T, Yegin A, Luleci E. Subintimal angioplasty of long superficial femoral artery occlusions. *J Vasc Interv Radiol* 2003; **14**(8): 997–1010.

7 Hirsch AT, Haskal ZJ, Hertzer NR *et al.* ACC/AHA 2005 guidelines for the management of patients with peripheral arterial disease (lower extremity, renal, mesenteric, and abdominal aortic). *J Am Coll Cardiol* 2006; **47**(6): 1239–1312.

8 Saha S, Gibson M, Magee TR, Galland RB, Torrie EP. Early results of retrograde transpopliteal angioplasty of iliofemoral lesions. *Cardiovasc Intervent Radiol* 2001; **24**(6): 378–382.

9 McLafferty RB. Patient selection: lesion characteristics and predictors of outcome. *Perspect Vasc Surg Endovasc Ther* 2006; **18**(1): 25–29.

10 Bolia A, Brennan J, Bell PR. Recanalization of femoropopliteal occlusions: improving success rate by subintimal recanalisation. *Clin Radiol* 1989; **40**: 325.

11 Nice C, Timmons G, Bartholemew P, Uberoi R. Retrograde vs. antegrade puncture for infra-inguinal angioplasty. *Cardiovasc Intervent Radiol* 2003; **26**(4): 370–374.

12 Nadal LL, Cynamon J, Lipsitz EC *et al.* Subintimal angioplasty for chronic arterial occlusions. *Tech Vasc Interv Radiol* 2004; **7**: 16–22.

13 Ingle H, Nasim A, Bolia A *et al.* Subintimal angioplasty of isolated infragenicular vessels in lower limb ischemia: long-term results. *J Endovasc Ther* 2002; **9**: 411–416.

14 Jacobs DL, Motaganahalli RL, Cox DE, Wittegen, Peterson GJ. True lumen re-entry devices facilitate subintimal angioplasty and stenting of total chronic occlusions: Initial report. *J Vasc Surg* 2006; **43**(6): 1291–1296.

15 Topaz O, Minisi AJ, Bernardo NL *et al.* Excimer laser effect on platelet aggregation. *Am J Cardiol* 2001; **87**: 849–855.

16 Balzer JO, Gastinger V, Thalhammer A *et al.* Percutaneous laser-assisted recanalization of long chronic iliac artery occlusions: primary and mid-term results. *Eur Radiol* 2006; **16**(2): 381–390.

17 Scheinert D, Laird JR, Schroder M *et al.* Excimer laser-assissted recanalization of long, chronic superficial femoral artery occlusions. *J Endovasc Ther* 2001; **8**: 156–166.

18 Laird JR. Late breaking clinical trials. LACI (laser angioplasty in chronic ischemia) trial. Paper presented at TCT Annual Meeting, September, 2002, Washington, DC.

19 Mossop PJ, Amukotuwa SA, Whitbourn RJ. Controlled blunt microdissection for percutaneous recanalization of lower limb arterial chronic total occlusions: a single center experience. *Catheter Cardiovasc Interv* 2006; **68**(2): 304–310.

20 Melzi G, Cosgrave J, Biondi-Zoccai GL *et al.* A novel approach to chronic total occlusions: the crosser system. *Catheter Cardiovasc Interv* 2006; **68**(1): 29–35.

21 Grube E, Sutsch G, Lim VY, Buellesfeld L. High frequency mechanical vibration to recanalize chronic total occlusions after failure to cross with conventional guidewires. *J Invasive Cardiol* 2006; 18: 85–91.

22 Laird J. Recanalization of peripheral artery CTOs using the CROSSER catheter system: The PATRIOT feasibility study results . Paper presented at TCT Annual Meeting, September, 2006, Washington, DC.

23 Morales PA, Heuser RR. Chronic total occlusions: Experience with fiber-optic guidance technology–optical coherence reflectometry. *J Interv Cardiol* 2001; 14: 611–616.

24 Kirvaitis RJ, Heuser RR, Das TS *et al.* Usefulness of optical coherent reflectometry with guided radiofrequency energy to treat chronic total occlusions in peripheral arteries (the GRIP trial). *Am J Cardiol* 2004; **94**(8): 1081–1084.

25 Wholey MH, Maynor MA, Wholey MH *et al.* Comparison of thrombolytic therapy of lower extremity acute, subacute and chronic arterial occlusions. *Cathet Cardiovasc Diagn* 1998; **44**: 159–169.

26 Motarjeme A. Thrombolysis and angioplasty of chronic iliac artery occlusions. *J Vasc Interv Radiol* 1995; **6**: 665–725.

27 Motarjeme A. Thrombolytic therapy in arterial occlusion and graft thrombosis. *Semin Vasc Surg* 1989; **2**: 155–178.

28 Atmakuri SR, Lev EI, Alviar C *et al.* Initial experience with a magnetic navigation system for percutaneous coronary intervention in complex coronary artery lesions. *J Am Coll Cardiol* 2006; **47**(3): 515–521.

29 Strauss BH, Goldman L, Qiang B *et al.* Collagenase plaque digestion for facilitating guide wire crossing in chronic total occlusions. *Circulation* 2003; **108**(10): 1259–1262.

30 Segev A, Nili N, Qiang B, Charron T, Butany J, Strauss BH. Human-grade purified collagenase for the treatment of experimental arterial chronic total occlusion. *Cardiovasc Revasc Med* 2005; **6**(2): 65–69.

31 Guttman MA, Lederman RJ, Sorger JM, McVeigh ER. Real-time volume rendered MRI for interventional guidance. *J Cardiovasc Magn Reson* 2002; **4**(4): 431–442.

32 Raval AN, Karmarkar PV, Guttman MA *et al.* Real-time magnetic resonance imaging-guided endovascular recanalization of chronic total arterial occlusion in a swine model. *Circulation* 2006; **113**(8): 1101–1107.

CHAPTER 20

High-Frequency Mechanical Revascularization

Eberhard Grube, MD *& Lutz Buellesfeld*, MD

Department of Cardiology & Angiology, HELIOS Heart Center, Siegburg, Germany

A prerequisite for successful percutaneous coronary interventions (PCI) of a chronic total occlusions (CTO) is the ability to cross the occlusion with a guidewire. A wide variety of techniques and devices to try and achieve this have been evaluated and used: specialized guidewires with hydrophilic or tapered tips [1,2], optical coherence reflectometry-guided radiofrequency ablation guidewires [3,4], mechanical approaches such as blunt microdissection [5], and ablative devices such as laser wires [6,7]. These varied methods have had variable success rates that may be somewhat dependent on experienced hands in tertiary centers, and may not be reproducible in the real world. The search for a simpler and reliably effective method continues unabated.

We report a new technology that utilizes mechanical vibrational energy to preferentially ablate plaque. The precedent for this technology came from the use of catheter-delivered therapeutic ultrasound to treat lesions in coronary and peripheral arteries. In biological tissues, high-energy ultrasound causes local effects of acoustic cavitation, microstreaming, thermal warming, and mechanical vibration. *In vivo* studies had shown that the results of ultrasound ablation of lesions were microscopic particulates, 90% of which were <20–25 μm in diameter [8,9]. It is hypothesized that the selective penetration of plaque is dependent on the difference in elasticity between the atherosclerotic plaque and the adjacent media. Collagen, the major determinant of tissue elasticity, is abundant in the media of muscular arteries, while the collagen in atherosclerotic plaque is abnormal, making the elasticity of plaque significantly lower than that of the media. When vibrational energy is applied, a given level of energy causes more deformation and a greater disintegrative effect on the less elastic atherosclerotic plaque as opposed to the more elastic arterial wall. The predominant effect that helps to disrupt the plaque is primarily mechanical as a result of the very rapid movement of the catheter tip on rigid plaque material. Normal segments of the arteries are not damaged by this action as they are elastic and therefore move out of the way of the oscillating probe tip. Previously, the use of this modality in coronary arteries was limited by the large catheter size and lack of deliverability of the device [10–12]. The new CROSSER system has a much smaller catheter tip size compared with the previous devices utilizing this modality.

The CROSSER™ system

The CROSSER System (FlowCardia, Inc., Sunnyvale, CA) uses high-frequency mechanical vibrational energy in a pulsed mode (30 ms on, 30 ms off) to penetrate both calcific and noncalcific atherosclerotic plaque material. The system consists of two components: a Generator and a catheter (Figure 20.1). The generator delivers high-frequency current to the transducer, which converts the current into high-frequency mechanical

Chronic Total Occlusions, 1st edition. Edited by R. Waksman and S. Saito. © 2009 Blackwell Publishing, ISBN: 978-1-4051-5703-2.

(a)   (b)

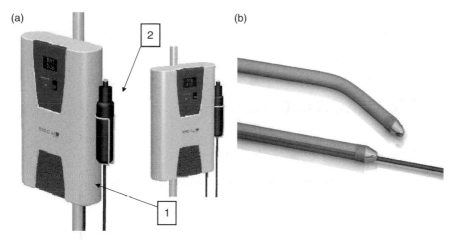

Figure 20.1 Components of the CROSSER system. (a) The CROSSER electronics includes generator (1) and transducer (2). (b) The CROSSER catheter in preshaped and straight (shown with a guidewire) configurations.

vibration that is propagated to the distal tip of the catheter. The transducer operates at a frequency of approximately 21 kHz. The monorail design of the catheter, however, allows the clinician, at any point in the procedure, to advance any conventional guidewire from the tip of the CROSSER catheter to facilitate guidewire placement through the CTO.

The generator is reusable and the CROSSER catheter is disposable. Both components are attached together and protected by a sterile drape during the interventional procedure.

Clinical study results

In a prospective registry, a total of 53 consecutive patients with 55 CTOs suitable for PCI were recruited from December 2002 through to January 2004 in four European centers. All patients entered into the study had a totally occlusive lesion that had been in existence for a minimum of 1 month, with associated TIMI 0 or 1 flow, and had a concurrent or previously documented failed conventional percutaneous procedure to cross the total occlusion.

The first 30 CTOs were chosen for the feasibility phase of the registry, while the subsequent 25 CTOs were chosen for the pivotal phase. The objective of the feasibility phase was to assess technology safety and identify possible opportunities for device improvement, while the objective

of the pivotal phase was to evaluate the efficacy of the device (after improvements in device flexibility and the addition of a hydrophilic coating to the catheter).

However, the primary difference between the early feasibility and the later pivotal phases was the device being studied. The initial design of the CROSSER catheter was uncoated and had a shaft diameter of 1.3 mm diameter. This version of the device often became stuck on proximal disease and tortuous anatomy. In the pivotal device, a hydrophilic coating was added to the distal end of the catheter and the profile was reduced to 1.1 mm, which dramatically improved deliverability.

Potential candidates for the study first underwent an attempt to cross the CTO with conventional percutaneous guidewire intervention for a minimum of 10 min of fluoroscopy time, unless they had a previously documented failed PCI attempt. If the attempt with a conventional technique was unsuccessful, the patient could then be recruited into the study at the physician's discretion. The CROSSER catheter was only used if conventional guidewires had failed to cross the CTO after this designated period of time. The CROSSER catheter was advanced over a guidewire of choice to the proximal cap of the CTO. The guidewire was then withdrawn into the catheter guidewire lumen and then the CROSSER catheter was energized and gently pushed forward against the proximal face of the lesion. In a majority of the cases, bilateral coronary injection was used to define coronary circulation proximal and distal to the CTO, to estimate the length of the CTO and to provide a roadmap for the recanalization procedure. The operator was able to utilize the guidewire at any time as necessary during the procedure. Successful guidewire placement in the true distal lumen was followed by balloon angioplasty and/or stenting. Each CROSSER catheter could be used for 5 min total activation time, and further catheters could be used as required to try and cross the CTO. If the CROSSER System was unsuccessful at crossing the occlusion within 15 min of catheter activation time, the procedure was considered a technical and procedural failure and the patient was managed per normal hospital procedures.

The technical success rate of the feasibility phase was 46.7% but the device efficacy was only 40.0%. No major adverse events or complications relating to vibrational energy, either clinical or angiographic, occurred during the procedure or within 30 days' follow-up. From the experience gathered during this phase, the limitations of the device were noted and redesigned accordingly, resulting in the final version of the CROSSER catheter that was used in the pivotal phase of the trial.

In the pivotal phase, using the improved version of the CROSSER device, the primary endpoint of device efficacy was 76.0% (Table 20.1). Overall, combining the results from both phases of the study, the device efficacy and clinical success were 56.4%. The procedure was quite safe in both arms

with a 30 day major adverse cardiac event (MACE) rate of 0%. In particular, no coronary perforation or pericardial tamponade occurred.

Table 20.2 summarizes the various reasons for which the CROSSER device was unsuccessful in crossing the CTO. The subintimal passage of either the guidewire or CROSSER device was the main reason for failure. The mean duration that the CROSSER was used during the study was 2 min 51 s.

Clinical impact and future perspective

This study demonstrated that high-frequency mechanical vibration is a feasible, well tolerated, and safe approach to facilitate the recanalization of CTOs where a standard guidewire approach had failed. Despite the relatively small number of cases, the success rate of 76.0% in the pivotal phase is very encouraging. Equally important is the observed safety of this system. No clinical complications have been described in any patient

Table 20.1 Summary of study endpoints (n = 55 lesions)

	Feasibility phase (n = 30)	Pivotal phase (n = 25)	Overall (n = 55)
Technical success, n (%)	14 (46.7)	19 (76.0)	33 (60)
Device efficacy, n (%)	12 (40.0)	19 (76.0)	31 (56.4)
Clinical success, n (%)	12 (40.0)	19 (76.0)	31 (56.4)

Table 20.2 Reasons for unsuccessful use of CROSSER device to cross chronic total occlusions (n = 55 lesions)

	No. of lesions
Unable to deliver CROSSER to occlusion	3
No progress of CROSSER through occlusion	5
Partial progress of CROSSER through occlusion	2
Guidewire or CROSSER subintimal	8
Procedure abandoned by physician for following reasons:	
Nontarget vessel spasm	1
Patient having chest pain throughout procedure	1
Aneurysm in distal cap	1
Inability to visualize distal target	1

that was a direct consequence of the vibrational energy itself, and no clinical sequelae of distal embolization such as bradycardia or vasospasm was observed. The deployment and application of the CROSSER catheter is simple and requires little training.

An important potential side-effect of high-frequency vibrational angioplasty is the local heating of tissues resulting from the dissipation of the catheter's mechanical energy. However, in the CROSSER system, 95% of this heating occurs at the proximal end of the catheter outside the body.

The CROSSER System, though much improved from previous generations of this technology, can still be further refined. The catheter tip had a tendency to move straight inside a vessel, which limits its tracking ability through CTOs located in tortuous vessels such as the proximal right coronary artery. The inability to redirect the catheter while navigating through a CTO may also cause the catheter to enter side branches or dissection planes inappropriately. A pre-shaped support catheter or a special access guidewire may be helpful. A CROSSER catheter with a pre-angled tip was used in some cases with the expectation that this would improve device steerability, but the difficulty in maneuvering the catheter and insufficient support from conventional guidewires led to minimal use of this version of the catheter in the study. Newer versions of the device may address these issues in order that a wider variety of CTOs may be treated.

References

1 Corcos T, Favereau X, Guerin Y *et al.* Recanalization of chronic coronary occlusions using a new hydrophilic wire. *Catheter Cardiovasc Diagn* 1998; **43**: 83–90.

2 Saito S, Tanaka S, Hiroe Y *et al.* Angioplasty for chronic total occlusion by using tapered-tip guidewires. *Catheter Cardiovasc Intervent* 2003; **59**: 305–311.

3 Chen WH, Ng W, Lee PY *et al.* Recanalization of chronic and long occlusive in-stent restenosis using optical coherence reflectometry-guided radiofrequency ablation guidewire. *Catheter Cardiovasc Intervent* 2003; **59**: 223–229.

4 Hoye A, Ondewater E, Cummins P *et al.* Improved recanalization of chronic total coronary occlusions using an optical coherence reflectometry-guided guidewire. *Catheter Cardiovasc Intervent* 2004; **63**: 158–163.

5 Whitbourn RJ, Cincotta M, Mossop P *et al.* Intraluminal blunt microdissection for angioplasty of chronic coronary total occlusions. *Catheter Cardiovasc Intervent* 2003; **58**: 194–198.

6 Hamburger J, Serruys PW, Scabra-Gomes R *et al.* Recanalization of total coronary occlusions using a laser guide-wire (the European TOTAL surveillance study). *Am J Cardiol* 1997; **80**: 1419–1423.

7 Hamburger JN, Gijsbers GHM, Ozaki Y *et al.* Recanalization of chronic total coronary occlusions using a laser guide wire: A pilot study. *J Am Coll Cardiol* 1997; **30**: 649–656.

8 Siegel RJ, Fishbein MC, Forrester J *et al.* Ultrasound plaque ablation. A new method of recanalization of partially or totally occluded arteries. *Circulation* 1988; **78**: 1443–1448.

9 Rosenscheim U, Bernstein JJ, Disegni E *et al.* Experimental ultrasound angioplasty: disruption of atherosclerotic plaques and thrombi *in vitro* and arterial recanalization *in vivo*. *J Am Coll Cardiol* 1990; **15**: 711–777.

10 Siegel RJ, Gunn J, Ahsan A *et al.* Use of therapeutic ultrasound in percutaneous coronary angioplasty: experimental *in vitro* studies and initial experience. *Circulation* 1994; **89**: 1587–1592.

11 Cannon LA, John J, LaLonde J. Therapeutic ultrasound for chronic total coronary artery occlusions. *Echocardiography* 2001; **18**: 219–223.

12 Siegel RJ, Gaines P, Crew JR *et al.* Clinical trial of percutaneous peripheral ultrasound angioplasty. *J Am Coll Cardiol* 1993; **22**: 480–488.

CHAPTER 21

Debulking of CTO

Etsuo Tsuchikane, MD, PhD

Department of Cardiology, Toyohashi Heart Center, Aichi, Japan

Higher patency and freedom from restenosis after successful recanalization of chronic total occlusions (CTOs) were greatly increased by the implantation of DES [1–4]. Despite its positive treatment outcomes, the delivery of DES in complex anatomy involving severely calcified and eccentric lesions still remains challenging. In this chapter, we discuss indications and techniques of plaque debulking in the DES era, illustrated by case examples. By the end of the chapter, the readers will have learned the role of plaque debulking in modern interventional cardiology.

Indications of plaque debulking

The management of heavily calcified lesions represents a formidable challenge for an interventional cardiologist. From a technical standpoint, the geometry and rigidity of these morphologies often prevent optimal device delivery and deployment. To overcome such unfavorable lesion subsets, a plaque debulking strategy should be considered. Rotational atherectomy (RA) and directional coronary atherectomy (DCA) are two of the most common devices used for plaque debulking in CTO-PCI (percutaneous coronary interventions). In addition, a newly introduced plaque debulking system, Silverhawk, is considered to be promising in the use of CTO-PCI.

RA involves the use of a high-speed diamond tip drill that pulverizes the thrombus into microscopic particles. DCA involves the use of a

Chronic Total Occlusions, 1st edition. Edited by R. Waksman and S. Saito. © 2009 Blackwell Publishing, ISBN: 978-1-4051-5703-2.

catheter tip equipped with a bladed rotor that cuts away the plaque and the debris is collected in a tiny container. The SilverHawk Plaque Excision System comprises an atherectomy device that is threaded through the lumen of the artery. It comprises a tiny rotating blade that scrapes the plaque from the lesion and the scraped material is collected in a chamber in the device's tip and is removed from the patient.

Rotational atherectomy

Rotational atherectomy (RA) is used to remove the plaque by debulking the atherosclerotic material producing millions of microparticles assumed to be smaller than red blood cells. It facilitates lesion and device success for a massive plaque with severe calcification. The massive plaque burden in CTO is considered to interfere with full stent expansion and/or accelerates in-stent neointimal proliferation after stent expansion.

Plaque debulking of CTO lesions requires careful case selection. For example, RA should be avoided if a conventional wire passes through the subintima. Intravascular ultrasound (IVUS) examination may be helpful in determining whether RA is suitable. Cases in which RA is contraindicated include patients with severe congestive heart failure or severe vessel tortuosity. Furthermore, the RA technique is considered to be an important factor for procedural success. Because CTO lesions have a massive plaque burden and insufficient pre-procedural antegrade flow, the rotating burr should be advanced carefully to prevent the no-reflow phenomenon. Careful case selection and an efficient procedural technique are essential to achieve successful results without major complications.

Optimal stent deployment may not be possible unless satisfactory dilatation of the lesion is achieved and the lesion is made more compliant. Such a lesion preparation of a severely calcified plaque is assumed to facilitate stent delivery and symmetrical stent expansion resulting in more homogeneous drug delivery. Since RA helps maximize lesion preparation, restenosis can be prevented by achieving the full expansion of the drug-eluting stents (DES) in highly calcified lesions.

To perform RA, a 1.5 mm over-the-wire balloon or a 3 Fr infusion catheter is used as a RotaWire (Boston Scientific, Natick, MA) instead of the conventional guidewire. Predilatation with a 1.5 mm balloon is performed when necessary. The Rotablator (RotaLink PLUS, Boston Scientific) burr size is determined and increased according to the vessel size if necessary. IVUS imaging should be used to determine the burr size. High-speed RA is preferred because drug-eluting stents should be implanted after the atherectomy. For a case example see Figure 21.1.

Directional coronary atherectomy

Directional coronary atherectomy (DCA), developed to excise obstructive coronary atheromas, is the only available device in which the operator decides the direction of plaque excision. Although pre-stent plaque debulking by DCA may reduce the rate of restenosis in complex cases [5,6], there have been few studies on debulking strategies with respect to CTO [6]. In addition, morphological characteristics of CTO are not always suitable for DCA. Hence, DCA plays a very limited role in the DES era. In current clinical practice, we consider DCA only for younger patients with ostial CTO of the left anterior descending artery (LAD). In this case, optimal plaque debulking is aimed at preventing DES implantation so as to terminate dual anti-platelet therapy within the first month.

To perform DCA, the use of an IVUS catheter is essential. Suitable lesions for DCA were selected on the basis of angiographic and IVUS findings, and the patient's clinical condition. DCA should not be performed in lesions located in vessels that are smaller than 2.8 mm as assessed by on-line quantitative coronary angiography, lesions with an arc of superficial calcium greater than 180° as assessed by IVUS, restenotic lesions after stenting or DCA, nonprotected left main trunk lesions, aorto-ostial lesions, bypass graft lesions, thrombotic lesions, or cases of acute myocardial infarction. For a case example see Figure 21.2.

The SilverHawk Plaque Excision System

The SilverHawk® Plaque Excision System recently received approval for peripheral application in the United States and for both coronary and peripheral applications in Europe. This device consists of two components: a low-profile catheter and a palm-sized drive unit. All device functionality is controlled by a single on/off thumb-switch that resides on the drive unit. A tiny blade on the tip of the catheter rotates when activated and removes the plaque from the arterial wall. After each pass, the cutter extends through the nose cone to pack the tissue and maximize the storage capacity of the collection chamber. The device can be used to treat very long segments of vessels and can remove 100–200 g or more of plaque. Because CTO presents with a massive plaque burden, the use of the device can be expected to optimize the treatment outcome in contemporary CTO-PCI. Unfortunately, the device has not received approval in Japan, but it will be applicable in the use of CTO-PCI.

Outcome of CTO-PCI

In the bare metal stent (BMS) era, plaque debulking plays a significant role in the reduction of restenosis by minimizing massive plaque burden in CTOs [7,8]. However, the role of plaque debulking in the DES era has been limited to facilitate device and lesion success. The higher incidence of procedure-related events may restrict the use of plaque debulking to certain lesion subsets, as demonstrated by the DOCTORS (Debulking of CTO with rotational or directional atherectomy before stenting) study conducted in Japan [9]. This study, which was conducted in the bare metal stent era, was a multicenter, prospective, randomized trial to evaluate the efficacy of pre-stent debulking of CTOs. The primary endpoint of this study was the angiographic restenosis rate at 6 months. Secondary endpoints were the procedure-related event rate and the major

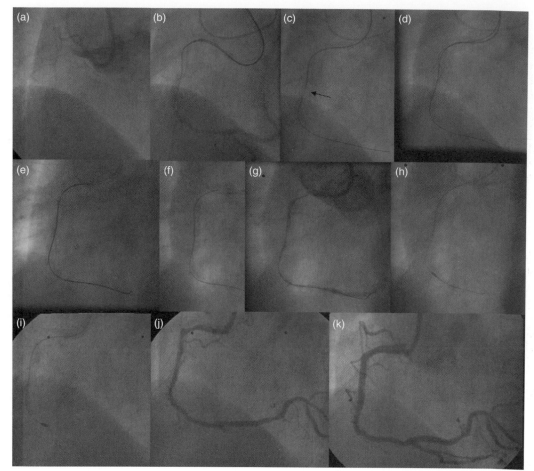

Figure 21.1 Long CTO in a severely calcified right coronary artery (a): Although the occlusion was successfully crossed using a tapered stiff wire (Confianza, Asahi Intecc, Japan), any 1.5 mm balloon may not cross the lesion (b). Penetration catheter (Tornus, Asahi Intecc, Japan) was introduced; however, it could not overcome the most constricted point of the vessel (arrow in c). Thus, to facilitate the passage of the balloon beyond this point, another stiff wire (Miraclebros 12, Asahi Intecc, Japan) was extended along the first wire to "crush" the tight plaque (d). After the successful passage of the second wire, a third stiff wire was introduced because the balloon was still not able to cross the constricted point even after the plaque was crushed by the second wire (three wires in e). After withdrawal of two wires, a 1.5 mm balloon finally crosses the lesion (f) and an antegrade flow was obtained (g). This technique should be called the "Crushing plaque technique." To ensure vessel dilatation and the passage of DES, RA was performed using a 1.25-mm burr (h) and a 1.75 mm burr (i). After vessel modification by RA (j), three Cypher stents were immediately delivered without any friction resistance along with full expansion leading to a successful angiographic result (k).

adverse cardiac event (MACE) rate at 1 year. Procedure-related events included MACEs within 30 days (death, Q-wave myocardial infarction, coronary arterial bypass grafting, target vessel revascularization, or sub-acute thrombosis), procedural failures (flow disturbance, residual stenosis, or failed device delivery), and procedural complications (perforation, temporary no-flow, or non-Q-wave myocardial infarction). In this study, the incidence of procedure-related events in the debulking group was significantly higher than that in the non-debulking group (18.1% versus 9.4%, $P = 0.04$), despite the fact that patients in the debulking group tended to have a lower binary restenosis rate than those in the nondebulking group (23.8% versus 34.6%, $P = 0.072$).

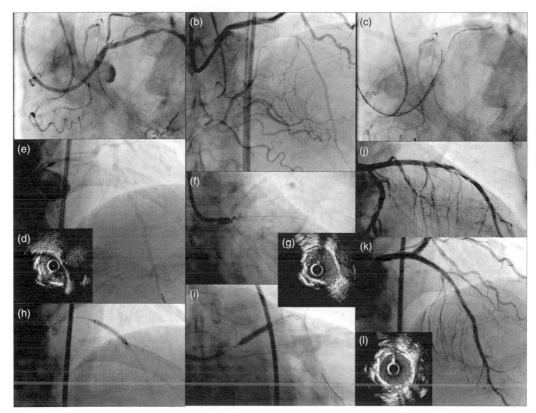

Figure 21.2 Ostial LAD CTO with mild calcification (a/b). After confirming the entrance of CTO using an IVUS catheter inserted into the left circumflex artery (LCx), the lesion was successfully crossed by an intermediate wire (Miraclebros 3) (c). The pre-dilatation IVUS image with a 1.5 mm balloon showed a mild calcified massive plaque burden at the ostium of the LAD that might allow plaque debulking by DCA (d); however, there was a superficial calcified plaque in the proximal LAD that could possibly obstruct the passage of the nose cone of the delivery (DCA) catheter. To facilitate its passage, RA using a 2.0 mm burr was performed prior to DCA (e). After RA, IVUS-guided DCA debulking was performed (f), and the plaque was successfully excised at the LAD ostium (g) to prevent its shift to LCx after DES implantation. A 3.0-mm Cypher was implanted in mid-LAD (h) and a 3.5-mm Cypher was implanted in the ostial LAD as a noncrossover stent to the left main trunk (j) with successful angiographic results (j/k). Final IVUS image confirmed fully expanded stent struts without any plaque shift to LCx (l).

Role of plaque debulking in CTO-PCI

Optimal stent deployment may not be possible unless satisfactory dilatation of the lesion is achieved and it is made more compliant [5]. In such cases, RA still plays a significant role in patients with severe calcification to facilitate success and achieve full expansion of the stent apposed to the vessel wall. The goal of lesion preparation in these patients is to facilitate stent delivery, reduce plaque shift, and allow optimal stent expansion [6]. Leaving an unexpanded stent in the arterial wall in a calcified lesion is likely to be associated with restenosis [10]. Clavijo *et al.* reported the effect of RA on heavily calcified coronary lesions treated with DES in 150 consecutive patients (69 patients who underwent DES implantation without atherectomy and 81 patients in whom atherectomy was required to facilitate DES implantation). The clinical success rates were equivalent in both patient groups, and no differences in in-hospital outcomes were observed between the groups. At 6 months, the target lesion revascularization rate was 4.9% in the DES-alone group and was 4.2% in the group that underwent

DES with RA (P = NS). Sirolimus-eluting stents performed well in patients with complex heavily calcified coronary lesions, with a relatively low event rate [11]. Although no significant differences were observed in this study, the results indicate a significant role of pre-stent lesion modification by RA in optimizing DES implantation in CTO with heavily calcified coronary lesions that otherwise do not permit full stent expansion.

To determine the efficacy of plaque removal by directional atherectomy before DES implantation for bifurcated lesions, a multicenter, nonrandomized, prospective trial was conducted in Japan in which 99 patients were enrolled. Angiographic follow-up was performed in 89 patients (90% follow-up rate) at a mean follow-up period of 259 ± 79 days. Restenosis rates of the main and side branch were 1.1% (1/89) and 3.4% (3/89), respectively, and the total restenosis rate, the primary endpoint of this study, was 4.5% (4/89). One-year clinical follow-up was accomplished in 96 patients (97% of the entire cohort). There were no incidences of death, coronary arterial bypass grafting or myocardial infarction in these patients. No stent thrombosis was observed. However, TLR was required in the main branch of one patient (1.0%) and in the side branch of another (1.0%) [12]. Directional atherectomy provides the best anatomical conditions for optimal and simple DES implantation because it removes the massive atherosclerotic plaque of CTOs located in the ostium of the LAD. In CTOs without a left main lesion, atherectomy enables implantation of a DES in the ostium of the LAD without plaque shift to the circumflex artery. In patients with a left main lesion, crossover stenting beyond the circumflex artery with the kissing balloon technique can be conducted after directional atherectomy for the distal left main LAD and its ostium. These simple DES implantations may reduce the higher restenosis rates of the side branch, which are commonly observed in the current stenting techniques.

Conclusion

In the DES era, the role of plaque debulking is limited to certain complex morphologies that are not satisfactorily treated with conventional angioplasty alone. Lesion preparation with plaque debulking before DES implantation may be an appropriate method for improving device and lesion success without compromising the clinical outcome.

References

1 Werner GS, Krack A, Schwarz G, Prochnau D, Betge S, Figulla HR. Prevention of lesion recurrence in chronic total coronary occlusions by paclitaxel-eluting stents. *J Am Coll Cardiol* 2004; **44**: 2301–2306.

2 Migliorini A, Moschi G, Vergara R, Parodi G, Carrabba N, Antoniucci Dl. Drug-eluting stent-supported percutaneous coronary intervention for chronic total coronary occlusion. *Catheter Cardiovasc Interv* 2006; **67**: 344–348.

3 Nakamura S, Muthusamy TS, Bae JH, Cahyadi YH, Udayachalerm W, Tresukosol D. Impact of sirolimus-eluting stent on the outcome of patients with chronic total occlusions. *Am J Cardiol* 2005; **95**: 161–166.

4 Hoye A, Tanabe K, Lemos PA *et al.* Significant reduction in restenosis after the use of sirolimus-eluting stents in the treatment of chronic total occlusions. *J Am Coll Cardiol* 2004; **43**: 1954–1958.

5 Palmer ND, Nair RK, Ramsdale DR. Treatment of calcified ostial disease by rotational atherectomy and adjunctive cutting balloon angioplasty prior to stent implantation. *Int J Cardiovasc Intervent* 2004; **6**(3–4): 134–136.

6 Moses JW, Carlier S, Moussa I. Lesion preparation prior to stenting. *Rev Cardiovasc Med* 2004; **5**(suppl 2): S16–S21.

7 Braden GA, Young TM, Love WM *et al.* Rotational atherectomy of chronic total coronary occlusion is associated with very low clinical rates: the treatment of choice. *J Am Coll Cardiol* 1999; **33**: 48A.

8 Tsuchikane E, Otsuji S, Awata N *et al.* Impact of pre-stent plaque debulking for chronic total occlusions on restenosis reduction. *J Invasive Cardiol* 2001; **13**: 584–589.

9 Tsuchikane E, Suzuki T, Asakura Y *et al.* and DOCTORS Investigators. Debulking of chronic coronary total occlusions with rotational or directional atherectomy before stenting. *Int J Cardiol* 2008; 125: 387–403.

10 Hadjimiltiades S, Tsikaderis D, Louridas G. Rotational ablation of unexpandable sirolimus-eluting stent. *J Invasive Cardiol* 2005; **17**: 116–117.

11 Clavijo LC, Steinberg DH, Torguson R *et al.* Sirolimus-eluting stents and calcified coronary lesions: clinical outcomes of patients treated with and without rotational atherectomy. *Catheter Cardiovasc Interv* 2006; **68**: 873–878.

12 Tsuchikane E, Aizawa T, Tamai H *et al.* PERFECT Investigators. Pre-drug eluting stent debulking of bifurcated coronary lesions. *J Am Coll Cardiol* 2007; **50**: 1941–1945.

CHAPTER 22

Vibrational Angioplasty

Lampros K. Michalis, MD, MRCP, FESC

Medical School, University of Ioannina, Ioannina, Greece

Introduction

Vibrational angioplasty is a technique that was initially presented in 1993 [1]. This technique facilitates the navigation of conventional coronary guidewires through recalcitrant lesions, thus allowing percutaneous interventions to be performed. Vibrational angioplasty has been shown to be successful in difficult chronic total coronary occlusions (CTOs), while the preliminary results in long femoropopliteal and infrapopliteal CTOs are encouraging.

Technology description

Vibrational angioplasty works as follows: a conventional coronary angioplasty guidewire (0.014 inch) is passed through an over-the-wire catheter so that 1–5 mm of the wire protrudes from the distal end, while the proximal end of the catheter and the guidewire are clamped to the vibrational angioplasty device (Figure 22.1).

The vibrational angioplasty device (Medical Miracles, UK) is a CE-marked handheld motorized device that generates a combination of reciprocal and lateral movements in the wire with frequencies of 16–100 Hz. The motion of the wire is transmitted through the catheter and produces a complex

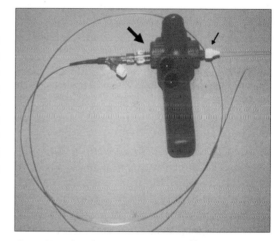

Figure 22.1 The vibrational angioplasty device, connected with an over the wire coronary angioplasty catheter and a coronary angioplasty guidewire. The proximal end of the balloon catheter is clamped to the front of the device (thick arrow), while the angioplasty wire is clamped to the distal part of the device after been fed through it (thin arrow).

motion (reciprocation, lateral movement at twice the reciprocation frequency and standing waves with nodal points) at the distal end of the wire, which protrudes from the distal end of the catheter. The degree of motion depends on the frequency of reciprocation (the device allows the operator to choose this frequency) and the length of the protruding wire (chosen also by the operator). When the protruding wire is short the main component of the wire movement is reciprocal, whereas longer protruding wires have more complex motions.

Chronic Total Occlusions, 1st edition. Edited by R. Waksman and S. Saito. © 2009 Blackwell Publishing, ISBN: 978-1-4051-5703-2.

The device can be attached to any angioplasty catheter–wire combination at any time during the procedure and can be activated for any length of time. Vibrational angioplasty is compatible with guiding catheters or sheaths of any size and for coronary cases both the femoral or radial approaches can be utilized. The device is compatible with any 0.014-inch conventional coronary guidewire. Reported data have shown that the use of the device in conjunction with stiff guidewires in the initial phase of the procedure causes less dissections and is related to a higher final success rate [2].

Vibrational angioplasty procedure

At the beginning of the procedure, when the wire is situated at the hard leading end of the occlusion, the wire usually protrudes 1 mm to facilitate entry into the lesion. After the wire has been advanced within the occlusion, the length can either remain the same or increase depending upon the type of lesion (shorter length is needed for hard parts to be penetrated, while longer lengths are needed for softer parts with channels). During activation of the device, the balloon catheter is pushed forward gently to enhance the penetrating effect of the reciprocal component while the lateral component searches for a path of least resistance. Frequent contrast injections at different radiographic projections are used to ensure that the guidewire progresses along the anticipated route. In case that the anticipated progression of the guidewire does not occur, the device is inactivated, the guidewire is slightly withdrawn and its tip is redirected manually. In case that the tip of the guidewire has lost its shape a different guidewire can be used with the same or slightly different tip (usually the tip of the guidewire should be small and shallow). It is not uncommon that after some progression within the chronically occluded lesion has occurred the combination of the balloon catheter and the guidewire cannot advance any further. In such cases the operator can choose to advance the same or a different wire manually within the lesion. Floppy wires with very good torque are quite often more successful in crossing the occlusion after the initial advancement within the occlusion of a stiff wire. Subsequently and after it has been ensured

that the position of the wire is within the lumen, mainly by using double contrast injections, the operator can try to cross the lesion either with the same balloon catheter or by using a lower profile monorail type of balloon. By the existing technology, roughly 8% of the cases that have been crossed successfully by a guidewire cannot be crossed by a balloon catheter (unpublished data).

Advantages and potential disadvantages

Vibrational angioplasty is a technique with a very short learning curve. It adds to the dexterity of the operator and uses conventional equipment (over the wire balloon catheters and coronary guidewires) that can be connected to the specific device. Vibrational angioplasty should not used as a device that will tackle occlusive lesions using high energy, but rather as an additional equipment that will enable a well-experience operator to tackle the different problems that appear during the process of CTO angioplasty. Unpublished data show that the utilization of the technique decreases the radiation exposure time and the amount of contrast media used.

The device at its present form is disposable and of rather low financial cost (≈200 euros). The way that chronic total occlusions are tackled when vibrational angioplasty technique is employed is by a combination of a controlled forward penetrating movement of the guidewire and a searching movement for low resistance channels. This combination of such movements is quite atraumatic and experimental research has shown that vibrational angioplasty causes less arterial damage compared to manual manipulation techniques [3].

The application of vibrational angioplasty is restricted in cases of extensive tortuosity and in cases where the occlusion is located after an acute bend, mainly because of the limited movement of the wire.

Experimental experience

The extend of damage caused by soft coronary guidewire manipulation was examined in normal sheep coronary arteries. Both manual and vibrating guidewire manipulation found to cause identifiable vascular damage, with the extend being less during vibrational manipulation (Table 22.1) [3].

Clinical experience

Chronic total coronary occlusions

Two-hundred and eight patients with CTOs have been treated by vibrational angioplasty in six cardiac centers by nine operators (Figures 22.2 and 22.3). In these patients vibrational angioplasty was used either in lesions in which conventional techniques had failed (115 lesions), or as a first-choice treatment (93 lesions).

The results of vibrational angioplasty in the 115 difficult chronic total occlusions (in which a

guidewire in conjunction with conventional techniques failed to cross the lesion) have been published previously [4–6] and the summarized results are presented in Table 22.2. The total experience in such cases shows technical and final success rates of 84.3% and 77.4% respectively, while no deaths have been reported. The tamponade and wire exit rates were 0.8% and 2.6% respectively.

A randomized multicenter study comparing the efficacy of vibrational angioplasty versus conventional techniques in consecutive chronic total coronary occlusions has recently concluded. The results of this study show that although the efficacy of vibrational angioplasty is not superior to conventional techniques, the use of vibrational angioplasty reduces radiation exposure and limits the use of contrast media (personal communication).

The predictors of failure of vibrational angioplasty in difficult chronic total occlusions are the duration of the occlusion (>6 months), the length of the occlusion (>15 mm), and the use of soft guidewires. The coronary artery in which the lesion is located, the presence of bridging collaterals, the calcification at the site of the occlusion and the morphology of the occlusion (abrupt versus tapered cutoff) are not predictors of failure. Should be noted also that young age is

Table 22.1 Histological damage caused by vibrational versus manual manipulation in normal sheep coronary arteries

	Vibrational angioplasty	Conventional manipulation	P
No. of sections been examined	62	50	
Damaged sections (%)	35.5	64.0	0.004
Sections with severe damage (%)	13.0	32.0	0.009

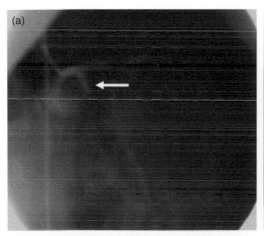

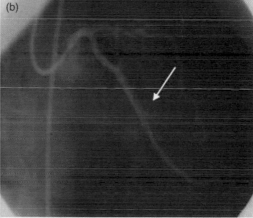

Figure 22.2 One of the first angioplasties attempted using the vibrational angioplasty technique. (a) A left circumflex artery (LCX) CTO (thick white arrow) with unfavorable characteristics (proximal LCX location, blunt stump, 2 small vessels starting at the site of the occlusion, estimated time of occlusion 7 months) been tackled with vibrational angioplasty. (b) The final result shows a fully recanalized LCX. A long dissection at the site of the recanalization left uncovered (thin white arrow) due to the difficulty of placing a J&J stent (the only existing at the time of the angioplasty).

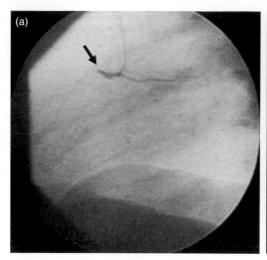 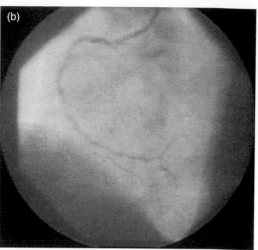

Figure 22.3 Recanalization of a right coronary artery (RCA) CTO with rather unfavourable characteristics (very proximal location, long occlusion, estimated time of occlusion 3 years) using vibrational angioplasty technique.
(a) A proximally totally occluded RCA (thick black arrow). (b) The final result shows a fully recanalized RCA. Angioplasty was successful, although the quality of the whole vessel was poor.

Table 22.2 Total experience in patients with CTOs in which vibrational angioplasty was attempted after conventional techniques had failed

Total number of patients	115
Technical success, n (%)	97 (84.3)
Final success, n (%)	89 (77.4)
Death, n (%)	0 (0)
Tamponade, n (%)	1 (0.8)
Vessel perforation, n (%)	3 (2.6)
Acute myocardial infarction, n (%)	1 (0.8)

the only independent predictor of peri-procedural complications [2,6].

In a retrospective study in which difficult chronic total coronary occlusions were tackled, vibrational angioplasty found to be superior to hydrophilic guidewires; the final success being 75.0% with vibrational angioplasty and 44.4% with hydrophilic guidewires [6].

Chronic total peripheral artery occlusions

In published studies, vibrational angioplasty has been shown to be effective in the treatment of patients with peripheral occlusive arterial disease (6 femoropopliteal and 21 infrapopliteal occlusions) [7,8].

Future directions for the use of vibrational angioplasty

Vibrational angioplasty is a low-cost and safe technique, shown to be effective in chronic total occlusions of both the coronary and the peripheral circulation. The technique, which has a short learning curve, mainly adds to the dexterity of the operator, helping him to increase the efficiency of existing conventional approaches. Unpublished results of a randomized trial comparing vibrational angioplasty to conventional techniques in the treatment of chronic total coronary occlusions reveal that vibrational angioplasty decreases the radiation exposure time and the amount of the utilized contrast agents. A new device compatible with bigger size (0.018 inch) guidewires is currently under evaluation, while an alternative vibrational device, which generates high-frequency vibrations (21.000 Hz) at a tip of a coronary guidewire, has recently shown promising results [9].

References

1 Rees MR, Michalis LK. Vibrational angioplasty in chronic total occlusions. *Lancet* 1993; 342: 999–1000.
2 Rees MR, Michalis LK, Pappa EC, Loukas S, Goudevenos JA, Sideris DA. The use of soft and flexible guidewires in the treatment of chronic total coronary occlusions

by activated guidewire angioplasty. *Br J Radiol* 1999; 72: 162–167.

3 Katsouras CS, Michalis LK, Malamou-Mitsi VD *et al.* Histologic comparison of vibrating guidewire with conventional guidewire technique in an experimental coronary *in vivo* model. *Cardiovasc Interv Radiol* 2003; 26: 454–458.

4 Rees MR, Michalis LK. Activated guide-wire technique for treating chronic coronary artery occlusion. *Lancet* 1995; 346: 943–944.

5 Michalis LK, Rees MR, Davis JAS *et al.* Use of vibrational angioplasty for the treatment of chronic total coronary occlusions: preliminary results. *Catheter Cardiovasc Interv* 1999; 46: 98–104.

6 Michalis LK, Rees MR, Davis JAS *et al.* Vibrational angioplasty and hydrophilic guidewires in the treatment of

chronic total coronary occlusions. *J Endovasc Ther* 2000; 7: 141–148.

7 Michalis LK, Tsetis DK, Katsamouris AN, Rees MR, Sideris DA, Gourtsoyiannis NC. Vibrational angioplasty in the treatment of chronic femoropopliteal arterial occlusions: preliminary experience. *J Endovasc Ther* 2001; 8: 615–621.

8 Tsetis DK, Michalis LK, Rees MR *et al.* Vibrational angioplasty in the treatment of chronic infrapopliteal arterial occlusions: preliminary experience. *J Endovasc Ther* 2002; 9: 889–895.

9 Meltzi G, Cosgrave I, Biondi-Zoccai G *et al.* A novel approach to chronic total occlusions. The Crosser system. *Cathet Cardiovasc Interv* 2006; 68: 29–35.

CHAPTER 23

Drug-Eluting Stents

David E. Kandzari, MD

Duke University Medical Center, Durham, NC, USA

Introduction

Compared with bare metal stents in randomized clinical trials, treatment with drug-eluting stents (DES) is associated with statistically significant and clinically meaningful reductions in angiographic restenosis and the need for repeat revascularization. Beyond the context of randomized trials with more restrictive inclusion criteria, however, observational studies evaluating outcomes among broad, unselected patient populations have extended the benefit of DES to those with more complex coronary lesion morphologies and in varied clinical settings. Despite these advances in the early and late procedural and clinical outcomes of percutaneous coronary revascularization, chronically occluded coronary arteries remain a formidable challenge and unresolved dilemma in interventional cardiology. Although a chronic total occlusion (CTO) is identified in approximately one-third up to one-half of diagnostic cardiac catheterizations, attempted revascularization accounts for approximately less than 10% of all percutaneous coronary interventions (PCI) [1,2]. Such a disparity between their frequency and treatment not only underscores the technical and procedural frustrations associated with these complex lesions, but also the clinical uncertainties regarding clinical benefits of CTO revascularization and the ongoing inadequacies of conventional PCI methods for sustaining restenosis-free patency following initial success. The purpose of this chapter

Chronic Total Occlusions, 1st edition. Edited by R. Waksman and S. Saito. © 2009 Blackwell Publishing, ISBN: 978-1-4051-5703-2.

therefore is to review the rationale for treatment with DES in CTO revascularization, summarize recent DES clinical trial results, and describe future directions for investigation.

Clinical rationale for DES in percutaneous revascularization of coronary occlusions

Unlike the widespread evaluation of DES beyond approved patient and lesion indications, until recently, few investigations have been performed to support the clinical benefit of DES in CTO revascularization. However, the appeal of DES to improve long-term vessel patency following CTO recanalization is related not only to the successes of DES in other complex lesion morphologies but also to the clinical inadequacies of bare metal stents in CTO revascularization. Although several previous trials comparing balloon angioplasty with bare metal stent placement [3–10] (Table 23.1) have varied considerably regarding trial design and methods, their results are remarkably consistent, demonstrating statistically significant reductions in angiographic restenosis, re-occlusion, and the need for repeat intervention associated with coronary stenting. Nevertheless, while demonstrating reduced angiographic and clinical adverse events compared with angioplasty, intermediate and long-term outcomes following successful stent placement were still inferior to those observed among patients treated for non-occlusive lesions. As an example, in the Total Occlusions Study of Canada-1 (TOSCA-1) trial, 6-month rates of restenosis and re-occlusion in complex lesions exceeded 50% and 10%, respectively [3]. At 3-year follow-up

Table 23.1 Randomized clinical trials of angioplasty versus stenting for chronic total coronary occlusions. NS, not significant

Trial	N	Reocclusion			Restenosis			Target vessel revascularization		
		PTCA (%)	Stent (%)	P value	PTCA (%)	Stent (%)	P value	PTCA (%)	Stent (%)	P value
Stenting in Chronic Coronary Occlusion (SICCO) [4]	114	26	16	0.058	74	32	<0.001	42	22	0.025
Gruppo Italiano di Studi sulla Stent nelle Occlusioni coronariche (GISSOC) [6]	110	34	8	0.004	68	32	0.0008	22	5	0.04
Mori et al. [7]	96	11	7	0.04	57	28	0.005	49	28	<0.05
Stent versus Percutaneous Angioplasty in Chronic Total Occlusion (SPACTO) [5]	85	24	3	0.01	64	32	0.01	40	25	NS
Total Occlusion Study of Canada (TOSCA) [3]	410	20	11	0.02	70	55	<0.01	15	8	0.03
Stents in Total Occlusion for Restenosis Prevention (STOP) [8]	96	17	8	NS	71	42	0.032	42	25	NS
Stent or Angioplasty After Recanalization of Chronic Coronary Occlusions (SARECCO) [10]	110	14	2	0.05	62	26	0.01	55	24	0.05
Primary Stenting of Occluded Native Coronary Arteries (PRISON) [9]	200	7	8	0.99	33	22	0.14	29	13	<0.0001

in this trial, the occurrence of re-occlusion was associated with a trend toward higher mortality and a significant increase in the need for repeat revascularization [11].

Considering the persistently high rates of target lesion failure in CTO revascularization involving bare metal stents, the potential for new stent designs to improve rates of restenosis and re-occlusion is considerable. Therefore, inferior clinical outcomes with conventional, bare metal stent placement in CTOs, combined with the observation that advances in the CTO technical and procedural success have been disproportionately low relative to an increasing number of PCI procedures involving non-acute occlusions mandate the need for systematic evaluation of DES safety and efficacy in CTOs. Further, failure to achieve or sustain patency after CTO recanalization has been associated with impairment in regional and global

left ventricular systolic function, recurrent angina and target vessel revascularization, and a greater need for late bypass surgery [12]. Considering the potential for DES to inhibit neointimal proliferation, the implications of improving long-term restenosis free patency in coronary occlusions therefore has potentially significant clinical impact.

Contemporary DES trials in CTO revascularization

Sirolimus-eluting stents

Against the background of several non-randomized, observational studies demonstrating improved angiographic and clinical outcomes with DES, only one randomized trial comparing DES with bare metal stents has been performed. In the primary stenting of occluded native coronary arteries (PRISON) II trial, 200 CTO patients were randomized in a single-blinded fashion at 2 centers in the Netherlands to treatment with either sirolimus-eluting stents (SES; Cypher, Cordis Corporation, Miami Lakes, FL) or the bare metal BX Velocity stent (Cordis Corporation) [13]. Patients enrolled in this study underwent 6-month angiographic follow-up to assess the primary endpoint of in-segment binary restenosis (≥50% reduction in minimal lumen diameter). Overall, diabetes mellitus was present in 13% of patients, 55% of patients had a total occlusion <3 months old, and the average lesion and stent lengths were approximately 16 mm and 30 mm, respectively. At 6 months, treatment with SES was associated with statistically significant reductions in both in-stent (36% versus 7%, $P < 0.0001$) and in-segment (41% versus 11%, $P < 0.001$) angiographic restenosis (Figure 23.1). Reocclusion was also significantly reduced with SES (13% versus 4%, $P < 0.04$), despite treatment in both groups with aspirin and clopidogrel for a minimum duration of 6 months. The clinical benefit with SES also paralleled the relative benefit observed with angiographic measures. Specifically, target lesion revascularization at 12 months occurred in 21% and 5% of bare metal and SES-treated patients respectively ($P = 0.001$ for comparison; Figure 23.2).

In addition to this randomized trial, several recent modest-sized observational studies examining clinical outcomes among patients treated with DES in CTO revascularization have supported the notion that DES may achieve similar reductions in the need for repeat target vessel revascularization as observed in less complex lesions (Table 23.2) [14–23]. In a retrospective study of 122 patients with chronic total occlusions

treated with SES ($N = 144$ lesions), clinical and angiographic outcomes were compared with a historical control of 259 patients treated with are metal stents ($N = 286$ lesions) [14]. At 6 months, overall major adverse cardiac events were significantly lower among SES-treated patients (16.4% versus 35.1%, $P < 0.001$), principally due to a significantly lower rate of repeat target lesion revascularization (7.4% versus 26.3%, $P < 0.001$) (Figure 23.3). Restenosis was identified in 9.2% of patients in the SES group and 33.3% in the bare metal stent group ($P < 0.001$). In multivariate analysis, significant predictors of 6-month major adverse events were the use of bare metal stents (hazard ratio 2.97; 95% confidence interval 1.80 to 4.89), lesion length (hazard ratio 2.02; 95% confidence interval 1.37 to 2.99) and reference vessel diameter >2.8 mm (hazard ratio 0.62; 95% confidence interval 0.42 to 0.92).

In the Rapamycin-Eluting Stent Evaluated at Rotterdam Cardiology Hospital (RESEARCH) Registry, among 56 patients treated with SES following CTO revascularization, the 1-year occurrence of repeat target vessel revascularization was 3.6%, compared with 17.9% among a historical control group of patients receiving bare metal stents [15]. Similarly, the 6-month rate of target lesion revascularization was only 1.4% for 360 patients with CTOs who were included in the prospective e-Cypher Registry [16]. Among

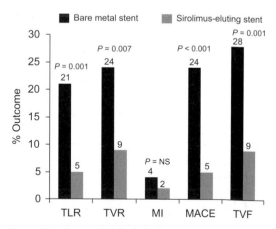

Figure 23.2 One-year clinical outcomes from the PRISON II trial. TLR denotes target lesion revascularization; TVR, target vessel revascularization; MI, myocardial infarction; MACE, major adverse cardiac events; TVF, target vessel failure.

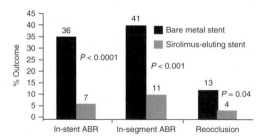

Figure 23.1 Six-month angiographic results from the PRISON II trial. ABR denotes angiographic binary restenosis.

Table 23.2 Clinical trials evaluating drug-eluting stents in total coronary occlusions

Trial	N	Angiographic restenosis (%)	Target vessel revascularization (%)	Major adverse cardiac events (%)	Target vessel revascularization (%)	Major adverse cardiac events (%)
		6 months			1 year	
SICTO [23]	25	0	8.0	12.0	12.0	12.0
e-Cypher Registry [16]	360	–	1.4*	3.1	–	–
RESEARCH Registry [15]	56	9.1	3.6	3.6	–	–
Werner et al. [19]	48	8.3	–	–	6.3	12.5
Nakamura et al. [18]	60	2.0	3.0	–	3.0	
Ge et al. [14]	122	9.2	9.0	16.4	–	–
WISDOM Registry [22]	65	–	–	–	6.7	1.7
TRUE Registry† [20]	183	17.0	16.9	17.1	–	–
Buellesfeld et al. [21]	45	13.2	13.2	15.6	–	–
ACROSS/TOSCA-4 [24]	200	7.5	6.0	6.5	–	–

*Denotes target lesion revascularization.

†7-month clinical and angiographic outcomes reported.

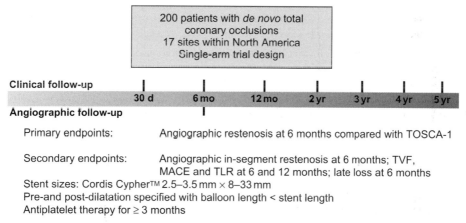

Figure 23.3 Study design of the Approaches to Chronic Occlusions with Sirolimus- eluting Stents (ACROSS)/Total Occlusion Study of Coronary Arteries-4 trial. TLR denotes target lesion revascularization; TVF, target vessel failure; MACE, major adverse cardiac events.

180 patients undergoing SES implantation for CTO revascularization in Asia, the 6-month occurrences of angiographic binary restenosis and target vessel revascularization were 1.5% and 2.3%, respectively [17].

As part of a multicenter Asian registry evaluating DES, clinical and angiographic outcomes among 60 patients who underwent SES implantation during CTO revascularization were compared with a matched control of 120 CTO patients treated with bare metal stents [18]. At 6-month clinical and angiographic follow-up, treatment with

SES was associated with significant reductions in in-stent late loss, restenosis, and reocclusion. Target lesion revascularization was significantly lower at 6 months (23.0% versus 2.0%, $P - 0.001$), and the left ventricular ejection fraction also significantly improved among the SES patients (51.8% baseline versus 57.0% at 6 months, $P < 0.01$), this latter finding implying that maintenance of vessel patency with DES may be an important predictor of the improvement in left ventricular function. At 1 year, treatment with SES was associated with sustained reductions

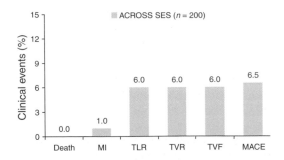

Figure 23.4 Six-month angiographic outcomes from the ACROSS/TOSCA-4 registry comparing treatment of CTOs with sirolimus-eluting stents (SES) versus a historical control group (TOSCA-1) treated with bare metal stents (BMS). TLR denotes target lesion revascularization; TVR, target vessel revascularization; NQMI and QMI, non-W-wave and Q-wave myocardial infarction; MACE, major adverse cardiac events.

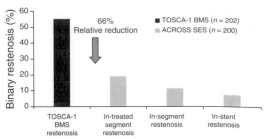

Figure 23.5 Six-month clinical outcomes from the ACROSS/TOSCA-4 registry evaluating treatment of CTOs with sirolimus-eluting stents (SES). TLR denotes target lesion revascularization; TVR, target vessel revascularization; MI, myocardial infarction; MACE, major adverse cardiac events; TVF, target vessel failure. (Note: In-treated segment refers to length of contiguous target segment exposed to balloon inflation. In-segment includes stented area plus 5 mm proximal and distal to stent.

in hierarchal major adverse events (3.0% versus 42.0%, $P = 0.001$) and target lesion revascularization (43.0% versus 3.0%, $P = 0.001$). In a related study of 226 patients undergoing CTO revascularization (SES 106, bare metal stents 120), treatment with SES was associated with a sustained, significant reduction in overall major adverse cardiac events through 4-year follow-up (7.5% versus 33.8%, $P < 0.001$) [24].

Most recently, the Approaches to Chronic Occlusions with Sirolimus-eluting Stents/Total Occlusion Study of Coronary Arteries-4 (ACROSS)/TOSCA-4 trial prospectively enrolled 200 patients undergoing CTO revascularization with SES using contemporary technique and crossing technologies (Figure 23.4) [25]. In this nonrandomized study, clinical and 6-month angiographic outcomes were compared with a historical control of patients receiving bare metal stents in the prior TOSCA-1 trial. Compared with the bare metal stent group, patients treated with SES had significantly older age, more chronic total occlusions (i.e., >6 weeks), smaller caliber vessels, a higher proportion of diabetes and longer lesion and stent lengths (Figure 23.5). However, despite higher complexity in the SES cohort, treatment with SES was associated with an unadjusted 66% relative reduction in the primary endpoint of angiographic binary restenosis within the treated segment (55% versus 19%, $P < 0.001$), defined as

the length of contiguous target segment exposed to balloon dilation prior to stent placement. Following adjustment for baseline characteristics predictive of restenosis, the treatment effect increased to an 84% relative reduction in treated segment restenosis. Rates of in-segment and in-stent restenosis were 11.5% and 6.5%, respectively. At 6-month clinical follow-up, rates of myocardial infarction and target lesion revascularization were 1% and 6%, respectively, contributing to a 6% occurrence of the composite endpoint of target vessel failure (cardiovascular death, myocardial infarction or repeat target vessel revascularization). While these findings further support the safety and efficacy of SES in following CTO recanalization, they also have implications regarding technique using DES in CTO revascularization. For example, given that restenosis in the treated segment (19% in-treated segment restenosis) occurred nearly twice as common beyond the margins of the stent than within the stent (7.5% in-stent restenosis), treatment with SES of the entire segment exposed to balloon predilatation angioplasty may yield further reductions in restenosis and subsequent repeat revascularization. These latter findings are consistent with a prior study of DES in CTOs in which treatment of diffuse atherosclerosis beyond the occluded segment with bare metal stents ("hybrid approach") was associated with significantly higher repeat target vessel revascularization than a strategy involving exclusive treatment with DES [26].

Paclitaxel-eluting stents

Compared with studies evaluating SES, relatively limited evidence exists to support the use of paclitaxel-eluting stents (PES) in CTO revascularization. Werner and others examined treatment with PES (Taxus, Boston Scientific Corporation, Natick, MA) in 48 patients undergoing CTO revascularization and compared these patients with a historical control group with similar clinical and angiographic characteristics [19]. At 6 months, both restenosis (8.3% versus 51.1%, $P < 0.001$) and reocclusion (2.1% versus 23.4%, $P < 0.005$) were significantly reduced among patients treated with PES. Due to significantly decreased rates repeat PCI or bypass surgery, overall major adverse events were also significantly lower in the paclitaxel group. One year following the index revascularization, repeat revascularization occurred in 3 patients in the PES group and 21 patients in the bare metal stent group (6.3% versus 43.8%, $P < 0.001$).

In the European TRUE Registry among 183 patients with total occlusions who were treated with PES, 7-month rates of restenosis and target vessel revascularization were 17.0% and 16.9%, respectively [20]. It is noteworthy that the mean ($\pm$ standard deviation) number of stents per patient (2.2 ± 1.2) total stent length (58 ± 33 mm) in this study were considerably greater than previous DES trials involving treatment of less

complex lesion subsets. Other studies evaluating PES in CTO revascularization have included fewer patients. Buellesfeld et al. [21] examined clinical and angiographic outcomes among 45 CTO patients treated with PES. At 6 months, the rates of angiographic restenosis and target vessel revascularization were 13.2%. Among 65 patients with CTOs in the international WISDOM registry, treatment with PES resulted in freedom from major adverse cardiac events and repeat intervention at 1 year in 93.3% and 98.3% of patients, respectively [22].

Comparative DES trials in CTO revascularization

Whether safety, clinical efficacy, and angiographic outcomes are similar between differing DES has only been recently examined [27,28]. Despite more predictable variance in measures of neointimal hyperplasia by angiography and intravascular ultrasound, demonstration of differences in clinical outcome across individual trials has been less consistent [29–35]. However, whether disparities in angiographic and clinical outcome emerge in more complex lesion morphologies is an issue of ongoing study and is particularly relevant to coronary total occlusions.

At present, four comparative trials of SES and PES have been performed (Table 23.3) [36–40]. In general, these studies have been limited by their small study populations that limit statistical comparisons, variability in trial design and limited clinical and angiographic follow-up. In

Table 23.3 Comparative drug-eluting stent trials in total coronary occlusions

Trial	N	Angiographic restenosis (%)		Target vessel revascularization (%)		Major adverse cardiac events (%)	
		SES	PES	SES	PES	SES	PES
RESEARCH/T-SEARCH Registry [36]*	76 SES, 57 PES	–	–	2.6	3.6	–	–
Nakamura et al., Asian Registry [37–39]*	396 SES, 526 PES	4.0	6.7	3.6	6.7	3.6	6.7
Suarez de Lezo et al. [41]†‡	60 SES, 58 PES	7.4	19.0	3.3	7.0	3.0	7.0
Jang et al. [40]	107 SES, 29 PES	9.4	28.6	3.7	6.9	4.2	14.2

P = Not significant for all comparisons unless otherwise noted.
*1-year outcomes.
†8-month outcomes.
‡Angiographic follow-up in only 48% of patients, P < 0.05.

the single center Rotterdam registry (RESEARCH and T-SEARCH) comparing clinical outcomes among CTO patients treated with bare metal stents ($N = 26$), SES ($N = 76$) and PES ($N = 57$), 1-year freedom from repeat target vessel revascularization was significantly greater with DES compared with bare metal stents (97.4% with SES, 96.4% with PES, 80.8% with bare metal stents, $P = 0.01$ for comparison), despite significantly greater stent number and length per patient with DES [36]. Similarly, the open-label, multicenter Asian chronic total occlusion registry reported no significant differences in the 1-year target vessel revascularization rates of 3.6% and 6.7% for SES- ($N = 396$) and PES-treated patients ($N = 526$) [37]. In a subgroup of patients with 3-year follow-up in this study, major adverse cardiac events were significantly lower in the SES group (10.9% SES versus 16.3% PES, $P = 0.03$), although rates of target lesion revascularization were statistically similar (7.7% SES versus 9.5% PES, $P = $ NS) [38]. Recently, these same investigators reported results from a prospective registry of 1149 CTO patients treated with SES ($N = 365$), PES ($N = 482$), zotarolimus-eluting stents ($N = 154$), tacrolimus-eltuing stents ($N = 109$), or endothelial progenitor cell (EPC) capture stents ($N = 39$) [39]. At 9 months, repeat target lesion revascularization was significantly lower with SES compared with ZES, TES and EPC stents, but did not statistically differ from PES. In another non-randomized comparison of CTO patients treated with SES ($N = 107$) and PES ($N = 29$), statistically significant differences were observed regarding angiographic restenosis (9.4% with SES versus 28.6% with PES, $P < 0.05$), although rates of target vessel revascularization did not statistically vary (3.7% with SES versus 6.9% with PES, $P = $ NS) [40]. Finally, a modest-sized randomized trial comparing SES ($N = 60$) and PES ($N = 58$) in CTO revascularization also demonstrated no significant difference in the 8-month target vessel revascularization rates of 3.3% and 7.0% in the SES and PES cohorts, respectively [41].

The ongoing PRISON III trial is intended to compare clinical and angiographic outcomes among 300 CTO patients randomized in a 1:1, open-label fashion to treatment with either the Cypher or zotarolimus-eluting Endeavor (Medtronic Corp., Santa Rosa, CA) stents [42]. The primary endpoint is in-segment late lumen loss at 8 month angiographic follow-up, in addition to assessment of secondary clinical endpoints including target lesion revascularization, target vessel failure and stent thrombosis.

Conclusion

Prior to recent evaluations detailing the clinical and angiographic outcomes observed with DES in CTO revascularization, our understanding of procedural and mid-term safety and efficacy of DES following CTO percutaneous revascularization was limited by the routine exclusion of such patients from major interventional cardiology clinical trials. Although several modest-sized studies evaluating both SES and PES in CTOs have demonstrated favorable improvements in angiographic and clinical measures compared with historical data with bare metal stents, there remains an ongoing need for further systematic, prospective evaluation of DES treatment in CTO revascularization. In addition to the variability among current trials in design, methods and duration of follow-up, because some patients who experience reocclusion or restenosis may remain asymptomatic, it is likely that angiographic follow-up should be included in a suitable cohort of patients to confirm the "proof of concept" efficacy of novel DES platforms in this complex lesion subset. Comparisons of both angiographic and clinical outcomes in CTOs will also be essential in the evaluation of next generation DES given that outcomes observed with newer DES in simple to moderate complexity lesions may differ markedly from those observed in CTOs. Finally, given that percutaneous revascularization of CTOs is routinely associated with more extensive stent placement, whether the improvement in restenosis is offset by a potentially higher risk of thrombotic occlusion or complications associated with stent fracture also is uncertain.

Chronic total occlusions have been routinely termed the "last great barrier to PCI success" not only due to the technical challenges of recanalization but also the inconsistencies in maintaining long-term patency with bare metal stents. Although restenosis and reocclusion do still occur, treatment with DES has been associated with considerable improvement in angiographic and clinical outcome.

However, as both lesion complexity and stent length and number increase, whether outcomes will vary for any given DES or between different DES is uncertain. Further, despite their common use in clinical practice, DES are not formally approved by the United States Food and Drug Administration for the treatment of total occlusions based on the absence of clinical trials that have rigorously and independently assessed safety and efficacy in addition to incorporating long-term (e.g., 5 years), post-approval surveillance. These issues, in addition to the need for expanded approval of DES in this lesion subset, inform the need for ongoing studies to not only confirm the benefit of currently approved DES but also to evaluate forthcoming novel antiproliferative agents and stent designs in coronary total occlusions.

References

1 Srinivas VS, Borrks MM, Detre KM et al. Contemporary percutaneous coronary intervention versus balloon angioplasty for multivessel coronary artery disease. A comparison of the National Heart, Lung, and Blood Institute Dynamic Registry and the Bypass Angioplasty Revascularization Investigation (BARI) study. Circulation 2002; 106: 1627–1633.

2 Christofferson RD, Lehmann KG, Martin GV, Every N, Caldwell JH, Kapadia SR. Effect of chronic total occlusion on treatment strategy. Am J Cardiol 2005; 95: 1088–1091.

3 Buller CE, Dzavik V, Carere RG et al. Primary stenting versus balloon angioplasty in occluded coronary arteries: the Total Occlusion Study of Canada (TOSCA). Circulation 1999; 100: 236–242.

4 Sirnes PA, Golf S, Myreng Y et al. Stenting in Chronic Coronary Occlusion (SICCO): a randomized, controlled trial of adding stent implantation after successful angioplasty. J Am Coll Cardiol 1996; 28: 1444–1451.

5 Hoher M, Wohrle J, Grebe OC et al. A randomized trial of elective stenting after balloon recanalization of chronic total occlusions. J Am Coll Cardiol 1999; 34: 722–729.

6 Rubartelli P, Niccoli L, Verna E et al. Stent implantation versus balloon angioplasty in chronic coronary occlusions: results from GISSOC trial. J Am Coll Cardiol 1998; 32: 90–96.

7 Mori M, Kurogane H, Hayashi T et al. Comparison of results of intracoronary implantation of Palmaz-Schatz stent with conventional balloon angioplasty in chronic total coronary arterial occlusion. Am J Cardiol 1996; 78: 985–989.

8 Lotan C, Rozenman Y, Handler A et al. for the Israeli Working Group for Interventional Cardiology. Stents in total occlusion for restenosis prevention (STOP). Eur Heart J 2000; 21: 1960–1966.

9 Rahel BM, Suttorp MJ, Laarman GJ et al. Primary stenting of occluded native coronary arteries: final results of the Primary Stenting of Occluded Native Coronary Arteries (PRISON) study. Am Heart J 2004; 147: e16–e20.

10 Sievert H, Rohde S, Utech A et al. Stent or angioplasty after recanalization of chronic coronary occlusions: the SARECCO trial. Am J Cardiol 1999; 84: 386–390.

11 Buller CE, Teo KK, Carere RG et al. Three year clinical outcomes from the Total Occlusion Study of Canada (TOSCA). Circulation 2000; 102: II–1885.

12 Stone GE, Kandzari DE, Mehran R et al. Percutaneous recanalization of chronically occluded coronary arteries: a consensus document: Part I. Circulation 2005; 112: 2364–2372.

13 Suttorp MJ, Laarman GJ, Braim MR et al. Primary Stenting of Native Totally Occluded Coronary Arteries II (PRISON II): A randomized comparison of bare metal stent implantation with sirolimus-eluting stent implantation for the treatment of total coronary occlusions. Circulation 2006; 114: 921–928.

14 Ge L, Iakovou I, Cosgrave J et al. Immediate and mid-term outcomes of sirolimus-eluting stent implantation for chronic total occlusions. Eur Heart J 2005; 26: 1056–1062.

15 Hoye A, Tanabe K, Lemos PA et al. Significant reduction of restenosis after the use of sirolimus-eluting stents in the treatment of chronic total occlusions. J Am Coll Cardiol 2004; 43: 1954–1958.

16 Holmes D. Complex lesions in the e-Cypher Registry. Presented at the Transcatheter Therapeutics 2004 Scientific Sessions, September 28–October 1, 2004, Washington, D.C.

17 Nakamura S, Selvan TS, Bae JH, Cahyadia YH, Pachirat O. Impact of sirolimus-eluting stents on the outcome of patients with chronic total occlusions: multi-center registry in Asia. J Am Coll Cardiol 2003; 43: 35A.

18 Nakamura S, Muthusamy TS, Bae JH, Cahyadi YH, Udayachalerm W, Tresukosol D. Impact of the sirolimus-eluting stent on the outcome of patients with chronic total occlusions. Am J Cardiol 2005; 95: 161–166.

19 Werner G, Krack A, Schwarz G, Prochnau D, Betge S, Figulla HR. Prevention of lesion recurrence in chronic total coronary occlusions by paclitaxel eluting stents. J Am Coll Cardiol 2004; 44: 2301–2306.

20 Grube E, Biondi Zoccai G, Sangiorgi G et al. Assessing the safety and effectiveness of TAXUS in 183 patients with chronic total occlusions: insights from the TRUE study. Am J Cardiol 2005; 96: 37H.

21 Buellesfeld L, Gerckens U, Mueller R, Schmidt T, Grube E. Polymer-based paclitaxel-eluting stent for treatment of chronic total occlusions of native coronaries: results of a Taxus CTO registry. Catheter Cardiovasc Interv 2005; 66: 173–177.

22 Abizaid A, Chan C, Lim YT *et al.* Twelve-month outcomes with a paclitaxel-eluting stent transitioning from controlled trials to clinical practice (WISDOM Registry). *Am J Cardiol* 2006; **98**: 1028–1032.

23 Lotan C, Almagor Y, Kuiper K, Suttorp MJ, Wijns W. Sirolimus-eluting stent in chronic total occlusion: the SICTO study. *J Interv Cardiol* 2006; **19**: 307–312.

24 Nakamura S, Nakamura S, Bae JH *et al.* Four-year durability of sirolimus-eluting stents in patients with chronic total occlusions compared with bare metal stents: multicenter registry in Asia. *Am J Cardiol* 2007; **100**: 93L.

25 Kandzari DE. Approaches to Chronic Occlusions with Sirolimus-eluting Stents/Total Occlusion Study of Coronary Arteries-4 (ACROSS)/TOSCA-4 trial. Presented at the Transcatheter Therapeutics 2007 Scientific Sessions, October 22, 2007, Washington, DC.

26 Werner GS, Schwarz G, Prochnau D *et al.* Paclitaxel-eluting stents for the treatment of chronic total coronary occlusions: a strategy of extensive lesion coverage with drug-eluting stents. *Cathet Cardiovasc Interv* 2006; **67**: 1–9.

27 Schomig A, Dibra A, Windecker S *et al.* A meta-analysis of 16 randomized trials of sirolimus-eluting stents versus paclitaxel-eluting stents in patients with coronary artery disease. *J Am Coll Cardiol* 2007; **50**: 1373–1380.

28 Stettler C, Wandel S, Allemann S *et al.* Outcomes associated with drug-eluting and bare-metal stents: a collaborative network meta-analysis. *Lancet* 2007; **370**: 937–948.

29 Windecker S, Remondino A, Eberli FR *et al.* Sirolimus-eluting and paclitaxel-eluting stents for coronary revascularization. *N Engl J Med* 205; **353**: 653–662.

30 Dibra A, Kastrati A, Mehillia J *et al.* ISAR-DIABETES Study Investigators. Paclitaxel-eluting or sirolimus-eluting stents to prevent restenosis in diabetic patients. *N Engl J Med* 2005; **353**: 663–670.

31 Goy JJ, Stauffer JC, Siegenthaler M, Benoit A, Seydoux C. A prospective randomized comparison between paclitaxel and sirolimus stents in the real world of interventional cardiology: The TAXI trial. *J Am Coll Cardiol* 2005; **45**: 308–311.

32 Kastrati A, Mehilli J, von Beckerath N *et al.* ISAR-DESIRE Study Investigators. Sirolimus-eluting stent or paclitaxel-eluting stent vs balloon angioplasty for prevention of recurrences in patients with coronary in-stent restenosis: a randomized controlled trial. *JAMA* 2005; **293**: 165–171.

33 Kastrati A, Dibra A, Eberle S *et al.* Sirolimus-eluting stents vs paclitaxel-eluting stents in patients with coronary artery disease: meta-analysis of randomized trials. *JAMA* 2005; **294**: 819–825.

34 Morice MC, Colombo A, Meier B *et al.* for the REALITY Trial Investigators. Sirolimus- versus paclitaxel-eluting stents in de novo coronary artery lesions: the REALITY Trial: A randomized controlled trial. *JAMA* 2006; **295**: 895–904.

35 de Lezo JS, Medina A, Pan M *et al.* Drug-eluting stents for complex lesions: latest angiographic data from the randomized rapamycin versus paclitaxel CORPAL study. *J Am Coll Cardiol* 2005; **45**(suppl A): 75A.

36 Hoye A, Ong ATL, Aoki J *et al.* Drug-eluting stent implantation for chronic total occlusions: comparison between the sirolimus- and paclitaxel-eluting stent. *Eurointerven* 2005; **1**: 193–197.

37 Nakamura S, Bae JH, Cahyadi YH, Udayachalerm W, Tresukosol D, Tansuphaswadikul S. Comparison of efficacy and safety between sirolimus-eluting stent and paclitaxel-eluting stent on the outcome of patients with chronic total occlusions: multicenter registry in Asia. *Am J Cardiol* 2005; **96**: 38H.

38 Nakamura S, Bae JH, Cahyadi YH *et al.* Comparison of efficacy and durability of sirolimus-eluting stents and paclitaxel-eluting stents in patients with chronic total occlusions: multicenter registry. *Am J Cardiol* 2007; **100**: 93L.

39 Nakamura S, Bae JH, Yeo HC *et al.* Drug-eluting stents for the treatment of chronic total occlusion: a comparison of sirolimus, paclitaxel, zotarolimus, tacrolimus-eluting and EPC capture stents: multicenter registry in Asia. *Am J Cardiol* 2007; **100**: 16L.

40 Jang JS, Hong MK, Cheol WL *et al.* Comparison between sirolimus- and paclitaxel-eluting stents for the treatment of chronic total occlusions. *J Invas Cardiol* 2006; **18**: 205–208.

41 Suarez de Lezo J, Medina A, Pan M *et al.* Drug-eluting stents for the treatment of chronic total occlusions: a randomized comparison of rapamycin- versus paclitaxel-eluting stents. *Circulation* 2005; **112**: II-477.

42 Suttorp MS, Laarman GJ. A randomized comparison of sirolimus-eluting stent implantation with zotarolimus-eluting stent implantation for the treatment of total coronary occlusions: rationale and design of the PRImary Stenting of Occluded Native coronary arteries III (PRISON III) study. *Am Heart J* 2007; **154**: 432–435.

CHAPTER 24

Laser for CTO Recanalization

On Topaz, MD

McGuire Veterans Affairs Medical Center, Richmond, VA, USA

Introduction

Laser was discovered and described as a spectacular physics phenomenon by Albert Einstein in 1917. The term laser represents an acronym for Light Amplification by Stimulated Emission of Radiation. Medical laser devices produce intense electromagnetic energy that is transferred as light photons through flexible catheters containing optic fibers for photoablation of biologic tissues. Most experience in cardiovascular applications of laser has been gained with the pulsed-wave, ultraviolet excimer laser that operates at the 308 nm wavelength of the light spectrum [1]. The Spectranetics cardiovascular CVX-300 excimer laser system (Spectranetics, Colorado Springs, CO, USA) is approved in the US and Europe for coronary and saphenous vein grafts and peripheral interventions and for pacemaker and AICD (Automatic Implanted Cardiac Defibrillator) lead removal. Absorption of excimer laser energy within the target biologic tissue creates effects on the non-aqueous components of the irradiated atherosclerotic plaque and its accompanying thrombus. It accounts for development of plaque-specific photochemical and photomechanical reactions including formation of gas vapor and acoustic shock waves. The vaporization of plaque content and concomitant propagation of acoustic resonance waves ultimately lead to debulking and removal of the lased tissue [2].

Chronic Total Occlusions, 1st edition. Edited by R. Waksman and S. Saito. © 2009 Blackwell Publishing, ISBN: 978-1-4051-5703-2.

Clinical applications of laser

The main clinical targets for laser angioplasty in coronary and peripheral interventions are symptomatic patients who sustain acute or chronic coronary syndromes and/or peripheral ischemic disease. These patients frequently present with complex atherosclerotic and thrombotic lesions that are considered either non-amenable or non-ideal for standard technologies of percutaneous or surgical revascularization [3]. Among the various indications for utilization of laser, recanalization of coronary and peripheral chronic total occlusions (CTO) constitutes an important application [4]. The CTO can consist of a *de novo* lesion (Figure 24.1) or in stent total restenosis (Figure 24.2). A growing interest in laser for recanalization of venous CTO has recently emerged. The fundamental merit of laser debulking in these types of CTO lesions stems specifically from its unique interaction each of the major histopathologic constituents of chronic total obstructions, i.e., atherosclerotic plaque, organized thrombus, fibrosis, and calcifications. Of note, both atherosclerotic plaque and accompanying thrombus are amenable to effects of the excimer laser energy and, therefore, can be targeted, debulked, and removed. In that regard, thrombus exhibits a specific challenge within the structure of CTO. Layers of thrombus of varying age and consistency are embedded within the CTO. Frequently, during attempts to recanalize a CTO, the thrombus becomes active and friable [5]. This is then accompanied by enhanced platelet aggregation, formation of new thrombus and localized discharge of vasoactive mediators.

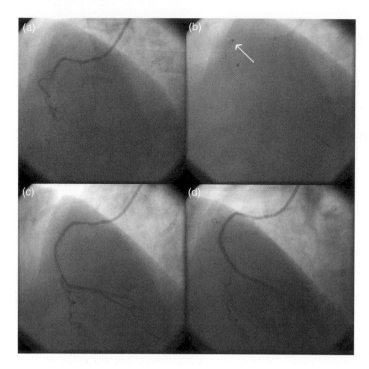

Figure 24.1 CTO laser treatment applied to diffuse 28 mm in-stent occlusion (a). Slow antegrade and retrograde lasing along the occluded stent with a 0.9 mm × 80 mm excimer catheter (b – tip of laser marked with an arrow) resulted in formation of adequate pilot recanalization (c). Final results show marked patency of the treated stent and vessel. (Courtesy of Nelson Bernardo M.D., Washington Hospital Center, Washington, DC.)

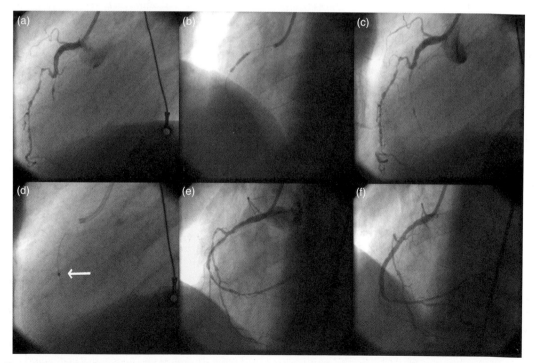

Figure 24.2 CTO of RCA (a). Rotablator failed to penetrate the lesion. Balloon dilation (b) failed (c). A 0.9 mm × 80 mm laser (d – arrow) was applied followed by a 1.4 mm COS excimer laser that expanded the recanalization (e). After adjunct balloon dilations and stenting the target CTO and vessel are patent (f). (Courtesy of Nelson Bernardo M.D., Washington Hospital Center, Washington, DC.)

The excimer laser induces unique effects on thrombi, with its ability to produce mechanical impact on the fibrin mesh within a clot leading to clot dissolution. Induction of a beneficial suppressive effect on platelet aggregability [6] has been demonstrated. This is a clinically important property for patients who cannot receive 2b/3a receptor antagonists or lack evidence of their effect [7].

Laser technology

Laser catheters provide mechanical support for advancement or exchange of guidewire into the CTO. Catheters can be advanced easily over the leading guidewire or exchange for a different size. In selected cases, the laser needs to be activated and advanced in front of the guidewire tip. Subsequent morphologic transformation of the target CTO lesions during and after such lasing technique enables safe guidewire advancement and penetration into the total occlusion. Adequate recanalization through the obstructive tissue ensues, leading to complete crossing of the lesion and facilitation of adjunct balloon and stenting. The speed of catheter advancement during lasing of CTO is of paramount importance. Slow advancement – less than 0.5 mm/s – is warranted because it increases absorption within the lased plaque [8]. The use of saline flush during lasing is in one aspect required as it reduces the synergistic effect of contrast media on acoustic shock waves, thereby reducing pressures within the lased CTO. On the other hand, many interventionalists maintain that the firm resistance of CTO calls for no saline injection, so the maximal effect of laser-induced acoustic phenomena that enhance target lesion debulking will be achieved.

Laser catheters contain a flexible fiber-optic cable made of high-purity silica fibers. A typical 2 mm excimer laser catheter has 240 fibers, each with a core diameter of 61 μm. The optical fibers are arranged around a guidewire lumen, and the distal tip is rounded and polished. The ultraviolet laser light emerges from individual fibers, penetrating approximately 40–50 μm onto the target tissue. A variety of over the wire and rapid exchange excimer laser catheters are available for CTO treatment. These laser catheters are as small as 0.7 mm [9] and as large as 2.5 mm. They include 1.4, 1.7, 2.0, 2.3, and 2.5 mm catheters with either concentric or eccentric optical fiber arrays, depending on the model. Most concentric laser catheters are built with the "optimally spaced" (90 μm space among individual fibers) arrangement of fibers which provides improved ablation in comparison to older catheters versions (77 μm space between fibers) [8]. The energy levels range from fluence of 25 mJ/mm^2 at 40 Hz to as high as 80 mJ/mm^2 at 80 Hz, depending on catheter specifications and the operators assessment of the degree of difficulty the occlusion will pose. The operator can use any preferred shape of guiding catheter for delivery of the desired guidewire and laser catheter to the total occlusion. The guiding catheter size is adjusted to accommodate the chosen laser catheter in accordance with instructions for use and recommendations from the laser manufacturer. The size of the first laser catheter selected for use is open to operator discretion. From a mechanical and safety viewpoint, a small catheter (such as the 0.9 mm) that creates a "pilot channel" is often preferred. However, the need to provide firm support and stable handling may require utilization of a larger size initial catheter, such as a 2.0 mm catheter for SFA (superficial femoral artery) applications. During CTO angioplasty, adjunct pharmacotherapy including thrombolytics, 2b/3a receptor antagonists, or direct thrombin inhibitor can be synergistically combined with delivery of excimer laser energy in coronary and peripheral interventions alike. This concept of enhanced or synergistic effect of laser energy on pharmacologic agents is termed "power thrombolysis" [10].

Coronary total occlusions

An important experience with a unique laser wire system for treatment of CTO in coronary vessels was gained during the TOTAL European multicenter study in the late 1990s. It incorporated a 0.018-inch laser wire for recanalization of these occlusions. This study [11] demonstrated that the laser wire was as effective and safe as standard guidewires. The cumulative crossing success rate was 61% when the laser wire preceded mechanical

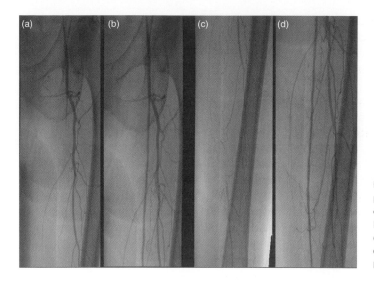

Figure 24.3 CTO of SFA. (a) Pre-laser proximal SFA (superficial femoral artery) occlusion. (b) Post turbo 2.0 mm excimer laser. (c) Pre-laser CTO of distal SFA. (d) Results post turbo 2.0 mm laser. Courtesy of Tony Das M.D., Presbyterian Heart Center, Dallas, TX.

wire and in about half of the patients less than 30 minutes of fluoroscopy time was needed for complete crossing. The investigators concluded that the laser wire is a useful tool for cases when a standard wire fails to cross and needs to be changed with a different mechanical modality. Perin and associates described [12] their experience with a "wireless" technique for laser recanalization of chronic total coronary and saphenous vein grafts occlusions.

SFA total occlusions

Excimer laser debulking in these lesions has been extensively studied and analyzed (Figure 24.3) [12–14]. These long lesions require careful navigation and manipulation of the revascularization equipment. The preferred laser technique for recanalization of these lesions was developed and introduced to the field by Biamino in Germany [14,15]. It incorporates laser activation in a "step-by-step" sequence whereby the guidewire is first advanced into the origin of the CTO and then the laser catheter is advanced over and beyond the tip of the wire into the first few millimeters of the occlusion. Then the laser catheter is activated and advanced stepwise for up to 5 mm followed by re-advancement of the guidewire toward the tip of the laser catheter. The sequence is repeated with the laser catheter

sequentially advanced and activated millimeter by millimeter ahead of the supporting guidewire until the entire total occlusion is crossed. Biamino and colleagues who gained extensive expertise in laser utilization in this type of lesions reported the results of laser angioplasty in 318 patients with 411 chronic SFA occlusions. The mean lesion length was 19.4 ± 6.0 cm. A 91% success rate was achieved with application of the step-by-step lasing technique. Subsequent stenting was needed in only 7% of treated lesions. After 1 year the primary patency rate was 65% and then re-intervention on re-occluded vessels resulted in a 75% secondary patency rate. The experience gained in total SFA lesions enables application of the laser with the above-mentioned techniques in total occlusions in other anatomic vascular locations such as the common iliac arteries and tibioperoneal arteries as well [16,17].

Total occlusions in critical limb ischemia

Critical limb ischemia (CLI) is frequently associated with severe atherosclerotic disease of the aortoiliac to infragenicular arteries. The disease is manifested by long total occlusions containing a large thrombus content [15–18]. A rescue revascularization strategy incorporating excimer laser in this clinical scenario carries several advantages including facilitation of lesion crossing, removal of the occlusive or resistant atherosclerotic burden, vaporization of underlying thrombus, and creation of a "pilot channel" which enables introduction of balloons for adjunct dilatations [19]. A substantial reduction of distal embolization from the total occlusion site and a reduced need for stenting in the infrapopliteal arteries are observed [16–19]. A subset of patients with CTOs refractory to guidewire canalization was selected for analysis from the LACI 2, the LACI CIS, and the LACI Belgium trials [20]. Altogether, 46 patients who experienced CLI with Rutherford category 4–6, with 47 limbs and 205 lesions (67% in SFA;11% in popliteal artery and 20% in infra-popliteal arteries) averaging 73.4 ± 7.3 mm in length (mean 4.4 lesions per limb) were treated with excimer laser angioplasty. The step-by-step lasing technique was utilized during attempts to cross the occlusions with a guidewire. Procedural success was 72%, a straight-line flow to the foot was established in 79%. Limb salvage was achieved in 95% of 42 surviving patients. The operators stressed the fact that this high rate of limb salvage was achieved in a group of patients with complex medical issues that otherwise would have had amputation.

Summary

Excimer laser is an ultraviolet, pulsed-wave laser that is uniquely suited for revascularization of CTO because of its selective debulking effect on atherosclerotic plaque and thrombus. Patients with acute and chronic ischemic coronary and peripheral syndromes who present with CTO that requires revascularization are candidates for treatment with this technology. The user-friendly over-the-wire or rapid-exchange catheters induce the plaque debulking and thrombus dissolution required for recanalization of complex CTO in the cardiovascular system. The excimer laser also facilitates stent delivery and deployment. Thus, utilizing proper lasing techniques, the excimer laser enables safe and effective coronary and peripheral debulking of

CTO associated with high success and low complications rates.

References

1 Topaz O, Bernardo NL, Shah R et al. Effectiveness of excimer laser coronary angioplasty in acute myocardial infarction or in unstable angina pectoris. *Am J Cardiol* 2001; **87**: 849–855.

2 Topaz O. Plaque removal and thrombus dissolution with pulsed wave lasers' photoacoustic energy-biotissue interactions and their clinical manifestations. *Cardiology* 1996; **87**: 384–391.

3 Topaz O. Laser. In: Topol EJ, ed. *Textbook of Interventional Cardiology*, 4th edn. WB Saunders, Philadelphia, 2003: 675–703.

4 Das T. Excimer laser angioplasty for CTOs. *Endovasc Today* 2003; **10**: 1–4.

5 Topaz O. On the hostile massive thrombus and means to eradicate it. *Cath Cardiovasc Intervent* 2005; **65**: 280–281.

6 Topaz O, Minisi AJ, Bernardo NL et al. Alterations of platelet aggregation kinetics with ultraviolet laser emission: the stunned platelet phenomenon. *Thromb Haemost* 2001; **86**: 1087–1093.

7 Topaz O. Ischemic coronary syndromes and SVG interventions – do 2b/3a inhibitors miss the target? *Cath Cardiovasc Interven* 2007; **69**: 630–631.

8 Topaz O, Lippincott R, Bellendir J, Taylor K, Reiser C. "Optimally spaced" excimer laser coronary catheters: performance analysis. *J Clin Laser Med Surg* 2001; **19**: 9–14.

9 Taylor K, Harlan K, Branan N. Small 0.7 mm diameter laser catheter for chronic total occlusions, small vessels, tortuous anatomy, and balloon resistant lesions-development and initial experience. *Euro Interv* 2006; **2**: 265–269.

10 Topaz O, Perin EC, Jesse RL, Mohanty PK, Carr ME, Rosenschein U. Power thrombolysis in acute coronary syndromes. *Angiology* 2003; **54**: 457–468.

11 Serruys PW, Hamburger JN, Kooler JJ et al. The TOTAL trial. *Euro Heart J* 2000; **21**: 1797–1805.

12 Perin EC, Leite-Sarmento R, Silva GV, Rogers MD, Topaz O. "Wireless" laser recanalization of chronic total coronary occlusions. *J Invas Cardiol* 2001; **13**: 401–405.

13 Steinkamp HJ, Wissgott C, Rademaker J et al. Short superficial femoral artery occlusions: results of treatment with excimer laser angioplasty. *Cardiovasc Intervent Radiol* 2002; **25**: 388–396.

14 Biamino G. The excimer laser: science fiction fantasy or practical tool? *J Endovasc Ther* 2004; **11**(suppl 2): 207–222.

15 Laird JR, Reiser C, Biamino G, Zeller T. Excimer laser assisted angioplasty for the treatment of Chronic total occlusions that cause critical limb ischemia such as complex tibial disease can be recanalized successfully as well critical limb ischemia. *J Cardiovasc Surg* 2004; **45**: 239–245.

16 Zeller T, Scheinert D. Laser angioplasty for critical limb ischemia. *Endovasc Today* 2004; **2**: 63–65.

17 Das TS. Percutaneous peripheral revascularization with excimer laser: equipment, technique and results. *Lasers Med Sci* 2001; **16**: 101–107.

18 Boccalandro F, Muench A, Sdringola S, Rosales OR. Wireless laser assisted angioplasty of the superficial femoral artery in patients with critical limb ischemia who have failed conventional percutaneous revascularization. *Cath Cardiovasc Intervent* 2004; **63**: 7–12.

19 Topaz O. Rescue excimer laser angioplasty for treatment of critical limb ischemia. *Cath Cardiovasc Intervent* 2004; **16**: 626.

20 Bosiers M, Peeters P, Elst FV *et al.* Excimer laser assisted angioplasty for critical limb ischemia; results of the LACI Belgium study. *Eur J Vasc Endovsc Surg* 2005; **29**; 613–619.

VI PART VI
Complications

CHAPTER 25

How to Handle Complications

Axel de Labriolle, MD *& Ron Waksman,* MD

Washington Hospital Center, Washington, DC, USA

Introduction

Chronic total occlusion (CTO) angioplasty constitutes a particular challenge for the interventional cardiologist. CTO patients are generally sicker, have more multivessel disease, and more comorbidity, such as renal insufficiency, low ejection fraction, and complex coronary anatomy when compared with patients subjected to percutaneous coronary intervention (PCI) without CTO. CTO lesions are particularly complex with small vessel sizes, calcifications, and absence of visualization of the vessel's distal bed. These features explain why CTO procedures are particularly difficult to recanalize, are lengthy in duration, are associated with multiple devices and wires, and require large amount of contrast agents and radiation exposure to the patient and the operator. The use of multiple wires and devices, such as directional or rotational atherectomy or lasers, increases the risk of complications such as dissection and perforation. Different types of complications have been reported in CTO angioplasty and are displayed in Table 25.1. These complications can be deleterious for the patient, are often life-threatening or are associated with decompensation of existing comorbidities. All potential complications must be considered before the procedure is initiated and should be discussed with the patient. This chapter will summarize potential complications, ways to prevent them, and how these complications should be managed once they occur.

Chronic Total Occlusions, 1st edition. Edited by R. Waksman and S. Saito. © 2009 Blackwell Publishing, ISBN: 978-1-4051-5703-2.

Preventative treatment

Despite the fact that the treatment of CTO is associated with prolonged radiation exposure and increased volume of contrast media (CM), there are few data published specifically in this setting. Some of the following considerations are extrapolated from data in non-CTO patients.

Radiation exposure

Fluoroscopic time

The complexity of CTO angioplasty in native coronary arteries is such that times of fluoroscopy are often longer than in non-CTO angioplasty. Furthermore, the risk for repeating procedures because of restenosis or thrombosis is not infrequent [1], potentially leading to high-radiation dose exposure. Mehran *et al.* reported at the fourth international chronic total occlusion summit in 2006 the experience of the Colombia University Medical Center. In that series of 245 CTO attempts between 08/2004 and 12/2006, the fluoroscopic time was 38 ± 28 min, with a procedure time of 75 ± 41 min. Fluoroscopic time was the same whether the procedure was successful or not. Suzuki *et al.* [2] confirmed these data. They observed that the total fluoroscopic time was significantly longer in CTO angioplasty (42.6 ± 17 min) versus multivessel disease PCI (25.1 ± 8 min) versus single-vessel PCI (14.6 ± 8 min). In another study of 39 patients, which sought to prospectively evaluate the performance of a laser guide wire in crossing chronic total coronary occlusions in patients with a failed previous mechanical guide wire attempt, the mean fluoroscopy time was 99 ± 43 min [3].

Table 25.1 Complications in chronic total occlusion percutaneous coronary intervention

Complication		Main causes	Treatment
Cardiac and vascular			
Myocardium	Myocardial infarction	Thrombus formation*	Depends on the cause
		Loss of collateral circulation	Medical
		Side branch occlusion	(anti platelet, anti coagulant vasodilatator agents)
		Air embolism*	Re-PCI ± stent
		Dissection*	CABG
		Distal embolization	
		Abrupt closure of the vessel in the first 24 hours*	
	Septal hematoma	Retrograde methods	Medical
		TRAC or CART techniques	
Pericardium	Pericardial effusion	Hydrophilic wire and stiff wire	Medical
	Tamponade	High-pressure inflation	Percutaneous pericardocentesis
		Directional or rotational atherectomy	Cardiac surgery
		Laser	
Rhythm	Ventricular arrythmia		Medical treatment
			Electrical defibrillation
Coronary arteries	Dissection	Guiding KT with strong back-up	Depends on grade and flow in artery
		Hydrophilic wire and stiffwire	Medical
		Can occur in the CTO or donor artery (ostium ++) according to the method used	Re-PCI using stents or CABG
	Thrombus	Length of the procedure	Medical
		Can occur in the CTO or donor artery according to the method used	(anti platelet agents, GP IIb/IIIa inhibitors)
			Re-PCI ± stent ± aspiration device
	Spasm	Length of the procedure	Medical
		Use of various intracoronary devices	(vasodilatators, antiplatelet agents)

	Perforation	Major risk with use of directional, rotational atherectomy devices, and laser	Medical PCI ± PTFE covered stent, plugs, coils, glue CABG
	Intramural hematoma	TRAC or CART techniques	Medical PCI + Stent (if vessel compression IVUS ++)
	Guidewire fracture with entrapment	Calcifications of the lesion Use of rotablator wire	PCI Cardiac surgery
Aortoiliac	Aortic root dissection		Medical Cardiac surgery
	Perforation of the sinus of valsalva		Cardiac surgery Percutaneous pericardiocentesis if tamponade
	Peripheric hematoma bleedings	Length of the procedure Size of device used Number of vascular access Antiplatelet therapy	Medical treatment Transfusions Vascular surgery
Others	Contrast media induced nephropathy		Hemodialysis
	Immoderate irradiation		Preventive treatment +++
	Stroke		Preventive treatment +++ Medical treatment or interventional treatment

*In the CTO or donor artery in case of retrograde methods being used.

Total radiation exposure

Monitoring the cumulative radiation dose received by the patient is possible with built-in ionizing chambers in most of the more recent angiographic systems [4–6] that give access to dose-area product, which is a decent reflection of the total radiation received by the patient. However, dose–area product does not reflect the patient's skin exposure because it does not take into account the skin exposure site and scattered radiation. In a series of 190 patients, Bell *et al.* [7] described that radiation entry exposure, calculated from fluoroscopy exposure times and using data from phantom studies, were increased in CTO angioplasty. Patients referred for CTO angioplasty ($n = 90$) had a mean dose of 53 roentgen while control patients ($n = 100$) with non-CTO angioplasty only received a mean dose of 34 roentgen. These procedures were performed using pulsed progressive fluoroscopy; radiation exposure would be considerably higher using conventional fluoroscopic systems. Cineangiographic radiation exposures were similar for each group and accounted for an average additional exposure of 14–22 roentgen for each procedure. Finally, the risk of neoplasms induced by procedure-related radiation exposure is quite low, equivalent to that incurred from 2 to 3 years of natural background radiation [8].

Skin exposure

Skin is the organ with the greatest risk of radiation injury at the site of direct beam penetration. Although not usually monitored, particular attention must be paid to the entrance skin dose (ESD). In their work, Suzuki *et al.* [2] showed a maximum ESD of 4.5 ± 2.8 Gy in CTO angioplasty versus 2.3 ± 0.7 in multivessel PCI versus 1.4 ± 0.9 in single-vessel PCI. Furthermore, during the procedure, the maximum ESD for CTO exceeded 5 Gy in 6/13 procedures. With such a dose, radiation skin injuries such as early transient erythema (2 Gy), permanent epilation (7 Gy), and delayed dermal necrosis (12 Gy) may occur [8–10] (Figure 25.1). Table 25.2, adapted from the ACCF/AHA/HRS/SCAI report [8] to optimize patient safety and image quality in fluoroscopically guided invasive cardiovascular procedures, summarizes

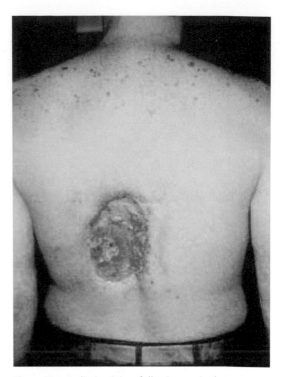

Figure 25.1 Radiation injury following angioplasty. This was the first reported case of radiation-induced skin necrosis from a coronary angioplasty procedure. The patient underwent three coronary angioplasty procedures, each of which lasted between 1 and 2 hours. The last two procedures were performed on the same day, 6 months after the first, and involved about 1 hour of fluoroscopy on-time. No data on the number of cine frames is available. Erythema was noted on the patient's back when the patient was removed from the table after the last procedure. One month later the patient reported erythema in the same area; this persisted. This image shows the appearance approximately 5 months after the procedures. (From Hirshfeld *et al.* [8].)

the main radiation skin injuries according to the X-ray dose received by patient. The International Commission on Radiological Protection (ICRP) [10] recommends recording the maximum skin dose and its location when the maximum cumulative skin dose is thought to be ≥3 Gy (≥1 Gy in repeated cases). Furthermore, when the presumed skin dose is ≥3 Gy, the ICRP recommends that a medical examination be performed 10–14 days postprocedure in order to check for any effects on the skin. In addition, patients should be informed

Table 25.2 Threshold skin entrance doses for various skin injuries

Single-dose effect	Threshold (Gy)	Onset
Early transient erythema	2	Hours
Main erythema	6	Approximately 10 days
Late erythema	15	Approximately 6–10 weeks
Temporary epilation	3	Approximately 3 weeks
Permanent epilation	7	Approximately 3 weeks
Dry desquamation	14	Approximately 4 weeks
Moist desquamation	18	Approximately 4 weeks
Secondary ulceration	24	Greater than 6 weeks
Ischemic dermal necrosis	18	Greater than 10 weeks
Dermal atrophy (1st phase)	10	Greater than 14 weeks
Dermal atrophy (2nd phase)	10	Greater than 1 yr
Induration (invasive fibrosis)	10	–
Telangiectasia	10	Greater than 1 yr
Late dermal necrosis	Greater than 12?	Greater than 1 yr
Skin cancer	Not known	Greater than 5 yr

Source: From Hirshfeld et al. [8].

about radiation injury before giving their consent for a procedure with possible high-radiation dose exposure. Although ESD is not monitored in clinical practice, it is important to pay attention to the patient's skin dose and thus make efforts to prevent radiation skin injuries during PCI for CTO. Reduction of the cumulative dose in the same area of skin during repeat procedures is important in PCI and could be obtained by regularly varying the incidence of the X-ray beam. Saito et al. [11] have proposed the following guidelines for procedure termination: ≤30 min time from arterial access to successful penetration of a guide wire through occlusion and ≤90 min for total procedure time. In our catheterization laboratory, the attempt to recanalize the CTO is ceased when 30 min of fluoroscopy is reached and the wire has still not crossed the lesion. Minimizing the distance between the image detector and the patient enables us to reduce the patient's irradiation.

Other risks

The risk of radiation-induced cataracts or alopecia is extremely rare after PCI since the X-ray beams are usually targeted from the back of the patient through the chest with no involvement of the head. In the same way, gonadal exposure or risk of solid tumors is not likely [8].

For physicians who perform numerous procedures, radiation exposure is a concern that must not be overlooked. Beyond the use of mobile radiation-shielding devices provided, physicians should use the following precautions: lead apron, thyroid lead collars, and lead glasses. Physicians must work as far away from the X-ray field as possible, and focus on angulations by which the procedure should be performed. By wearing badges, operators can monitor their overall radiation exposure. By measuring radiation exposure in real time, operational dosimetry can be a useful tool to help physicians limit the received dose. The main radiation safety principle is referred to as ALARA (as low as reasonably achievable).

Contrast-induced nephropathy exposure

Iodinated contrast media may result in iatrogenic renal function deterioration. The incidence of contrast-induced nephropathy (CIN) depends on its definition. The most common definition for CIN is an increase of ≥25% or ≥0.5 mg/dL in pre-PCI serum creatinine at 48 hours after PCI [12]. CIN inducing the need for dialysis was reported in 0.3–0.7% of patients undergoing PCI [13]. The risk of CIN also depends on the iodinated contrast volume used and on the cardiovascular risks of the patient, such as age, diabetes history, or previous renal insufficiency [14] – all of which are prominent in CTO patients. Usually the rise in serum creatinine occurs within the first 24 hours after CM exposure, while the peak is reached at 72 hours. CIN constitutes an important independent factor for morbidity and mortality [15].

In CTO angioplasty, the risk of CIN is probably more important than in other angioplasty cases, thus some rules should be kept in mind to improve the prognosis of patients undergoing CTO procedures [16,17] (Table 25.3).

Iodinated contrast media

Volume

Among the major risk factors identified for CIN is iodinated CM volume [13]. The main randomized clinical trials [18–23] dealing with the prevention of clinical contrast CIN where the volume of CM was well monitored, report the mean use of 130 to 260 mL of CM in PCI. In these studies, different PCI cases, such as single-vessel PCI, multivessel PCI, and bypass graft PCI were reported, but most excluded patients who underwent CTO recanalization. In CTO, the CM volume used is more important because of the difficulty of the procedures previously named. Thus, in their series of 245 CTO patients treated

Table 25.3 Hydration regimen and contrast media characteristics used to avoid contrast-induced nephropathy

Volume	Bolus 3 mL/kg 1 hour before procedure Infusion 1 mg/kg 6 hours postprocedure
Produit	Sodium bicarbonate
N-acethylcysteine	*Needs more clinical investigation*
Ionic/non-ionic	*Needs more clinical investigation*
CM osmolarity	Iso-osmolar
Tonicity	Isotonic hydration

between August 2004 and December 2006 at Colombia University Medical Center, Mehran et al. (4th summit of CTO) reported a mean CM volume of 432 ± 315 cm^3. There was no difference between successful or failed procedures (448 mL versus 429 mL, respectively; $p = 0.58$). In another work studying a laser guidewire for recanalization of CTO [3], the volume of CM used was 515 ± 154 mL. According to the studies of Saito et al. and Kini et al. [11,24], a relatively safe cut off point of CM volume is around 220 mL. Finally, the key message is that the use of small amounts of CM is the best measure to prevent CIN [11], and efforts should be made to not exceed 300 mL of total dye volume. Moreover, the total dye volume should be calculated based on the baseline creatinine clearance.

Osmolarity

Aspelin et al. [19] demonstrated in a series of 129 diabetic patients with increased creatinine (1.5–3.5 mg/dL) randomized between iodixanol and iohexol that CIN were less likely to develop with use of an iso osmolar (300 mOsm/kg H_2O) CM iodixanol (visipaque) than with a low osmolar (600 mOsm/kg H_2O) CM – iohexol (omnipaque). The CIN rate was 3% in the iodixanol group versus 26% in the iohexol group; $p = 0.002$. Thus, the odds of nephropathy were 11 times less with iodixanol. Jo et al. [20] confirmed in a study comparing the nephrotoxicity of iodixanol (non-ionic, dimeric, iso-osmolar – 300 mOsm/kg H_2O – CM) with ioxaglate (ionic, dimeric, low-osmolar – 600 mOsm/kg H_2O – CM) in patients with renal impairment undergoing coronary angiography that the use of CM with an osmolality close to the plasma osmolality was much more important that ionicity or viscosity for preventing the occurrence of CIN.

Hydration regimen

It is well known that a vigorous hydration regimen is needed in patients who undergo PCI for CTO treatment [25], but the best regimen remained a matter of debate until recently.

Isotonic hydration

Mueller et al. [18] have shown that isotonic hydration (NaCl 0.9%) is superior to half-isotonic hydration (0.45%) in the prevention of CIN. In their series of 1620 unselected patients undergoing PCI, the incidence of CIN was 0.7% in the isotonic hydration group versus 2% in the half-isotonic hydration group; $p = 0.04$.

Sodium bicarbonate

Most hydration protocols to prevent CIN use sodium chloride, whereas in animal models, pretreatment with sodium bicarbonate is more effective than sodium chloride. The alkalinization of the renal tubular fluid with bicarbonate may allow for a decrease in free radical formations, which are responsible for the renal injury. Merten et al. [21] have compared the effect of these two hydration regimens – 154 meq/L of sodium chloride versus 154 meq/L of sodium bicarbonate – on the incidence of CIN. Infusions were started 1 hour before CM injection as a bolus of 3 mL/kg and 6 hours after the procedure at an infusion rate of 1 mL/kg. The CIN rate was 13.6% in the sodium chloride group versus 1.7 % in the sodium bicarbonate group (OR = 11.9 [2.6 – 21.2]; $p = 0.02$).

N-acetylcysteine

Because free radical formations are considered important pathophysiological causes of CIN, many studies, without great success to date, have tried to prevent CIN using antioxidant molecules. Among the substances tested, only N-acetylcysteine (NAC) seems to confer a clinical gain as demonstrated by Briguori et al. [22] Recent works, however, were neither conclusive nor provided proof of the benefit of NAC to prevent CIN [23,26].

Prophylactic hemodialysis

In selected patients with advanced renal failure, some works show that prophylactic hemodialysis could allow for a decrease in the incidence of CIN. Recently, Lee et al. have demonstrated that prophylactic hemodialysis is effective in improving renal outcome in chronic renal failure patients undergoing coronary angiography [27].

Curative treatment

Although the literature is profuse with procedural complications during CTO angioplasty, few

focus on their management. PCI of a CTO has traditionally been considered a low-risk procedure. The risk of such a procedure has been evaluated between that of coronary angiography and that of non-occluded coronary artery angioplasty [28]. In-hospital major adverse event rates, however, may exceed 5%, periprocedural myocardial infarction can occur in >2%; and death may occur in 1% of patients [29–32]. The severity and nature of these complications vary and depend on operator experience. These complications and the treatment observed during CTO treatment are listed in Table 25.1.

Medical treatment

Numerous complications observed in CTO are non specific and require the same medical treatment that would have occurred in different setting. Therefore, Q-wave or non-Q-wave myocardial infarction, transient ischemic attack, or intracoronary thrombus needs an anti-ischemic treatment with anticoagulants and/or antiplatelet therapy. Transfusions may be useful in case of hematoma or important decreases in hemoglobin level. Halting glycoprotein IIb/IIIa inhibitor or bivalirudin use and reversal of anticoagulation may be particularly useful in cases of perforation by intravenous sulfate protamine (1 mg/100 U heparin), with ultimate dose titration guided by the activated clotting time. Arrhythmias can be treated medically or with external defibrillators if tolerance is low. In the few cases of septal hematoma described when retrograde methods are used for opening occlusions [33], careful medical monitoring is needed. Hemodialysis could be useful in cases of severe CIN.

Percutaneous pericardiocentesis

Tamponade is one of the most serious perforation complications observed in CTO angioplasty. Patients deteriorate quickly and develop cardio respiratory arrest within a few minutes. The delay for surgery, however minimal, may be fatal. In these cases, life-threatening cardiac tamponade can be effectively treated by percutaneous pericardiocentesis (Figure 25.2), using a dedicated kit. In cases of unsuccessful pericardiocentesis or to complement the percutaneous pericardiocentesis, surgical pericardiocentesis is required at the time of the surgical repair.

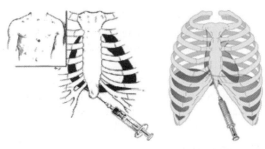

Figure 25.2 Pericardiocentesis requires the use of a needle to withdraw fluid from the pericardial sac. The insertion site just below the sternum is cleansed, and a local anesthetic given. A pericardiocentesis needle is then inserted and guided into the pericardial sac. Once the needle has reached the pericardial sac, a guide wire is inserted. The needle is removed and replaced with a catheter. The fluid is withdrawn through this catheter and put into containers. Usually this pericardial catheter is left in place to continue the draining for several hours. Echocardiography may be useful to monitor drainage but must not delay the treatment.

Repeat angiography and Repeat PCI

Abrupt closure of the vessel within the first 24 hours of successful CTO PCI is not uncommon and can occur in 8% of cases. Furthermore, re-occlusion may be clinically silent [34]. Therefore careful attention to the patient, his/her ECG, and biology is required within the 24–48 hours after PCI CTO to detect these silent and delayed events.

Surgical treatment

Many complications in CTO-PCI that would not have been fixed during the PCI procedure by using stents, plugs, coils, glue, antiplatelet agents or vasodilatators may require an emergent coronary artery bypass grafting (CABG) or other surgical repair (Table 25.1). Thus, occlusive dissection of the CTO artery, retrograde dissection of left main coronary artery, guidewire fracture with entrapment, or side-branch occlusion can be treated by CABG [29]. Others complications such as coronary perforation, aortic root dissection, or valsalva sinus perforation may need other types of surgical repairs.

Perforations

Coronary perforation is the dreaded complication in CTO-PCI. It represents a complete disruption

Table 25.4 Types of perforations

Type I	Extraluminal crater without extravasation
Type II	Pericardial or myocardial blush without contrast jet extravasation
Type III	Extravasation through a frank (≥1 mm) perforation or cavity spilling into an anatomic cavity chamber

including that to the three layers of the vessel wall. A classification for perforations has been proposed on the basis of angiographic appearance (Table 25.4), indicating the severity of the perforation. The perforation can occur at the site of the CTO or distal to the vessel. A few series have described the incidence of such complications in CTO lesions. According to Olivieri *et al.* [31], the incidence of perforation in CTO-PCI is approximately 2%. Although the nature of the CTO lesion accounts for a perforation risk factor, coronary perforation may be secondary to the coronary wire and particularly to the hydrophilic or stiff wire used [34–36]. High-pressure inflation on these ACC/AHA (American College of Cardiology/American Heart Association) type C lesions can also increase the risk of perforation. However, most perforations are related to the specific technology used, such as rotational or directional atheroablative devices or excimer laser [37,38]. In a series of 72 perforation cases, Javaid *et al.* [35] showed that 87% of wire-induced perforations were with hydrophilic wires, whereas 67% of atheroablative device perforations were due to the use of Rotablator. Most wire perforations were grades I or II, whereas most of post-atheroablative perforations were grades II or III. Also, some techniques used in CTO-PCI, such as the Subintimal Tracking And Re-Entry (STAR) technique or the Retrograde Subintimal Tracking Technique (CART) technique can increase the risk of perforations. Clinical presentations of perforations vary and can be either well tolerated or directly life threatening with occurrence of a tamponade. Clinical events depend on the grade of the perforation. Sometimes the clinical manifestations of a perforation are delayed and can occur within 24 hours after dismissal from the catheterization laboratory [39], Coronary perforation can carry a high mortality. The prognosis of perforations depends on the grade [35,39], the presence of renal insufficiency, and on the prescription of IIb/IIIa platelet inhibitors [40] at the time of the event. In the study by Javaid et al. [35], no patient with grade I perforation had a tamponade or in-hospital death. Emergent CABG was required in only 7% of cases. Among patients with grade II perforation, 12% developed tamponade, 3% died during the hospital stay, and emergent CABG was required in 27% of these patients. In patients with grade III perforation, 40% developed tamponade, 60% required emergency CABG, and 44% died during the index hospitalization.

Treatment of these perforations is determined by the type of perforation and by the clinical tolerance by the patient. Different, more or less complex, algorithms have been proposed [39,41]. If the perforation is grade I and due to the wire, prolonged balloon inflation seems to be sufficient. If the perforation is grade II, prolonged balloon inflation with perfusion balloons [41,42] is required. Plugs, coil embolization [43], and local infusion of thrombogenic molecules [44] are usually reserved for grades I and II when the hole in the wall artery is not too large. In grades I and II, we advise reversing the anticoagulation and monitoring the patient clinically and by serial echocardiography for careful examination of the pericarde and right cavities (tamponade). A percutaneous pericardiocentesis must be done if there are clinical and/or echographic signs of tamponade.

If the perforation is grade III with a tamponade, prolonged balloon inflation is mandatory. At the same time, a percutaneous pericardiocentesis [41] should be performed. In addition, another catheter should be placed at the ostium of the CTO artery through a second vascular access for the purpose of aterial perforation treatment, possibly with a polytetrafluoroethylene (PTFE)-covered stent [45]. After disengaging the first catheter and placing the second catheter at the ostium, a slight deflation of the first balloon is done. The second wire is advanced, it crosses the lesion, and goes to the distal bed. Then, the first balloon is removed and the stent is implanted. PTFE-covered stents must be used in larger arteries (product is available from 3.0–5.0 mm in diameter with stent lengths of 9–26 mm). Sometimes open heart surgery with or without CABG is required if the PCI procedure does not fix the perforation. Late stent thrombosis after implantation of PTFE-covered stents remains a concern and requires prolonged dual antiplatelet therapy, including aspirin and thienopyridines, for ≥12 months after stent implantation [46].

Conclusion

The complication rate during CTO recanalization is often higher when compared to non-CTO angioplasty. These complications must be considered prior to the procedure and the risk/benefit rate should be calculated for every case. A plan to minimize potential complications, along with a set of rules regarding radiation exposure and CM volume, should be in place prior to the procedure. Equipment such as covered stents, a pericardiosynthesis kit, aspiration devices, and a surgical backup should be available. A rule of when to stop should also be in place prior to the procedure, to which the physician should adhere. See Plates 25 through 28 in the color plate section.

References

1 Buller CE, Dzavik V, Carere RG et al. Primary stenting versus balloon angioplasty in occluded coronary arteries: the Total Occlusion Study of Canada (TOSCA). *Circulation* 1999; **100**: 236–242.

2 Suzuki S, Furui S, Kohtake H et al. Radiation exposure to patient's skin during percutaneous coronary intervention for various lesions, including chronic total occlusion. *Circ J* 2006; **70**: 44–48.

3 Hamburger JN, Gijsbers GH, Ozaki Y, Ruygrok PN, de Feyter PJ, Serruys PW. Recanalization of chronic total coronary occlusions using a laser guide wire: a pilot study. *J Am Coll Cardiol* 1997; **30**: 649–656.

4 Bashore TM. Radiation safety in the cardiac catheterization laboratory. *Am Heart J* 2004; **147**: 375–378.

5 Neofotistou V, Vano E, Padovani R et al. Preliminary reference levels in interventional cardiology. *Eur Radiol* 2003; **13**: 2259–2263.

6 Tsapaki V, Kottou S, Kollaros N et al. Comparison of a conventional and a flat-panel digital system in interventional cardiology procedures. *Br J Radiol* 2004; **77**: 562–567.

7 Bell MR, Berger PB, Menke KK, Holmes DR Jr. Balloon angioplasty of chronic total coronary artery occlusions: what does it cost in radiation exposure, time, and materials? *Catheter Cardiovasc Diagn* 1992; **25**: 10–15.

8 Hirshfeld JW Jr, Balter S, Brinker JA *et al.* ACCF/AHA/ HRS/SCAI clinical competence statement on physician knowledge to optimize patient safety and image quality in fluoroscopically guided invasive cardiovascular procedures. A report of the American College of Cardiology Foundation/American Heart Association/American College of Physicians Task Force on Clinical Competence and Training. *J Am Coll Cardiol* 2004; **44**: 2259–2282.

9 Wagner LK, Eifel PJ, Geise RA. Potential biological effects following high X-ray dose interventional procedures. *J Vasc Interv Radiol* 1994; **5**: 71–84.

10 International Commission on Radiological Protection. Avoidance of radiation injuries from medical interventional procedures (ICRP Publication 85). *Ann ICRP* 2000; **30**: 25–43.

11 Saito S, Tanaka S, Hiroe Y *et al.* Angioplasty for chronic total occlusion by using tapered-tip guidewires. *Catheter Cardiovasc Interv* 2003; **59**: 305–311.

12 Mehran R, Aymong ED, Nikolsky E *et al.* A simple risk score for prediction of contrast-induced nephropathy after percutaneous coronary intervention: development and initial validation. *J Am Coll Cardiol* 2004; **44**: 1393–1399.

13 McCullough PA, Wolyn R, Rocher LL, Levin RN, O'Neill WW. Acute renal failure after coronary intervention: incidence, risk factors, and relationship to mortality. *Am J Med* 1997; **103**: 368–375.

14 Rihal CS, Textor SC, Grill DE *et al.* Incidence and prognostic importance of acute renal failure after percutaneous coronary intervention. *Circulation* 2002; **105**: 2259–2264.

15 Levy EM, Viscoli CM, Horwitz RI. The effect of acute renal failure on mortality. A cohort analysis. *JAMA* 1996; **275**: 1489–1494.

16 Naidu SS, Selzer F, Jacobs A *et al.* Renal insufficiency is an independent predictor of mortality after percutaneous coronary intervention. *Am J Cardiol* 2003; **92**: 1160–1164.

17 Stacul F, Adam A, Becker CR *et al.* CIN Consensus Working Panel. Strategies to reduce the risk of contrast-induced nephropathy. *Am J Cardiol* 2006; **98**(6A): 59K–77K.

18 Mueller C, Buerkle G, Buettner HJ *et al.* Prevention of contrast media-associated nephropathy: randomized comparison of 2 hydration regimens in 1620 patients undergoing coronary angioplasty. *Arch Intern Med* 200; **162**: 329–336.

19 Aspelin P, Aubry P, Fransson SG, Strasser R, Willenbrock R, Berg KJ. Nephrotoxicity in high-risk patients study of iso-osmolar and low-osmolar nonionic contrast media study investigators. Nephrotoxic effects in high-risk patients undergoing angiography. *N Engl J Med* 200; **348**: 491–499.

20 Jo SH, Youn TJ, Koo BK *et al.* Renal toxicity evaluation and comparison between visipaque (iodixanol) and hexabrix (ioxaglate) in patients with renal insufficiency undergoing coronary angiography: the RECOVER study: a randomized controlled trial. *J Am Coll Cardiol* 2006; **48**: 924–930.

21 Merten GJ, Burgess WP, Gray LV *et al.* Prevention of contrast-induced nephropathy with sodium bicarbonate: a randomized controlled trial. *JAMA* 2004; **291**: 2328–2334.

22 Briguori C, Airoldi F, D'Andrea D *et al.* Renal Insufficiency Following Contrast Media Administration Trial (REMEDIAL): a randomized comparison of 3 preventive strategies. *Circulation* 2007; **115**: 1211–1217.

23 Zagler A, Azadpour M, Mercado C, Hennekens CH. N-acetylcysteine and contrast-induced nephropathy: a meta-analysis of 13 randomized trials. *Am Heart J* 2006; **151**: 140–145.

24 Kini AS, Mitre CA, Kim M, Kamran M, Reich D, Sharma SK. A protocol for prevention of radiographic contrast nephropathy during percutaneous coronary intervention: effect of selective dopamine receptor agonist fenoldopam. *Catheter Cardiovasc Interv* 2002; **55**: 169–173.

25 Morcos SK, Thomsen HS, Webb JA. Contrast-media-induced nephrotoxicity: a consensus report. Contrast Media Safety Committee, European Society of Urogenital Radiology (ESUR). *Eur Radiol* 1999; **9**: 1602–1613.

26 Ozcan EE, Guneri S, Akdeniz B *et al.* Sodium bicarbonate, N-acetylcysteine, and saline for prevention of radiocontrast-induced nephropathy. A comparison of 3 regimens for protecting contrast-induced nephropathy in patients undergoing coronary procedures. A single-center prospective controlled trial. *Am Heart J* 2007; **154**: 539–544.

27 Lee PT, Chou KJ, Liu CP *et al.* Renal protection for coronary angiography in advanced renal failure patients by prophylactic hemodialysis. A randomized controlled trial. *J Am Coll Cardiol* 2007; **50**: 1015–1020.

28 Meier B. Total coronary occlusion: a different animal? *J Am Coll Cardiol* 1991; **17**(6 Suppl B): 50B–57B.

29 Stone GW, Reifart NJ, Moussa I *et al.* Percutaneous recanalization of chronically occluded coronary arteries: a consensus document: Part II. *Circulation* 2005; **112**: 2530–2537.

30 Suero JA, Marso SP, Jones PG *et al.* Procedural outcomes and long-term survival among patients undergoing percutaneous coronary intervention of a chronic total occlusion in native coronary arteries: a 20-year experience. *J Am Coll Cardiol* 2001; **38**: 409–414.

31 Olivari Z, Rubartelli P, Piscione F *et al.* TOAST-GISE Investigators. Immediate results and one-year clinical outcome after percutaneous coronary interventions in

chronic total occlusions: data from a multicenter, prospective, observational study (TOAST-GISE). *J Am Coll Cardiol* 2003; **41**: 1672–1678.

32 Ruocco NA Jr., Ring ME, Holubkov R, Jacobs AK, Detre KM, Faxon DP. Results of coronary angioplasty of chronic total occlusions (the National Heart, Lung, and Blood Institute 1985–1986 Percutaneous Transluminal Angioplasty Registry). *Am J Cardiol* 1992; **69**: 69–76.

33 Lin TH, Wu DK, Su HM, Chu CS, Voon WC, Lai WT, Sheu SH. Septum hematoma: a complication of retrograde wiring in chronic total occlusion. *Int J Cardiol* 2006; **113**: e64–e66.

34 Favereau X, Corcos T, Guerin Y *et al*. Early reocclusion after successful coronary angioplasty of chronic total occlusions. *J Am Coll Cardiol* 1995; **25**: 139A (Abstract).

35 Javaid A, Buch AN, Satler LF *et al*. Management and outcomes of coronary artery perforation during percutaneous coronary intervention. *Am J Cardiol* 2006; **98**: 911–914.

36 Wong CM, Kwong Mak GY, Chung DT. Distal coronary artery perforation resulting from the use of hydrophilic coated guidewire in tortuous vessels. *Catheter Cardiovasc Diagn* 1998; **44**: 93–96.

37 Bittl JA, Ryan Jr TJ, Keaney JF, Jr *et al*. Coronary artery perforation during excimer laser coronary angioplasty. *J Am Coll Cardiol* 1993; **21**: 1158–1165.

38 Gruberg L, Pinnow E, Flood R *et al*. Incidence, management, and outcome of coronary artery perforation during percutaneous coronary intervention. *Am J Cardiol* 2000; **86**: 680 682 A8.

39 Ellis SG, Ajluni S, Arnold AZ *et al*. Increased coronary perforation in the new device era. Incidence, classification, management, and outcome. *Circulation* 1994; **90**: 2725–2730.

40 Gunning MG, Williams IL, Jewitt DE, Shah AM, Wainwright RJ, Thomas MR. Coronary artery perforation during percutaneous intervention: incidence and outcome. *Heart* 2002; **88**: 495–498.

41 Dippel EJ, Kereiakes DJ, Tramuta DA *et al*. Coronary perforation during percutaneous coronary intervention in the era of abciximab platelet glycoprotein IIb/IIIa blockade: an algorithm for percutaneous management. *Catheter Cardiovasc Interv* 2001; **52**: 279–286.

42 Flynn MS, Aguirre FV, Donohue TJ, Bach RG, Caracciolo EA, Kern MJ. Conservative management of guidewire coronary artery perforation with pericardial effusion during angioplasty for acute inferior myocardial infarction. *Catheter Cardiovasc Diagn* 1993; **29**: 285–288.

43 Gaxiola E, Browne KF. Coronary artery perforation repair using microcoil embolization. *Catheter Cardiovasc Diagn* 1998; **43**: 474–476.

44 Storger H, Ruef J. Closure of guide wire-induced coronary artery perforation with a two-component fibrin glue. *Catheter Cardiovasc Interv* 2007; **70**: 237–240.

45 Briguori C, Nishida T, Anzuini A, Di Mario C, Grube F, Colombo A. Emergency polytetrafluoroethylene-covered stent implantation to treat coronary ruptures. *Circulation* 2000; **102**: 3028–3031.

46 Mulvihill NT, Boccalatte M, Sousa P *et al*. Rapid scaling of coronary perforations using polytetrafluoroethylene-covered stents. *Am J Cardiol* 2003; **91**: 343–346.

CHAPTER 26

How to Minimize Contrast Nephropathy

Robin Mathews, MD *& Luis Gruberg,* MD, FACC

Stony Brook University Medical Center, Stony Brook, New York, NY, USA

Introduction

The number of diagnostic and therapeutic cardiac angiograms performed annually in the US has markedly increased over the past two decades. These procedures require administration of iodinated contrast media that can be an important source of nephrotoxicity. Contrast-induced nephropathy (CIN) is a serious complication of coronary angiography and contrast-based procedures [1–4]. CIN is the third leading cause of hospital acquired renal failure (after decreased renal perfusion and nephrotoxic drugs) and accounts for approximately 11% of cases [3,4]. Multiple studies have established that post procedure rises in serum creatinine have been associated with increased mortality, myocardial infarction, and target vessel revascularization [5,6].

Percutaneous coronary intervention (PCI) is now the preferred method for revascularization in many patients with coronary artery disease. Technological and pharmacological advances, have paved the way for the widespread used of percutaneous coronary artery revascularization including increasing use of PCI in more complex and multi-vessel lesions. Recent data have shown that up to one-third of patients with significant coronary artery disease on angiography have at least one chronic total coronary occlusion (CTO) [7–13]. Although percutaneous revascularization of CTOs

is a well established procedure accounting for up to 10% of patients undergoing PCI, it still remains one of the most demanding procedures in interventional cardiology [8–10,14]. It requires extensive effort and experience with newer equipment and techniques as well as higher contrast administration and greater radiation exposure time [14].

Definition

Many definitions of contrast-induced nephropathy are available in the literature, but the two most common include a rise in serum creatinine ≥25% from baseline or an absolute increase of >0.5 mg/dL from baseline. In the majority of patients, this rise occurs within the first 24 hours, peaking 3–5 days after the procedure, and is coupled with a reduction in creatinine clearance [1–4,15–18]. Unfortunately, serum creatinine measurement is an insensitive method to monitor renal function, as >50% reduction in glomerular filtration rate may occur before any increase is observed. A more accurate way to assess the renal function is to calculate the creatinine clearance by applying the Cockcroft–Gault formula or by calculating the glomerular filtration rate using the Modification of Diet in Renal Disease (MDRD) formula.

Pathophysiology

CIN can be caused by multiple pathologic processes that include vasoconstriction, direct toxicity,

Chronic Total Occlusions, 1st edition. Edited by R. Waksman and S. Saito. © 2009 Blackwell Publishing, ISBN: 978-1-4051-5703-2.

reactive oxygen specifies and impaired nitric oxide production [4,19,20]. It is currently believed that disturbances in renal hemodynamics and direct tubular cell toxicity are primarily responsible [19]. After injection of contrast medium, there is a transient increase followed by a more prolonged decrease in renal blood flow [19–21], with the outer medulla at greatest risk for ischemic damage [20]. A direct toxic effect by contrast media was initially suggested by pathologic changes such as cellular necrosis, interstitial inflammation, and epithelial cell vacuolization [4,19,20]. Oxygen free radicals that may cause apoptosis in renal tubular and glomerular cells have also been implicated in animal models [2].

Risk factors

Recent studies have found that incidence of CIN varies from 3.3% to 14.4% [1,17]. Multiple studies using multivariate analysis have shown that the presence of baseline renal dysfunction, diabetes mellitus, congestive heart failure and increased doses of contrast media increase the risk of CIN [4,5,22]. In the absence of risk factors, the overall incidence is low at 2–5% [23], but in those with the identified risk factors, the incidence has been reported from 11% to 50% [22–24]. Mehran and colleagues [24] retrospectively examined 8357 patients who underwent PCI and developed a risk score assessment after identifying eight variables (hypotension, IABP (intra-aortic balloon pump), heart failure, age >75 years, anemia, diabetes, contrast media volume, and serum creatinine >1.5 mg/dL or GFR (glomerular filtration rate) <60 mL/min/1.73 m^2) that were independent predictors of CIN. The rate of CIN increased exponentially with increasing risk score (8.4% and 55.9% for low and high-risk score, respectively) [24].

Pre-existing renal disease is the greatest independent predictor of CIN and the severity of renal impairment appears to be directly correlated with the incidence of CIN [1,6,25]. Rihal and others retrospectively studied 7586 patients undergoing coronary intervention and found that CIN developed in 22.4% of patients with a baseline serum creatinine of 2.0 to 2.9 mg/dL and 30.6% of patients with creatinine higher than

3.0 m/dL, compared to a 2.4% incidence in those with creatinine levels <2.0 mg/dL [1].

Diabetes mellitus is another strong predictor of CIN after coronary intervention. Rihal and colleagues found that diabetic patients with normal or mild renal impairment (serum creatinine <2.0 mg/dL) had a significantly higher risk of CIN than non diabetic patients [1]. However, with baseline serum creatinine levels above 2.0 mg/dL, higher proportions of both diabetics and non diabetics experienced similar incidence of CIN without statistically significant differences. These results were confirmed by other investigators that showed that diabetic patients with mean serum creatinine level of 1.3 mg/dL had a higher rate of CIN compared to non diabetics patients [17].

Several studies have shown that congestive heart failure is also an independent risk factor for CIN [1,15,25]. The risk associated with CHF may be caused by alterations in renal blood flow due to the low flow state of heart failure and by the use of medications including angiotensin converting enzyme inhibitors and diuretics [2]. Other reported risk factors for CIN include reduced arterial volume, concurrent use of nephrotoxic medications (nonsteroidal anti-inflammatory drugs, aminoglycosides), hypertension, hyponatremia, blood transfusion, older age, and hypoalbuminemia [4,22,26,27].

Prophylactic measures

Currently there is no treatment to reverse contrast induced nephropathy, but only prophylaxis. Many preventative measures, including diuretics, mannitol, dopamine, atrial natriuretic peptide, and endothelin receptor antagonists have failed to show benefit in randomized, controlled trials. At present, few measures have shown consistent benefit in the prevention of CIN [28].

Hydration

Volume expansion can reduce the risk of CIN. The beneficial effects of saline hydration before and after contrast administration are thought to be due to increased renal flow and glomerular filtration, which may counteract hemodynamic changes caused by contrast media [2,18,28]. In a study of 1620 patients randomized to either

0.9% saline or 0.45% saline intravenous fluid at 1 mL/kg/hour for 24 hours starting on the morning of angioplasty [29], Mueller and others found that the incidence of CIN after hydration with 0.9% saline was significantly lower (0.7% versus 2%, $p = 0.04$), with the greatest benefit in women, diabetics, and those receiving >250 mL of contrast (Figure 26.1). A recent study by Clavijo and others showed that rapid administration of 1 liter of 5% dextrose 5 minutes before coronary angiography through the common femoral artery sheath reduced the incidence of CIN from 5.7% to 1.4% ($p = 0.03$) (Figure 26.2) [16]. After review of six protocols that have been used in trials of volume expansion, the CIN working panel has suggested the optimum protocol to reduce CIN risk to be 1–1.5 mL/kg/hour of isotonic crystalloid 12 hours before and 6–24 hours after the procedure [28].

Evidence suggesting prolonged reductions in renal blood flow of up to 50% for 4 hours postcontrast, have highlighted the importance of post procedure volume resuscitation [21]. If volume overload is a concern in cardiac patients, consideration may be given to right heart catherization for hemodynamic monitoring [28].

A recent study by Merten *et al.* [30] assessed the benefit of sodium bicarbonate hydration for the prevention of CIN in patients undergoing diagnostic or interventional procedures. A total of 119 patients were randomized to either a sodium chloride solution or to sodium bicarbonate in dextrose and water. The initial dose was a 3 mL/kg bolus 1 hour immediately before the procedure, followed by 1 mL/kg/hour during the procedure, and for 6 hours after the procedure. Despite a higher mean baseline serum creatinine level in patients randomized to the bicarbonate arm, only 1.7% of these patients developed CIN compared with 13.6% in patients treated with sodium chloride ($p = 0.02$) (Figure 26.3). Based on these results, it is possible that prophylactic hydration with sodium bicarbonate is a more efficient way to prevent CIN due to its potential to neutralize free radicals in the distal tubule. This single center study in a limited number of patients needs to be corroborated by further studies.

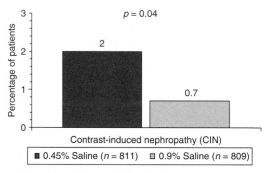

Figure 26.1 The in-hospital rates of contrast-induced nephropathy (CIN) in patients treated with 0.45% saline (black bar) versus those treated with normal saline 0.9% (grey bar). (Data abstracted from reference [29] by Mueller *et al.*)

Antioxidants

There have been over 25 studies evaluating the role of *N*-acetylcysteine, an acetylated amino acid with sulfhydryl groups antioxidant, in CIN prophylaxis. There have also been nine published meta-analyses

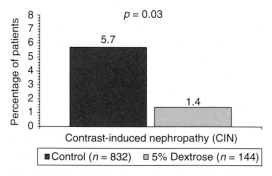

Figure 26.2 The in-hospital rates of contrast-induced nephropathy (CIN) in patients in the control arm (black bar) versus those treated with Dextrose 5% (gray bar). (Data abstracted from reference [16] by Clavijo *et al.*)

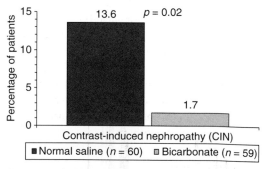

Figure 26.3 The in-hospital rates of contrast-induced nephropathy (CIN) in patients treated with 0.9% saline (black bar) versus those treated with bicarbonate (gray bar). (Data abstracted from reference [30] by Merten *et al.*)

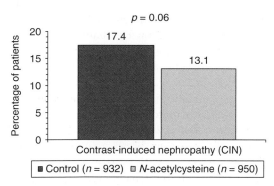

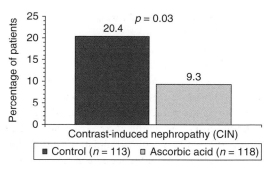

Figure 26.4 The in-hospital rates of contrast-induced nephropathy (CIN) in the control arm (black bar) versus those treated with *N*-acetylcysteine (gray bar). (Data abstracted from reference [31] by Zagler *et al.*)

Figure 26.5 The in-hospital rates of contrast induced nephropathy (CIN) in patients in the control arm (black bar) versus those treated with ascorbic acid (gray bar). (Data abstracted from reference [32] by Spargias *et al.*)

documenting the heterogeneity between the studies and limits the conclusions to be drawn. A recent meta-analysis of 13 trials with 1892 randomized patients showed a possible but statistically nonsignificant 32% reduction in the risk for CIN in patients treated with *N*-acetylcysteine (RR 0.68, 95% CI 0.46–1.01) (Figure 26.4) [31]. Most studies have used a standard oral regimen of 600 mg twice daily for 24 hrs the day before and the day of the procedure. Despite the lack of compelling evidence of the benefit of *N*-acetylcysteine in the prevention of CIN, its low cost, ease of administration, and lack of severe side-effects are all legitimate reasons for the routine use of this drug for the prevention of CIN in high-risk patients, particularly diabetic patients with chronic renal insufficiency.

The antioxidant ascorbic acid has been shown to attenuate renal damage caused by a variety of insults. A randomized, double-blind, placebo-controlled trial in 231 patients treated with either 3 g of ascorbic acid or placebo administered orally at least 2 hours before the start of the index procedure followed by 2 g of ascorbic acid or placebo the night and the morning after the procedure showed a significant reduction in the incidence of CIN in patients treated with ascorbic acid (Figure 26.5) [32]. These results are encouraging, but deserve confirmation.

Contrast media

Contrast media are composed of a monomer or dimer of triiodobenzene units with varying numbers of iodine molecules that provide the "contrast" effect [2,6]. Increased iodine content allows for better radiographic visualization and water solubility, but also increases the osmolality. Contrast media characteristics such as osmolarity might influence the likelihood of CIN in patients at risk [2,20]. Multiple compounds with varying properties and physiologic effects have been created in an attempt to create radio contrast media with high attenuation while limiting side effects. Initial high-osmolar contrast media (HOCM) (approximately 2,000 mOsm/kg) were followed by low-osmolar contrast media (LOCM) that had an osmolarity 2–3 times lower than HOCM (approximately 600–800 mOsm/kg) but still remained hyperosmolar in comparison to serum [23]. Most of these compounds are nonionic (iohexol and iopamidol) with ioxaglate as the only ionic compound [20]. In a pooled analysis of 25 randomized trials, Barrett and others noted that HOCM posed a greater risk of CIN than LOCM in patients with pre-existing renal dysfunction [33]. There has been evidence that iso-osmolar contrast media (IOCM) (290 mOsm/kg) (iodixanol) reduces the risk of CIN in high-risk patients [34]. A recent meta-analysis of sixteen randomized, controlled trials compared creatinine changes after administration of the IOCM iodixanol versus various LOCM, found the overall incidence of CIN in the IOCM patients at 1.4% versus 3.5% in the LOCM group [23]. The largest absolute difference existed between those patients with chronic kidney disease or diabetics or the combination of both [23].

The volume of contrast medium administered during coronary angiography has been found in some studies to correlate with the incidence of CIN but with varying degrees of significance [1,2,4,17,22,25,26,35,36]. In a study of 183 patients undergoing cardiac catheterization, Rich and others found that contrast volume >200 mL was an independent risk factor for nephrotoxicity (RR 2.1, $p = 0.005$) [22]. Often though, total contrast volume is not found to be a univariate predictor of CIN with statistical significance. This is likely due to the dose-dependent nature of contrast as a function of body weight and creatinine clearance. Cigarroa and others derived a formula to calculate a contrast material "limit": 5 mL of contrast multiplied by body weight in kg divided by serum creatinine (mg/dL). This study found that the incidence of CIN is rare when adhering to this formula [37]. Morcos proposes that with the administration of less nephrotoxic LOCM, the limit as per the Cigarroa formula can be expanded by a factor of 1.5 based on the extent of reduction of renal function by HOCM [38]. Other studies noted the odds ratio for contrast dose and nephropathy requiring hemodialysis is very low [17,39]. Rihal and others noted in a study of 7586 patients that each contrast volume of 100 mL correlated with an odds ratio of 1.12 of acute renal failure after PCI [1]. More recently, a retrospective analysis of nearly 17,000 coronary interventions were reviewed to evaluate the role of weight- and creatinine-adjusted maximum radiographic contrast dose (MRCD) [26]. After adjustment of baseline risk factors, MRCD was the strongest independent predictor of nephropathy requiring dialysis (OR 6.2, 95% CI, 3.0–12.8). In addition, in-hospital mortality was significantly higher in patients who exceeded MRCD compared with those who did not. This "threshold" effect, rather than a linear dose effect, has been noted other studies as well [37,40]. Taliercio and others [40] found that those patients who received greater than 125 mL of contrast were at almost ten times more likely top develop contrast nephropathy.

Hemofiltration

Continuous veno-venous hemofiltration is a form of renal-replacement therapy used in acute renal failure patients that may be used as an alternative strategy for the prevention of CIN in high-risk patients. In a randomized study by Marenzi and colleagues, 114 consecutive patients with chronic renal failure who were undergoing coronary interventions were randomly assigned to either hemofiltration ($n = 58$, mean serum creatinine 3.0 ± 1.0 mg/dL) or isotonic-saline hydration ($n = 56$, mean serum creatinine 3.1 ± 1.0 mg/dL) 4–8 hours before PCI and 18–24 hours after PCI. CIN occurred less frequently among patients in the hemofiltration group than among the control patients (5% versus 50%, $p < 0.001$) [41]. These data was corroborated by other studies in high-risk populations by the same group of investigators.

Future directions

Most of the contrast medium injected into the coronary arteries during coronary angiography is thought to drain into the coronary sinus. Novel methods are being devised to be able to cannulate the coronary sinus, detect, capture, and remove the contrast material before it enters the systemic circulation and reaches the kidneys [42]. These systems are still in the experimental phase.

The Be*nephi*t® Infusion System is a selective infusion catheter system that may deliver therapeutic agents for the prevention of CIN directly into the renal arteries through a dedicated infusion catheter while allowing simultaneous coronary procedures through a single vessel access site in the femoral artery. Preliminary data with different agents, such as fenoldopam, sodium bicarbonate, and alprostadil has shown promising results in the prevention of CIN [43].

Chronic total occlusions

Anatomically, CTOs consist of a hard fibrocalcific proximal cap, a distal cap with less fibrotic material, and an area of organized thrombus centrally [7]. The highly calcific nature of these occlusions accounts for the increased difficulty in successful recanalization. Traditionally, when compared to non occlusive lesions, PCI of a CTO is associated with lower procedural success rates (70–80% compared to 95–98%) predominately related to difficulty in crossing the lesion. However, technical advances such as specialty wires have improved success rates [7,36,44]. These procedures still differ from sub total occlusion interventions in multiple factors including time commitment of the operator, equipment used, and total volume of contrast administered. The amount of contrast used during CTO interventions average 200 ± 96 mL compared to 162 ± 65 mL used in simpler lesions [14]. Although there are no documented trials that have examined incidence of CIN in CTO revascularization, the increased contrast volumes administered and the role of contrast dosage as a risk factor in high risk patients, has been well established as outlined above. Injection of contrast media should be limited to the lowest possible dose of IOCM or LOCM. As noted above, because contrast volumes exert a dose dependant effect on the risk of CIN based on pre existing renal impairment as well as weight, the formula proposed by Cigarroa and others [37] may be a useful reference point.

The use of intravascular ultrasound-guided PCI without the use of contrast media has been reported [45]. Although technically more demanding, intravascular ultrasound can be used to assess the course of the procedure and can limit the amount of contrast used. Non invasive assessment of left ventricular function in patients at high risk for CIN by echocardiography or nuclear scanning before angiography is common practice is some institutions [40]. This allows left ventriculography to be avoided and reduces the contrast load by up to 50 mL. In addition, repeat radio contrast studies if necessary should be spaced with adequate time between them [18].

Summary

Contrast nephropathy is a major cause of morbidity and mortality in patients undergoing coronary angiography. In addition to patient-related risk factors for CIN, it is clear that CTO revascularization may hold additional procedural-related risks such as total contrast volume and recent contrast administration for other non-CTO interventions. Therefore, every effort should be made to identify patients at high risk and implement all current available measures for the prevention of CIN and its dire consequences.

References

1 Rihal CS, Textor SC, Grill DE et al. Incidence and prognostic importance of acute renal failure after percutaneous coronary intervention. Circulation 2002; 105: 2259–2264.

2 Gami AS, Garovic VD. Contrast nephropathy after coronary angiography. Mayo Clin Proc 2004; 79: 211–219.

3 McCullough PA, Adam A, Becker CR et al. on behalf of the CIN consensus working panel. Epidemiology and prognostic implications of contrast induced nephropathy. Am J Cardiol 2006; 98: 5K–13K.

4 McCullough PA, Soman SS. Contrast induced nephropathy. Crit Care Clin 2005; 21: 261–280.

5 Lindsay J, Apple S, Pinnow EE et al. Percutaneous coronary intervention associated nephropathy foreshadows increased risk of late adverse events in patients with normal baseline serum creatinine. Catheter Cardiovasc Intervent 2003; 59: 338–343.

6 Gruberg L, Weissman NJ, Waksman R et al. Comparison of outcome after percutaneous coronary revascularization with stents in patients with and without mild chronic renal insufficiency. Am J Cardiol 2002; 89: 54–57.

7 Braden GA. Chronic total occlusions. Cardiol Clin 2006; 24: 247–254.

8 Christofferson RD, Lehmann KG, Martin GV, Every N, Caldwell JH, Kapadia SR. Effect of chronic total coronary occlusion on treatment strategy. Am J Cardiol 2005; 95: 1088–1091.

9 Suero JA, Marso SP, Jones PG et al. Procedureal outcomes and long term survival among patients undergoing percutaneous coronary intervention of a chronic total occlusion in native coronary arteries: a 20 year experience. J Am Coll Cardiol 2001; 38: 409–414.

10 Puma JA, Sketch MH, Tcheng JE et al. Percutaneous revascularization of chronic total occlusions: an overview. J Am Coll Cardiol 1995; 26: 1–11.

11 Hoye A, Domburg RT, Sonnenschein K, Serruys PW. Percutaneous coronary intervention for chronic total occlusions: the Thoraxcenter experience 1992–2002. Euro Heart J 2005; 26: 2630–2636.

12 Drazod J, Wojcik J, Opalinska E, Zapolski T, Widomska-Czekajska T. Percuntaneous angioplasty of chronically occluded coronary arteries: Long term clinical follow up. Kardiol Pol 2006; 64: 667–673.

13 Baks T, Geuns RJ, Duncker DJ et al. Prediction of left ventricular function after drug-eluting stent implantation for chronic total coronary occlusions. J Am Coll Cardiol 2006; 47: 721–725.

14 Bell MR, Berger PB, Menke KK, Holmes DR. Balloon angioplasty of chronic total coronary occlusions: What does it cost in radiation exposure, time and materials? Cathet Cardiovasc Diag 1992; 25: 10–15.

15 Jo SH, Youn TJ, Koo BK *et al.* Renal toxicity evaluation and comparison between visipaque (iodixanol) and hexabrix (ioxaglate) in patients with renal insufficiency undergoing coronary angiography. The RECOVER study: a randomized control trial. *J Am Coll Cardiol* 2006; **48**: 924–930.

16 Clavijo LC, Pinto TL, Kuchulakanti PK *et al.* Effect of a rapid intra-arterial infusion of dextrose 5% prior to coronary angiography on frequency of contrast induced nephropathy in high risk patients. *Am J Cardiol* 2006; **97**: 981–983.

17 McCullough PA, Wolyn R, Rocher LL, Levin RN, ONeill WW. Acute renal failure after coronary intervention: incidence, risk factors, and relationship in mortality. *Am J Med* 1997; **103**: 368–375.

18 Rudnick MR, Kesselheim A, Goldfarb S. Contrast induced nephropathy: how it develops, how to prevent it. *Cleaveland Clinic J Med* 2006; **73**: 75–86.

19 Rudnick MR, Goldfarb S. Pathogenesis of contrast induced nephropathy: experimental and clinical observations with an emphasis on the role of osmolality. *Rev Cardio Med* 2003; **4**: S29–S33.

20 Tumlin J, Stacul F, Adam A, Becker CR, Davidson C, Lameire N *et al.* on behalf of the CIN consensus working panel. Pathophysiology of contrast-induced nephropathy. *Am J Cardiol* 2006; **98**: 14K–20K.

21 Tumlin JA, Wang A, Murray PT, Mathur VS. Fenoldopam mesylate blocks reductions in renal plasma flow after radiocontrast dye infusion: a pilot trial in the prevention of contrast nephropathy. *Am Heart J* 2002; **143**: 894–903.

22 Rich MW, Crecelius CA. Incidence, risk factors, and clinical course of acute renal insufficiency after cardiac catherization in patients 70 years of age or older. A prospective study. *Arch Int Med* 1990; **150**: 1237–1242.

23 McCullough PA, Bertrand ME, Brinker JA, Stacul F. A meta-analysis of the renal safety of isosmolar iodixanol compared with low-osmolar contrast media. *J Am Coll Cardiol* 2006; **48**: 692–699.

24 Mehran R, Aymong ED, Nikolsky E *et al.* A simple risk score for prediction of contrast induced nephropathy after percutaneous coronary intervention. *J Am Coll Cardiol* 2004; **44**: 1393–1399.

25 Gruberg L, Mintz GS, Mehran R *et al.* The prognostic implications of further renal function deterioration within 48 hours of interventional coronary procedures in patients with pre-existent chronic renal insufficiency. *J Am Coll Cardiol* 2000; **36**: 1542–1548.

26 Freeman RV, ODonnell M, Share D *et al.* for the Blue Cross Blue Shield of Michigan Cardiovascular Consortium (BMC2). *Am J Cardiol* 2002; **90**: 1068–1073.

27 Morocos SK. Prevention on contrast media nephrotoxicity- the story thus far. *Clin Radiology* 2004; **59**: 381–389.

28 Stacul F, Adam A, Becker CR *et al.* on behalf of the CIN consensus working panel. Strategies to reduce the risk of contrast induced nephropathy. *Am J Cardiol* 2006; **98**: 59K–77K.

29 Mueller C, Buerkle G, Buettner HJ *et al.* Prevention of contrast media associated nephropathy. Randomized comparison of 2 hydration regimens in 1620 patients undergoing coronary angioplasty. *Arch Intern Med* 2002; **162**: 329–336.

30 Merten GJ, Burgess WP, Gray LV *et al.* Prevention of contrast induced nephropathy with sodium bicarbonate A randomized control trial. *JAMA* 2004; **291**: 2328–34.

31 Zagler A, Azadpour M, Mercado C, Hennekens CH. N-Acetylcysteine and contrast induced nephropathy: A meta analysis of 13 randomized trials. *Am Heart J* 2006; **151**: 140–145.

32 Spargias K, Alexopoulos E, Kyrzoppulos S *et al.* Ascorbic acid prevents nephropathy in patients with renal dysfunction undergoing coronary angiography or intervention. *Circulation* 2004; **110**: 2837–2842.

33 Barrett BJ, Carlisle EJ. Meta analysis of the role of relative nephrotoxicity of high and low osmolality iodinated contrast media. *Radiology* 1993; **188**: 171–178.

34 Aspelin P, Aubry P, Fransson SG, Strasser R, Willenbrock R, Berg KJ for the NEPHRIC Investigators. Nephrotoxic effects in high risk patients undergoing angiography. *N Eng J Med* 2003; **348**: 491–499.

35 Rudnick MR, Golfarb S, Wexler L *et al.* Nephrotoxicity of ionic and nonionic contrast media in 1196 patients: a randomized trial. The Iohexol cooperative study. *Kidney Int* 1995; **47**(1): 254–261.

36 Migliorini A, Moschi G, Vergara R, Parodi G, Carrabba N, Antoniucci D. Drug eluting stent supported percutaneous coronary intervention for chronic total coronary occlusion. *Catheter Cardiovasc Interven* 2006; **67**: 344–348.

37 Cigarroa RG, Lange RA, Williams RH, Hillis D. Dosing of contrast material to prevent contrast nephropathy in patients with renal disease. *Am J Med* 1989; **86**: 649–652.

38 Morcos SK. Prevention of contrast media induced nephrotoxicty after angiographic procedures. *J Vasc Interv Radiol* 2005; **16**: 13–23.

39 Gruberg L, Mehran R, Dangas G *et al.* Acute renal failure requiring dialysis after percutaneous coronary interventions. *Catheter Cardiovasc Intervent* 2001; **52**: 409–416.

40 Taliercio CP, Vlietstra RE, Fischer LD, Burnett JC. Risks of renal dysfunction with cardiac angiography. *Ann Int Med* 1986; **104**: 501–504.

41 Marenzi G, Marana I, Lauri G *et al.* The prevention of radiocontrast-agent-induced nephropathy by hemofiltration. *N Engl J Med* 2003; **349**: 1331–1338.

42 Michishita I, Fujii Z. A novel contrast removal system from the coronary sinus using an adsorbing column during coronary angiography in a porcine model. *J Am Coll Cardiol* 2006; **47**(9): 1866–1870.

43 Rogers CDK. Real-World Use of Targeted Renal Therapy – Results from the Be-RITe! International Registry. Presented at Transcatheter Cardiovascular Therapeutics, October 18, 2005, Washington, DC.

44 Ge L, Iakovou I, Cosgrave J *et al.* Immediate and mid term outcomes of sirolimus-eluting stent implantation for chronic total occlusions. *Euro Heart J* 2005; **26**: 1056–1062.

45 RezKalla SH. Successful direct stenting guided by intravascular ultrasound without contrast in a patient with renal dysfunction. *J Interv Cardiol* 2003; **5**: 449–451.

VII PART VII
Interesting Cases

CHAPTER 27

Interesting Cases I, II

Takafumi Tsuji, MD *& Hideo Tamai,* MD

Kusatsu Heart Center, Shiga, Japan

Case I

A 67-year-old diabetic male presented with chronic stable angina and breathlessness. Coronary angiography revealed a severe stenosis of the right coronary artery (RCA) and a total occlusion of the left circumflex artery (LCX) with collateral vessels from left anterior descending artery (LAD). He underwent percutaneous coronary intervention (PCI) for RCA and two Cypher stents (Cordis, Miami, FL, USA) were inserted in proximal and mid-RCA.

Six months later, follow-up coronary angiography revealed no restenosis of stented segment in RCA. So, he was decided to open the occluded LCX because he still had some effort angina. An 8 F Amplatz Left-1 guiding catheter with side holes was deployed to the left coronary artery via the right femoral artery, and a 6 F Amplatz Left-1 catheter was deployed to the RCA via the left femoral artery to perform contralateral angiography. The LCX was occluded just after the first obtuse marginal branch (OM1) (Figure 27.1a). Collateral vessels mainly came up from LAD and slowly filled an irregular, heavily diseased distal vessel (Figure 27.1b). The estimated occlusion length was 10 mm. A 0.014 inch floppy guide wire was advanced to the OM1 and the intravascular ultrasound (IVUS) imaging was performed to confirm the ostium of occluded vessel.

A Neos Miracle 6 g wire (Asahi Intecc, Nagoya, Japan) was advanced to the occlusion through a

Chronic Total Occlusions, 1st edition. Edited by R. Waksman and S. Saito. © 2009 Blackwell Publishing, ISBN: 978-1-4051-5703-2.

1.5 mm diameter, 20 mm long Ranger over-the-wire balloon (Boston Scientific, Natrick, MA, USA). In spite of careful manipulation, the wire was advanced to subintimal space just beside the distal true lumen (Figure 27.1c). The balloon was withdrawn leaving the wire there. Another Neos miracle 6 g wire was loaded into the Ranger balloon and advanced along with the former wire (Figure 27.1d). This is so-called "parallel-wire technique," ensuring the direction to the distal true lumen and reducing dye contrast consumption by leaving the former failed wire as a landmark. In this case, the latter wire was advanced to the distal of the LCX through the occluded lesion (Figure 27.2a). The Ranger balloon passed the lesion and was then inflated to 12 atm. A 2.5-mm-diameter, 30-mm-long Vento balloon (Invatec, Roncadelle, Italy) was inflated throughout the diseased lesion to 14 atm (Figure 27.2b). The artery was then revealed as being very large, with numerous branches, but there was very hard plaque in mid LCX (Figure 27.2c).

The balloon was changed to a 2.5 mm diameter, 20 mm long Quantum Maverick high-pressure balloon (Boston Scientific, Natrick, MA, USA) and inflated throughout the diseased lesion to 20 atm. There still remained a balloon indentation at mid LCX even at 24 atm (Figure 27.2d). The IVUS imaging revealed severe calcium around the lesion. To dilate this solid lesion, another Miracle 6 g wire was also inserted in the distal LCX and balloon inflation was attempted to cut the hard plaque using the wire shaft beside the balloon, but failed to dilate the lesion (Figure 27.3a). Then, a Neos Miracle 12 g wire (Asahi Intecc, Aichi, Japan) was advanced to the solid lesion

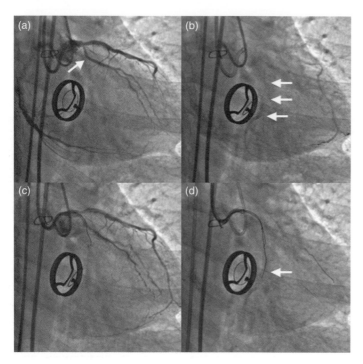

Figure 27.1 (a) In the control angiogram, the left circumflex artery (LCX) was occluded just after the first obtuse marginal branch (OM1; arrow). (b) Collateral vessels mainly came up from left anterior descending artery (LAD) and slowly filled an irregular, heavily diseased distal vessel (arrows). (c) A Neos Miracle 6 g wire was advanced to subintimal space just beside the distal true lumen. (d) The second Neos miracle 6 g wire (arrow) was loaded into the Ranger balloon and advanced along with the former wire.

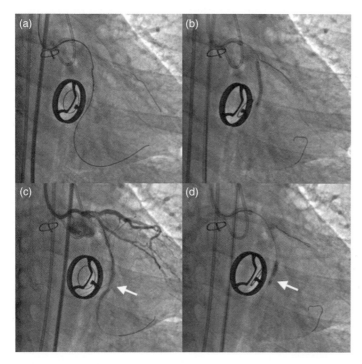

Figure 27.2 (a) The wire was advanced to the distal of the LCX through the occluded lesion. (b) A 2.5 mm x 30 mm balloon was inflated throughout the diseased lesion to 14 atm. (c) After 2.5 mm balloon dilatation, the artery was revealed as being very large, with numerous branches, but there was very hard plaque in mid LCX (arrow). (d) A balloon indentation at mid LCX still remained even at 24 atm (arrow).

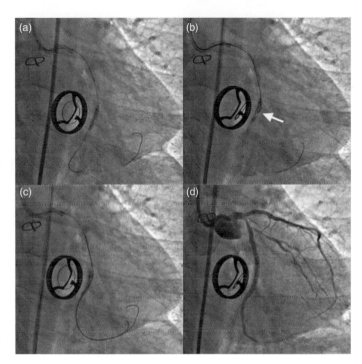

Figure 27.3 (a) Another Miracle 6 g wire was also inserted in the distal LCX and balloon inflation was attempted to cut the hard plaque using the wire shaft beside the balloon, but failed to dilate the lesion (arrow). (b) A Neos Miracle 12 g wire was advanced to the solid lesion and carefully repeated stabbing into the hard plaque from the subintimal space to crack the calcium while the balloon was inflated in the lumen (arrow). (c) After the wire cracking, the solid lesion was dilated at 26 atm. (d) The final angiographic result was excellent.

and carefully repeated stabbing into the hard plaque from the subintimal space to crack the calcium while the balloon was inflated in the lumen (Figure 27.3b). After that, the solid lesion was dilated at 26 atm (Figure 27.3c). The IVUS imaging revealed cracked calcified plaque and enough vessel size to put stents. A 3 mm × 33 mm Cypher stent (Cordis, Miami, FL, USA) was inserted to mid LCX and fully expanded at 16 atm. A 3 mm × 23 mm Cypher stent (Cordis, Miami, FL, USA) was then inserted to occluded proximal LCX at 20 atm. The final angiographic result was excellent (Figure 27.3d).

Case II

A 73-year-old diabetic and hypertensive female presented to another hospital with unstable angina. Coronary angiography demonstrated a severe stenosis of proximal left anterior descending artery (LAD), a moderate stenosis of mid left circumflex artery (LCX) and a total occlusion of mid right coronary artery (RCA) with preserved left ventricular function. She underwent percutaneous coronary intervention (PCI) in which two Cypher stents (Cordis, Miami, FL, USA) were implanted in proximal and mid-LAD, but the wire failed to cross the occluded lesion in RCA.

Two months later, she admitted to this hospital to treat the occluded RCA. Coronary angiography revealed a diffuse severe stenosis of ostial and proximal RCA and a total occlusion of mid RCA with good collateral vessels from septal branches of LAD (Figure 27.4a). An 8 F Judkins Right-4 guiding catheter with side holes was deployed to the RCA via the right femoral artery, and a 6 F Amplatz Left-1 guiding catheter was deployed to the LAD via the left femoral artery to perform contralateral angiography. In this case, the retrograde approach technique that is a novel PCI method to penetrate the wire into the chronic total occlusion (CTO) retrogradely via collateral vessels was selected. A Runthrogh floppy wire (Terumo, Tokyo, Japan) was carefully advanced through a septal branch to the distal end of CTO (Figure 27.4b and c). A 1.25-mm-diameter,

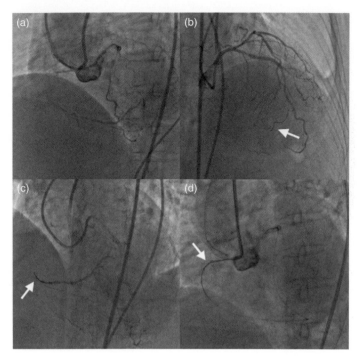

Figure 27.4 (a) The control coronary angiography revealed a diffuse severe stenosis of ostial and proximal right coronary artery (RCA) and a total occlusion of mid RCA with good collateral vessels from septal branches of LAD. (b) A Runthrogh floppy wire was carefully advanced through a septal branch (arrow). (c) A Runthrogh floppy wire was advanced to the distal end of CTO (arrow). (d) A miracle 6 g wire was slowly advanced into the CTO, but followed a subintimal path nearly to the ostial RCA (arrow).

10-mm-long Speeder balloon (Invatec, Roncadelle, Italy) crossed the collateral vessel and was inflated throughout the collateral vessel at 2 atm to allow larger balloons to cross this retrograde path. After that, a 2.5 mm diameter, 20 mm long Ranger over-the-wire balloon (Boston Scientific, Natrick, MA, USA) was advanced to just distal site of occlusion via collateral vessel and the wire was changed to a Neos Miracle 6 g wire (Asahi Intecc, Nagoya, Japan) through the balloon. The wire was slowly advanced into the CTO, but followed a subintimal path nearly to the ostial RCA (Figure 27.4d). Then, the balloon was advanced to proximal RCA and inflated in the subintimal place at proximal and mid RCA at 8 atm to create subintimal dissections in the CTO portion (Figure 27.5a).

A Neos Miracle 12 g wire (Asahi Intecc, Aichi, Japan) was antegradely advanced from the ostial RCA to occluded lesion and slowly penetrated into the plaque. The retrograde balloon was inflated several times in the subintimal space beside the antegrade wire (Figure 27.5b). After deflation of the balloon, the wire was advanced to the subintimal space made by the balloon that was connected to the distal true lumen. The wire was easily crossed to the posterodescending branch (Figure 27.5c). The occluded lesion was dilated with the 2.5 mm × 20 mm Ranger balloon and two 3.0 mm × 33 mm Cypher stent (Cordis, Miami, FL, USA) was inserted at proximal and mid RCA at 16 atm. The final angiographic result was excellent (Figure 27.5d).

Discussion

Percutaneous coronay intervention for CTO lesions is so complicated that it is difficult to achieve high procedural success rate. To improve the recanalization success rate, various wire techniques have been invented. In the Case I, the parallel wire technique was very effective to cross the occlusion adjusting the second wire tip to the correct direction without dye injection. The technique was also used to crack a very hard calcified plaque which led the balloon to

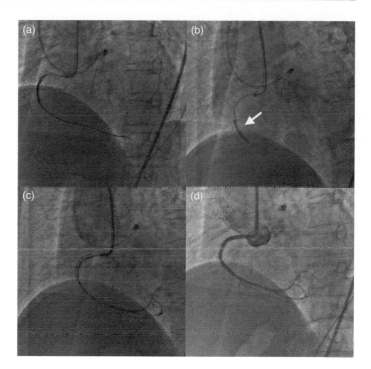

Figure 27.5 (a) The balloon was advanced to proximal RCA and inflated in the subintimal place at proximal and mid RCA at 8 atm to create subintimal dissections in the CTO portion.
(b) The retrograde balloon was inflated several times in the subintimal space beside the antegrade wire (arrow).
(c) The wire was easily crossed to the posterodescending branch. (d) The final angiographic result was excellent.

fully expand. In Case II, the lesion was treated with the retrograde approach that is a novel method of retrogradely penetrating a wire into the CTO lesion through the collateral vessel. The author attempts this technique as below:
• Retrograde approach is attempted if the collateral vessels are confirmed with contralateral dye injection.
• A floppy guidewire is advanced to the distal end of CTO through a collateral vessel, which become a good landmark to antegrade wiring.

• If a balloon catheter retrogradely crosses to the distal CTO, the guidewire is changed to harder one to retrogradely penetrate into CTO.
• When the antegrade wire is getting close to distal end of CTO, retrograde balloon is dilated to open the distal cap of CTO.
• All stent procedures are performed by antegrade approach.

These techniques may be helpful to improve the success rate of CTO treatment and reduce contrast dye injection.

Index